Handbook of Obstetric Management

SYLVIA K. ROSEVEAR
MD, MRCOG
Consultant Obstetrician and Gynaecologist

Blackwell
Science

© 1996 by
Blackwell Science Ltd
Editorial Offices:
Osney Mead, Oxford OX2 0EL
25 John Street, London WC1N 2BL
23 Ainslie Place, Edinburgh EH3 6AJ
250 Main Street, Malden,
    MA 02148 5018, USA
54 University Street, Carlton,
    Victoria 3053, Australia
10, rue Casimir Delavigne
    75006 Paris, France

Other Editorial Offices:

Blackwell Wissenschafts-Verlag GmbH
Kurfürstendamm 57
10707 Berlin, Germany

Blackwell Science KK
MG Kodenmacho Building
7–10 Kodenmacho Nihombashi
Chuo-ku, Tokyo 104, Japan

The right of the Author to be identified as
the Author of this Work has been asserted in
accordance with the Copyright, Designs
and Patents Act 1988.

First published 1996
Reprinted 1999

Set in 8pt Trump Mediaeval
by DP Photosetting, Aylesbury, Bucks
Printed and bound in the UK at the
University Press, Cambridge

The Blackwell Science logo is a trade mark
of Blackwell Science Ltd, registered at the
United Kingdom Trade Marks Registry

DISTRIBUTORS

Marston Book Services Ltd
PO Box 269
Abingdon
Oxon OX14 4YN
(*Orders:* Tel: 01235 465500
          Fax: 01235 465555)

USA
Blackwell Science, Inc.
Commerce Place
350 Main Street
Malden, MA 02148 5018
(*Orders:* Tel: 800 759 6102
          781 388 8250
          Fax: 781 388 8255)

Canada
Login Brothers Book Company
324 Saulteaux Crescent
Winnipeg, Manitoba R3J 3T2
(*Orders:* Tel: 204 837 2987
          Fax: 204 837 3116)

Australia
Blackwell Science Pty Ltd
54 University Street
Carlton, Victoria 3053
(*Orders:* Tel: 03 9347 0300
          Fax: 03 9347 5001)

A catalogue record for this title
is available from the British Library

ISBN 0–632–05457–3

Library of Congress
Cataloging-in-Publication Data
Rosevear, Sylvia K.
    Handbook of obstetric
    management/Sylvia K. Rosevear
        p. cm.
    Includes bibliographical references and
    index.
    ISBN 0–632–05457–3 (pbk. : alk. paper)
    1. Obstetrics—Handbooks, manuals,
    etc. I. Title
    [DNLM: 1. Pregnancy Complications—
    therapy—handbooks. 2. Obstetrics—
    handbooks.   WQ 39 R8175h   1995]
    RG531.R65   1995
    618.2—dc20
    DNLM/DLC
    for Library of Congress   95-21394
                                          CIP

For further information on
Blackwell Science, visit our website:
www.blackwell-science.com

For
Anna, Jacob, Kyle & Patrick Rosevear

Contents

Preface

This book collates for ready reference obstetric information about good clinical practice and for giving informed advice to women for whom we care. As well as covering general obstetric conditions, it also gives details on management of complicated problems where appropriate action in difficult situations may make a great deal of difference. Of course appropriate advice from experts must always be sought when indicated. I hope that it results in the thoughtful and appropriate use of tests and explanations to women patients. Occasionally, opinion may differ, but I hope that the information provides an appropriate guide for improved care of women.

Note: This book should not be used as a prime source of prescribing and dispensing drugs. The Author and Publishers have undertaken reasonable endeavours to check medicines information and content for accuracy. Because the science of clinical pharmacology is continually advancing, our knowledge base continues to expand. Therefore, the reader should always check the manufacturer's product information before administering any medication.

Acknowledgements

Dr Heather Andrews, Consultant Radiologist, United Bristol Healthcare Trust (UBHT).

Dr Gary Bryan, Senior Registrar, Anaesthetics UBHT

Mr Mathew Eagle, Department of Statistics, University of Oxford.

Dr Peter Harrison, Consultant in Renal Medicine, Southmead Health Services.

Dr Margaret Honeyman, Consultant Psychiatrist, Mercy Hospital, Auckland, New Zealand.

Dr Carolyn Heaf, SHO UBHT.

Dr Peter Lunt, Consultant Clinical Geneticist, UBHT.

Dr Neil Marlow, Consultant Senior Lecturer in Neonatal Medicine, University of Bristol.

Dr Paul Newrick, Senior Registrar, Department of Medicine (Endocrinology) UBHT.

Dr Alfred Roome, Clinical Lecturer, Public Health Laboratory Service, University of Bristol.

Dr John Smoleniec, Lecturer/Senior Registrar in Obstetrics & Gynaecology, University of Bristol.

Professor David Spence, Emeritus Professor of Mathmatics, Imperial College, London.

Dr Patrick Taylor, Consultant in Genito-urinary Medicine, UBHT

Dr Trevor Thomas, Consultant in Anaesthesia, UBHT

Dr Rupert Vessey, Research Registrar, Nuffield Department of Medicine, John Radcliffe Hospital, Oxford.

Mr Peter Wardle, Consultant Senior Lecturer in Obstetrics & Gynaecology, University of Bristol.

Dr Michael Woolridge, Lactation Research Fellow, University of Bristol Department of Child Health.

Abbreviations

AC	abdominal circumference
ACE	angiotensin converting enzyme
AChR	acetylcholine receptor
AFP	alphafetoprotein
AIDS	acquired immune deficiency syndrome
ALP	alkaline phosphatase
AP	antero-posterior
APCK	adult polycystic kidney disease
APL	antiphospholipid
APTT	activated partial thromboplastin time
ARM	artificial rupture of the membranes
AST	aspartate transaminase
ATIII	antithrombin III
ATP	alloimmune thrombocytopenia
AV	atrioventricular
b.d.	*bis in diem* (twice a day)
BFPR	biological false positive reaction
BMD	Becker muscular dystrophy
BP	blood pressure
BPD	bi-parietal diameter
BPP	biophysical profile
BW	birthweight
CCT	controlled cord traction
CF	cystic fibrosis
CGA	cytosine adenosine
CGG	cytosine guanine
CHD	congenital heart defect
CHM	complete hydatidiform mole
CK	creatinine kinase
CLASP	collaborative low dose aspirin (randomised trial)
CMT	Charcot–Marie–Tooth (syndrome)
CMV	cytomegalovirus
CNS	central nervous system

COC	combined oral contraceptive
CPR	cardiopulmonary resuscitation
CRL	crown–rump length
CSF	cerebrospinal fluid
CT	computerised tomography
CTG	cardiotocograph
CVP	central venous pressure
CVS	chorionic villus sampling
DPB	diastolic blood pressure
DI	diabetes insipidus
DIC	disseminated intravascular coagulation
DM	myotonic dystrophy
DMD	Duchenne muscular dystrophy
DPG	diphosphoglycerate
dRVVT	dilute Russell viper venom time
DVT	deep vein thrombosis
DZ	dizygous
ECG	electrocardiogram
EDTA	ethylenediamine tetraacetic acid
EEG	electroencephalograph
ELISA	enzyme-linked immunosorbent assay
ERPF	effective renal plasma flow
ESR	erythrocyte sedimentation rate
ETT	endotracheal tube
FBC	full blood count
FDP	fibrin degradation products
FFP	fresh frozen plasma
FHR	fetal heart rate
FISH	fluorescent *in situ* hybridisation
FL	femur length
FSH	follicle stimulating hormone
FTA	fluorescent treponemal antibody
FVW	flow velocity waveform
GA	gestational age
GBS	Group B streptococcus
GFR	glomerular filtration rate

GGT	gamma-glutamyl transferase
GIFT	gamete intrafallopian transfer
GPL/MPL	IgG and IgM antiphospholipid antibody units
GnRH	gonadotrophin releasing hormone
GTD	gestational trophoblastic disease
GTN	glyceryl trinitrate

hAS	human albumin solution
HBIg	hepatitis B immunoglobulin
HBV	hepatitis B virus
HC	head circumference
HC	Huntington chorea
Hct	haematocrit
hCG	human chorionic gonadotrophin
HDN	haemolytic disease of the newborn
HELLP	haemolysis, elevated liver function tests and low platelets
HIE	hypoxic ischaemic encephalopathy
HIV	human immunodeficiency virus
HLA	human leucocyte antigen
HM	hydatidiform mole
hMG	human menopausal gonadotrophin
HOCM	hypertrophic obstructive cardiomyopathy
HSV	herpes simplex virus

IgG	immunoglobulin G
IgM	immunoglobulin M
i.m.	intramuscular(ly)
IM	invasive mole
INR	international normalised ratio
IPPV	intermittent positive pressure ventilation
ISSHP	International Society for the Study of Hypertension of Pregnancy
ITP	immune (idiopathic) thrombocytopenia
ITU	intensive therapy unit
IUCD	intrauterine contraceptive device
IUGR	intrauterine growth retardation
IUI	intrauterine insemination
i.v.	intravenous(ly)
IVF	in vitro fertilisation

IVIg	intravenous immunoglobulin
JVP	jugular venous pressure
KCT	kaolin clotting time
LA	lupus anticoagulant
LDH	lactate dehydrogenase
LE	lupus erythematosus
LFT	liver function test
LH	luteinising hormone
LHRH	LH-releasing hormone
LMP	last menstrual period
LMWH	low molecular weight heparin
LSCS	lower segment caesarean section
MCHC	mean cell haemoglobin concentration
MCKD	multicystic dysplastic kidney disease
MCV	mean cell volume
MEN	multiple endocrine neoplasia
MoM	multiples of the median
MSU	mid-stream urine
MZ	monozygous
NAIT	neonatal autoimmune thrombocytopenia
NF	neurofibromatosis
NSAID	non-steroidal anti-inflammatory drug
NTD	neural tube defect
OD	optical density
OFD	occipito-frontal diameter
OP	occipito-posterior
PAIgG	platelet-associated immunoglobulin G
PCOD	polycystic ovarian disease
PCR	polymerase chain reaction
PCV	packed cell volume
PG	prostaglandin
PGE	prostaglandin E
PGF	prostaglandin F

PGI	prostacycline
PHM	partial hydatidiform mole
PKU	phenylketonuria
POP	progestogen only containing pill
PPF	plasma protein fraction
PPH	post-partum haemorrhage
PTU	propylthiouracil
q.d.s.	*quater die sumendum* (four times a day)
RIA	radioimmunoassay
SAG-M	sodium chloride, adenine, glucose and mannitol
SBP	systolic blood pressure
s.c.	subcutaneous(ly)
SLE	systemic lupus erythematosus
SRP	short rib-polydactyly (syndrome)
t.d.s.	*ter die sumendum* (three times a day)
TFT	thyroid function test
TIBC	total iron binding capacity
TOP	termination of pregnancy
TORCH	toxoplasmosis, rubella, cytomegalovirus, herpes
TPA	tissue plasminogen activator
TPHA	*Treponema pallidum* haemagglutination
TRH	thyrotrophin-releasing hormone
TSH	thyroid stimulating hormone (thyrotrophin)
TTT	tissue thromboplastin time
TX	thromboxane
UTI	urinary tract infection
VDRL	venereal disease reference laboratory
VSD	ventricular septal defect
VZIg	*Varicella zoster* immunoglobulin
WBC	white blood cell

1 Early Pregnancy

ESTABLISHING A DIAGNOSIS OF PREGNANCY

Pregnancy tests

A pregnancy test detects human chorionic gonadotrophin (hCG). hCG is a glycoprotein consisting of an alpha and beta sub unit produced by the trophoblast. The beta sub unit of hCG shares amino acid sequences with luteinising hormone and follicle stimulating hormone. A luteinising hormone (LH) peak occurring at ovulation or an increase in pituitary gonadotrophins towards the menopause may account for a false positive pregnancy test if the test is very sensitive to hCG levels. About three per cent of blood samples give serum concentrations of hCG of 5–25 IU/L.

By 11 days after the LH peak hCG should be detectable in all normal pregnancies.

The concentration at the time of the first missed period is about 100 IU/L. It then rises to a peak of about 100 000 IU/L between 8–10 weeks' gestation from the last menstrual period. It falls to about 10 000 IU/L by 20 weeks and remains at this level.

Types of pregnancy test

1 Slide or tube agglutination inhibition test. A urine specimen is mixed with a solution of hCG antibody which will bind any hCG present in the test specimen. A suspension of hCG coated latex beads or erythrocytes is then added. If hCG is present in the test specimen, the binding of hCG coated latex particles or erythrocytes to the

antibody will be blocked and the agglutination reaction is inhibited.

- No agglutination indicates that the pregnancy test is positive.
- Agglutination (i.e. the presence of fine flocular precipitant) indicates that the woman is not pregnant.

The test lacks sensitivity, requiring a concentration of at least 1000 IU/L. Therefore, it ought to be repeated after an interval.

2 Haemagglutination techniques take one to two hours and are more sensitive than agglutination inhibition tests. With the use of sub unit specific monoclonal antibodies the sensitivity of the assay is 75–150 IU/L.

3 Radioimmunoassays, which are rapid and are highly specific for hCG, have a sensitivity of 40 IU/L.

4 The blue colour change on a dipstick test in urine is only observed if the woman is pregnant. Tests are sensitive to 25–50 IU/L and therefore can give a positive pregnancy test result as early as 8–10 days after fertilisation. False negative rates range from 0 to less than 2 per cent.

Quantitative estimation of beta hCG

- At levels of 1500 IU/L an intrauterine sac should be seen on ultrasound scanning.
- Levels of 6000 IU/L should be associated with a visible intrauterine pregnancy.
- Abnormally high levels (> 20 000 IU/L) may be found in gestational trophoblastic disease and multiple pregnancy.
- In early pregnancy the hCG concentration increases exponentially up to the sixth week. This means that the time taken for the hCG concentration to double is constant (approximately 48 hours).
- Most women with an ectopic pregnancy will have hCG levels of < 66 per cent or a doubling time of more than three days.

Ultrasound imaging of early pregnancy (abdominal)

Weeks' gestation	Ultrasound observation
5	Decidual reaction
6	Gestation sac
6–7	Fetal pole
7	Fetal heart
9	Morphological fetal features

- Vaginal scanning is able to image a 1 mm gestational sac at 4 weeks 2 days from the last menstrual period (LMP) of a regular cycle. Early gestational structures can usually be seen about 1 week earlier by transvaginal rather than transabdominal ultrasound.
- In normal pregnancy the sac diameter increases by 1.2 mm/day. Growth of less than 0.7 mm/day is a poor prognostic sign. The sac diameter should be greater than 30 mm at 6–7 weeks' gestation.
- Gestational age by sac size in the first 30–50 days of pregnancy can be calculated by the formula:

[age (days from LMP) = mean sac diameter (mm) + 30]. (see Table 1.1)

- The yolk sac is the first structure that can be accurately identified within the gestational sac. Initially it is much larger than the embryo.
- A diagnosis of an anembryonic pregnancy is suggested when a gestational sac is larger than 20 mm in diameter with no yolk sac or greater than 25 mm without a fetus. A large yolk sac (greater than 10 mm in diameter) is also associated with poor outcome.
- Fetal cardiac activity can be first identified at 41–3 days of gestation using a 2.5 MHz transabdominal sector transducer.
- Fetal heart activity should be visible in a normally developing embryo of 5–6 mm and the sac diameter should be greater than 30 mm at about 6.5 weeks from the LMP.
- Over 90 per cent of embryos with cardiac activity identified on ultrasound have a normal outcome. The risk of miscarriage is reduced from about 40–50 per cent to between 1 and 3 per cent, depending on the gestational age when the fetal heart is first imaged and the age of the woman. If the heart rate is less than 85 beats/minute miscarriage is likely.

Table 1.1 Gestational sac sizes.

Weeks from LMP	Size in mm
4	2
5	5
6	10
7	20
8	25

MISCARRIAGE

1

Definition

The World Health Organisation definition of miscarriage is 'The expulsion or extraction from its mother of an embryo or fetus weighing 500 g or less' (see Fig. 1.1). This corresponds to a gestational age of 20–22 weeks which was considered to be pre-viable.

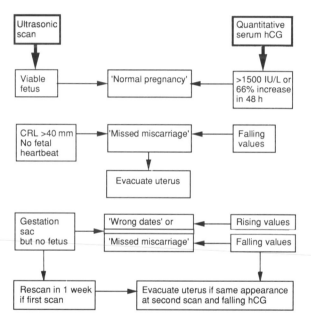

Fig. 1.1 Management of bleeding in early pregnancy. (Reproduced with permission from Rosevear, S.K. (1994) Bleeding in early pregnancy, In: *High Risk Pregnancy, Management Options* (Ed. by D.K. James, P.J. Steer, C.P. Weiner & B. Gonik) W.B. Saunders, London.)

Incidence of miscarriage

- Early loss among clinically recognised pregnancy is between 12 and 15 per cent. At least a further 15 per cent of fertilised ova are lost before implantation. Most miscarriages occur before 14 weeks' gestation. The expected outcome of pregnancy in a variety of circumstances is shown in Table 1.2.

- *Even after three or more consecutive losses the chance of a successful pregnancy is still at best 75 per cent and at worst about 50 per cent.*

- The greatest predictor of outcome is the history of previous pregnancies (see Tables 1.3 and 1.4).

RECURRENT MISCARRIAGE

- Defined as three or more consecutive early pregnancy losses.

- The incidence of recurrent miscarriage is about 1 per cent of women who become pregnant.

Table 1.2 Expected outcome of pregnancy.

	Miscarriage rate (per cent)
Primigravida	5
Multigravida	14
Successful	4
Unsuccessful	24
The last pregnancy:	
Successful	5
Unsuccessful	19
Two previous miscarriages:	
Probability of a third	17–35
More than three miscarriages	25–46

Table 1.3 The risks of miscarriage in successive pregnancies according to previous outcomes. (Adapted from Regan *et al.* (1989) with permission.)

	Percentage risk of miscarriage with gravidity of			
	1	2	3	4
Whatever previous outcome	12	4	7	9
When each successive pregnancy ends in miscarriage	12	15	38	60
When last pregnancy was livebirth		3	6	8
When all previous pregnancies ended in livebirth		3	9	8

Table 1.4 Comparison of risk of miscarriage with those women who have had one livebirth at any stage. (Adapted from Regan *et al.* (1989) with permission.)

Number of miscarriages	Percentage risk of subsequent miscarriage
1	5.2
2	5.8
3	15.1
4	16.3
	Percentage risk after consecutive losses
1	11.5
2	20.4
3	36.4

- Primary recurrent miscarriage is where a woman has lost all previous pregnancies.
- Secondary recurrent miscarriage is where one successful pregnancy is followed by consecutive losses.

Causes and associations

1 Genetic disorders

The most common cause of recurrent miscarriage is probably sporadic genetic disorders (e.g. aneuploidy) in the fetus often occurring consecutively by chance. Therefore **check the fetal karyotype** in the products of conception after recurrent miscarriage if possible.

Parental balanced translocation accounts for about 4 per cent of cases. Therefore **check parental karyotypes** in all cases and refer to clinical geneticist if abnormal.

Molecular mutations are probably very important but cannot yet be determined. DNA analysis may become available.

2 Endocrine factors

Elevated luteinising hormone (LH) levels around conception and implantation usually associated with polycystic ovarian syndrome are associated with recurrent early pregnancy loss. Therefore **check LH levels on day six**: if elevated (> 10 IU/L) repeat in another cycle. If still elevated refer to a gynaecological endocrinologist for advice. Low levels of progesterone in the luteal phase are most frequently the result of a failing pregnancy rather than its cause. Progestogen or hCG therapy are of no proven benefit.

3 Anatomical defects of the cervix or uterus

A too pessimistic view has arisen about the risk of pregnancy loss in women with uterine malformations. They may be present in 15 to 30 per cent of women with recurrent losses. Identify any anatomical defect by vaginal ultrasound and if a uterine defect is suspected proceed to hysterosalpingography or hysteroscopy. Uterine septae are probably best divided hysteroscopically by someone experienced in the technique.

Cervical incompetence typically presents with sudden rupture of membranes in the second trimester followed by painless miscarriage. The reported incidence is 13 to 20 per cent. Diagnosis is too frequently based on clinical history alone. A cervical os measuring over 9 mm at vaginal ultrasound suggests incompetence.

Treatment is by cervical cerclage at 12 to 14 weeks. The status of the cervix should be checked every two to four weeks by vaginal ultrasound. If the cervix is opening insertion of a second suture may be justified. The suture is removed at 38 weeks or earlier if labour supervenes.

4 Infection

There is no good evidence that any microbial infection is associated with recurrent pregnancy loss as distinct from sporadic miscarriage.

5 Immune causes

Women with systemic lupus erythematosus have an increased risk of recurrent miscarriage.

The presence of lupus anticoagulant is also an association. Women with recurrent miscarriage should be screened for it by checking their activated partial thromboplastin time (APTT) and kaolin clotting time (KCT). The typical history is of pregnancies failing earlier and earlier and personal and family history of thrombosis or autoimmune diseases. However, miscarriage may be the first manifestation. Treatment is described in Section 4.2. Other immune causes are far less certain and routine investigation for them is not justified.

6 Diabetes or thyroid disorders

Women with poorly controlled diabetes are more likely to miscarry but there is no increased incidence of subclinical diabetes in women with recurrent loss. Screening is therefore not necessary. The evidence to date implicating subclinical thyroid disorders is very poor but the possibility cannot yet be ruled out.

7 *Psychological stress*

Too much has been made of the poorly controlled research on the influence of psychological stress on the success of pregnancy. All pregnant women, particularly those at high risk of a poor outcome, deserve all the tender loving care that can be given.

Investigation of recurrent miscarriage (see Table 1.5)

Table 1.5 gives the colour of the test tube top for universal containers (used in the UK) necessary for blood taken for the investigation of recurrent miscarriage.

ECTOPIC PREGNANCY (See Fig. 1.2)

Clinical symptoms and signs

- Irregular vaginal bleeding
- Symptoms of pregnancy
- Abdominal pain/peritonism
- Shoulder tip pain
- Collapse

Diagnosis

Carry out an abdominal or vaginal ultrasound scan and check serum level of hCG. If a serum hCG level is 6500 IU/L or over an intrauterine sac should be detectable on abdominal ultrasound. (Pseudogestational sacs that can be seen with ectopic pregnancy rarely occur above this level.) If an intrauterine pregnancy cannot be seen an ectopic pregnancy should be excluded. The definitive diagnosis is made by laparoscopy.

Treatment

The definitive treatment is conservative surgery but expectant treatment may be indicated in some cases (see Table 1.6).

Table 1.5 Investigations for recurrent miscarriage.

Universal container		Colour coding equivalent (UK)
Serum separation tube		Yellow
Fluoride tube		Grey
Citrate tube		Light blue
Heparin tube		Green
EDTA tube		Purple
Plain tube (cross match)		Pink
1 Opportunistic screening		
Full blood count		1 Purple tube
Rubella status		1 Pink tube
Hepatitis B		1 Yellow tube
'TORCH' screen		1 Yellow tube
Random blood glucose		1 Grey tube
2 Routine tests		
Parental karyotype	Woman	1 Green tube
	Partner	1 Green tube
LH levels day 6 (repeat if > 10 IU/L)		
APTT		
Clotting time	}	5 mL Blue tube
Prothrombin time		
KCT		1 Yellow tube
3 More specific investigation		
Lupus anticoagulant		2 Blue tubes
Anti-DNA antibodies		1 Yellow tube
Anti-cardiolipin antibody		1 Yellow tube
Autoimmune profile		1 Yellow tube
Anti Ro		1 Yellow tube
Thyroid function tests		1 Yellow tube
Liver function tests		1 Yellow tube
Urea and electrolytes		1 Yellow tube
Complement		1 Yellow tube

On some occasions it may be possible to use intrapregnancy injection of a variety of drugs (e.g. prostaglandins or methotrexate) either by ultrasound or laparoscopic control (see Table 1.7).

Surgical management

Every attempt should be made to remove the tubal pregnancy without

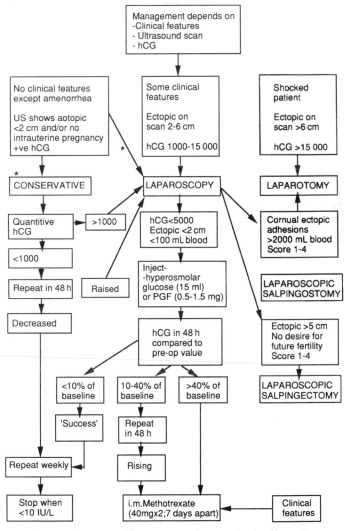

Fig. 1.2 Management of ectopic pregnancy. (Reproduced with permission from Rosevear, S.K. (1994) Bleeding in early pregnancy, In: *High Risk Pregnancy, Management Options* (Ed. by D.K. James, P.J. Steer, C.P. Weiner & B. Gonik) W.B. Saunders, London.)

sacrificing the fallopian tube. Techniques (either at laparotomy or laparoscopy) are linear salpingotomy (primary surgical closure), salpingostomy (delayed spontaneous closure), or segmental tubal resection with immediate or delayed surgical closure (Table 1.8).

Table 1.6 Criteria for expectant management of an ectopic pregnancy.

hCG > 75 IU
Ultrasound scan showing an empty uterus
Absence of fluid in the pouch of Douglas
Haematosalpinx < 2 cm
Haematoperitoneum < 50 ml
hCG < 1000 IU/L

Table 1.7 Criteria for treatment of ectopic pregnancies by local injection.

Serum beta hCG of less than 1000 IU/L,
Tubal pregnancy not exceeding 2 cm in diameter
Absence of chorionic tissue in currettage material from the uterus and
    haemodynamically stable
Suitable substances for injection of tubal pregnancies
PGF2-alpha in contrast to other prostaglandins invariably causes marked
    contractions of smooth muscle fibres and pronounced constriction of the tubal
    artery. It may be administered in the form of 250 micrograms of 15 methyl PGF2-
    alpha (hemabate) diluted in 10 mL of normal saline into the fallopian tube via 4–5
    sites or
Hyperosmolar glucose (10–20 mL of a 50% solution)

Table 1.8 A scoring system for determining whether to do a laparoscopic salpingostomy or laparoscopic salpingectomy.

Infertility	2
Previous ectopic pregnancy	2
Tuboplasty	2
Tubal occlusion	2
Localisation	
Isthmic	1
Ampullary	0
Fimbria	−1
Tubal rupture	1

If the score was 1–4 a laparoscopic conservative procedure would be suitable; if 6 or above a radical (salpingectomy) procedure should be done.

Laparoscopic salpingostomy

This is the treatment of choice if continuing fertility is desired. Up to 90 per cent of all ectopic pregnancies may be treated laparoscopically either by linear salpingostomy or salpingectomy if absolutely necessary.

Conservative surgery (laparoscopic salpingostomy) gives subsequent intrauterine pregnancy rates of up to 85 per cent, reduced by half if there has been a history of infertility. Even when the pregnancy is in a woman's only remaining tube it is at least twice as likely as *in vitro* fertilisation to result in a livebirth. If conception occurs, a term pregnancy is at least twice as likely as another ectopic pregnancy. The contraindications to salpingostomy, therefore, are shown in Table 1.9.

Table 1.9 Absolute contraindications to laparoscopic treatment of ectopic pregnancies.

Haematoperitoneum > 2000 mL
Shock or haemodynamic instability
Ectopic pregnancies > 5 cm
Cornual (interstitial) gestation, whether ruptured or unruptured, should never be treated laparoscopically because of the high risk of uncontrollable haemorrhage
hCG > 15 000 IU/L

Technique of laparoscopic surgery for the treatment of ectopic pregnancies

- Laparoscopic surgery involves triple puncture of the abdominal wall. A 10 or 11 mm laparoscope is introduced subumbilically and via 2 × 5 mm suprapubic portals.
- Atraumatic forceps are introduced through the suprapubic site and used to stabilize the tube, close to the ectopic site.
- The antemesenteric border of the tubal gestation is incised with either a fine needle electrode or an operative laser. The incision then is extended to 1–2 cm over the gestation sac.
- The products of conception will extrude spontaneously, or can easily be removed with Semm spoon forceps.
- Alternatively, special devices can be used for aspirating blood and/or products of conception and for irrigating the implantation site with Hartmann's solution at the end of the procedure.
- Primary closure of the tubal wall is unnecessary.

Laparoscopic salpingectomy

Salpingectomy may be needed in up to 60 per cent of cases. Relative indications include: chronic lesions; thick ampullary wall; large gestation sac; previous tuboplasty; homolateral relapse; immediate failure of conservative treatment; and failure of the hCG to come down to normal levels two weeks after conservative surgery.

Laparoscopic resection (and not linear salpingostomy) of the fallopian tube is the procedure of choice for a ruptured isthmic or ampullary gestation.

• Two 5 mm trocars are introduced suprapubically for atraumatic grasping forceps and diathermy forceps and scissors as required to successively coagulate and cut the tube and mesosalpinx. The tube proximal and distal to the ectopic pregnancy is coagulated with bipolar forceps and then divided with hook scissors or laser. The mesosalpinx is then coagulated and cut in a similar fashion.

• Alternatively, the mesosalpinx is coagulated and cut to mobilise the tube and an endoloop is placed around the tube before it is cut and removed through the abdominal portal.

Laparoscopic treatment of ectopic pregnancies will not be possible in appproximately 10 per cent of cases, mostly due to rupture. Technical failure occurs in under 0.5 per cent of cases. Post-operative morbidity should be less than 1 per cent with a laparoscopic approach.

Follow up hCG and ectopic pregnancy

• Measure hCG at weekly intervals, after any conservative operation to identify persistent trophoblastic activity at an asymptomatic stage. Symptoms (of pregnancy or pain or bleeding) following conservative surgery may occur 10 or more days after surgery.

• The post-operative decline in beta hCG is very important. Levels of 10 per cent of the admission value on the second day after operation suggest successful treatment. If levels are about 25 per cent, the patient should be watched carefully until the hCG is negative. If 35 per cent, on the second day, then success of treatment is doubtful and if greater than 40 per cent, failure is likely.

• Methotrexate (50 mg intramuscularly) may be given for a persisting ectopic pregnancy without symptoms.

Adverse factors for subsequent pregnancy outcome

• Nulliparity;
• previous pelvic inflammatory disease;

- previous history of an ectopic pregnancy or tubal surgery;
- tubal rupture.

GESTATIONAL TROPHOBLASTIC DISEASE (GTD)

Hydatidiform mole (HM)

The worldwide range of incidence is 0.2 to 2.0 per 1000 pregnancies. The incidence in the UK and in the USA, is about 1.5 per 1000 live-births.

There are two types of hydatidiform mole, complete and partial.

Complete mole (CHM)

The conceptus consists solely of hyperplastic, hydropic chorionic villi; no fetus is present. It usually results from fertilisation of an ovum which then loses its nucleus. The haploid sperm duplicates its own chromosomes by meiosis. The results are that: the chromosome complement is usually homozygous 46XX derived solely from the father (androgenetic) or that only one pair of paternal HLAs is expressed.

About 10 per cent of CHMs are heterozygous – usually 46XY but sometimes 46XX. They arise from fertilisation of an anucleate egg by two sperm. CHMs uniquely combine paternal nuclear DNA with maternal mitochondrial DNA. Women with CHMs have an increased incidence of balanced translocations and this could explain the loss of the ovum nucleus.

Partial mole (PHM)

There is focal hyperplasia of trophoblast with varying degrees of hydropic villous degeneration; a fetus is present. Chromosomal abnormalities (particularly triploidy-69, XXX or XXY) are often found. The source of the extra set of chromosomes may be double fertilisation (dispermy) or failure of the first paternal meiotic division.

Clinical features of HM

Most symptoms are related to excessive production of hCG.
- Amenorrhoea combined with exaggerated pregnancy symptoms, e.g. hyperemesis gravidarum.
- Irregular vaginal bleeding and the loss may contain the classical vesicles; often presenting as incomplete miscarriages.

- Pre-eclampsia may develop unusually early.
- Hyperthyroidism develops in about 5 per cent of women with CHM.
- The uterus may be large for dates.
- Ovaries may be palpably enlarged due to presence of theca-lutein cysts.

Diagnosis

- Beta hCG can be markedly raised in serum and urine, but most patients have values within the normal range for pregnancy.
- Ultrasound – the characteristic 'snowstorm' appearance is not pathognomonic. In CHM fetal parts are absent. PHM and missed abortion can be confused.

Invasive mole (IM)

This is a histological diagnosis usually made after hysterectomy which has become necessary because vaginal bleeding has continued and hCG levels have remained raised after initial attempts to empty the uterus.

There is local invasion of the myometrium and it is therefore much less readily removed by evacuation. The tumour may perforate the uterus. Vaginal metastases may also occur but more distant spread is uncommon. There is usually a good response to chemotherapy.

Gestational choriocarcinoma

This is a highly malignant tumour characterised by disordered growth of syncytio- and cytotrophoblast and invasion of the myometrium causing necrosis and haemorrhage. Metastasis is common. It usually arises within two years of the causal pregnancy.

The incidence is about 1 in 20 000 to 1 in 40 000 pregnancies in Western countries, increasing to about 1 in 13 000 pregnancies in the Far East.

Only about 1 in 30 hydatidiform moles develop into choriocarcinoma. However, the risk of subsequent choriocarcinoma is 1000 times greater after a mole than after a normal pregnancy. Thus, as many cases follow moles as follow other pregnancies (Hetero zygous CHM have a greater malignant potential than do homozygous CHM.)

The risk of choriocarcinoma is increased when the woman and her partner have different ABO groups. Groups B and AB patients have a worse prognosis. HLA compatibility between partners may be associated with increased risk of developing choriocarcinoma.

Pathology

Local extension is frequent but ovarian spread is uncommon. The predominant route of spread is vascular. Lymphatic spread is rare. Pulmonary metastases occur in about 70 per cent of cases. They may have a 'cannon-ball' or 'snowstorm' appearance on chest X-ray. Haemoptysis is a common symptom.

Staging of GTD

Stage 0   Molar pregnancy.

Stage I   Persistently elevated hCG titres (i.e. six months or more after evacuation) and tumour confined to body of uterus.

Stage II   Pelvic and/or vaginal metastasis.

Stage III   Pulmonary metastasis.

Stage IV   All other distant metastases.

A prognostic scoring system can be used in Stages I to IV to determine the appropriate treatment for each patient. For details see Tables 1.10 and 1.11.

Management of GTD (Fig. 1.3)

Once a firm diagnosis of molar pregnancy is made the mole needs to be removed, preferably by suction evacuation and curettage. This may need to be repeated if irregular bleeding persists or hCG levels are still elevated six weeks after initial evacuation. Hysterectomy can be carried out in older women whose family is complete. In the UK, patients should be registered with one of the three reference laboratories.

Follow up

Serum beta hCG estimations should be carried out weekly until levels are normal (< 5 IU/L), monthly for a year and then three-monthly during the second year.

The woman may begin to try to become pregnant 6 months after hCG values have become and remain normal. A barrier method of contraception should be used until hCG levels are normal: then oral

Table 1.10 Categorisation of women with gestational trophoblastic tumours. (Reproduced with permission from Newlands, E.S. (1983) Treatment of trophoblastic disease. In *Progress in Obstetrics* Vol. 3 (Ed. by J. Studd), p. 162, Churchill Livingstone, London.)

Risk factors	Score			
	0	10	20	40
Age (years)	< 39	> 39		
Parity	1, 2, > 4	3 or 4		
Antecedent pregnancy	Mole	Abortion	Term	
Interval (AP-chemotherapy) in months	< 4	4–7	7–12	> 12
hCG (plasma mIU/mL or urine IU/day)	10^3–10^4	10^4	10^4–10^5	10^5
ABO	$A \times A$ $\times B$ $\times AB$	$O \times O$ $A \times O$ –	$B \times$ $AB \times$ –	
Number of metastases	0	1–4	4–8	> 8
Site of metastases	Not detected Lungs Vagina	Spleen Kidney	GI tract Liver	Brain
Largest tumour mass	< 3 cm	3–5 cm	> 5 cm	
Lymphocytic infiltration	Marked	Moderate	Slight	
Immune status	Reactive	Unknown	Unreactive	
Previous chemotherapy	Nil		Single drug	Two drugs or more

Scores for individual risk factors are added and risk group determined by the total score as follows: low risk 50 or less; medium risk 55–95; high risk > 95.

Table 1.11 Survival of women by their prognostic score on admission (analysis up to 1973). Reproduced with permission from Newlands, E.S. (1983) Treatment of trophoblastic disease. In *Progress in Obstetrics* Vol. 3 (Ed by J. Studd), p. 163, Churchill Livingstone, London.

	0–40	40–80	90–120	130–180	> 180
Total	94	90	68	45	15
Deaths	0	2	16	24	15
% Alive	100	98	76	47	0

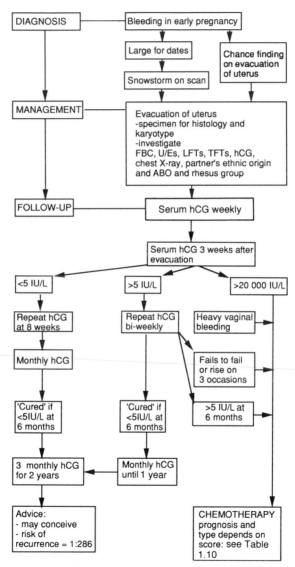

Fig. 1.3 Management of gestational trophoblastic disease. (Reproduced with permission from Rosevear, S.K. (1994) Bleeding in early pregnancy, In: *High Risk Pregnancy, Management Options* (Ed. by D.K. James, P.J. Steer, C.P. Weiner & B. Gonik) W.B. Saunders, London.)

contraception can be used. There may be a higher incidence of subsequent choriocarcinoma if oral contraception is started before hCG levels fall. hCG levels should be checked three weeks after the end of any pregnancy subsequent to a molar pregnancy.

Chemotherapy is not necessary unless the disease progresses. Among the signs of this are:

- Serum beta hCG level > 20 000 IU/L four weeks after evacuation;
- Any elevation of hCG levels six months after evacuation;
- Persistent or recurrent uterine bleeding with raised hCG levels.

Management of Stages I–IV should be confined to specialised centres.

Results of therapy

Remission can be expected in all women adequately treated in Stages I to III and in up to 70 per cent of women with Stage IV disease.

Subsequent pregnancies

A normal outcome can be expected. The incidence of congenital malformation is not increased in women who have received chemotherapy.

INFERTILITY

In the normal population there is a range of fertility with the chance of conception related to time. The peak conception rate in normal fertile couples is about 33 per cent in the first three cyles of 'trying' which falls subsequently to about 20 per cent and by 12 months to below 10 per cent per cycle. The average is 25 per cent per cycle.

Infertility affects 1.2 couples/1000 population and one in six couples needs specialist help at some stage for infertility.

Treatment of infertility – indications and results

The main causes of infertility and their incidence are given in Table 1.12. Fig. 1.4 shows cumulative conception rates of some of the commonest single causes of infertility in a complete population of infertile couples treated by conventional methods, over a 24 month period, compared with normal.

Table 1.12 Main causes of infertility and their incidence.

Cause	Incidence (per cent)
Unexplained	28
Sperm defects	24
Failure of ovulation (amenorrhoea or dysmenorrhoea)	21
Endometriosis	6
Coital failure	6
Tubal damage	4
Cervical mucus defects	3
Obstructive oligospermia or 1° spermatic failure	2
Hormonal causes of male infertility	rare

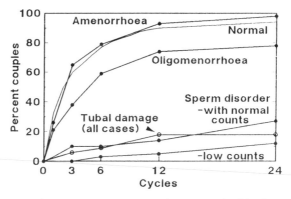

Fig. 1.4 Cumulative pregnancy rates in single groups with subfertility with conventional treatment. (Courtesy Professor M.G.R. Hull.)

Table 1.13 and Fig. 1.5 show the cumulative pregnancy rate after IVF treatment (maximum nine months).

Amenorrhoea with polycystic ovarian disease resistent to clomiphene

After treatment with gonadotrophin therapy the pregnancy rate is approximately 23 per cent per cycle with a 17 per cent miscarriage rate.

Tubal surgery

The two year cumulative pregnancy rate is approximately 20 per cent depending on the extent of damage prior to surgery and whether the serum is positive or negative for chlamydia infection. In vitro fertili-

Table 1.13 Pregnancy rates after IVF.

13–28 per cent first cycle
35–51 per cent after 3 cycles
54 66 per cent after 6 cycles
71–79 per cent after 9 cycles

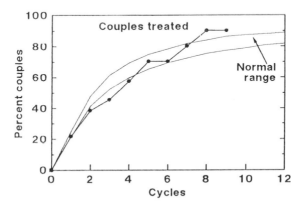

Fig. 1.5 Cumulative pregnancy rates in couples with subfertility treated by IVF over 9 months. (Courtesy Professor M.G.R. Hull.)

sation (IVF) should be considered after 1–2 years if the patient is not pregnant.

Endometriosis

Untreated, this can be associated with marked subfertility. Controlled studies have shown no benefit of danazol or progestogen treatment in mild endometriosis.

Sperm disorders

Sperm disorders are the most common cause of infertility and are heterogeneous in origin. They can occur in men with normal sperm 'counts' on standard semen microscopy.

In couples with prolonged 'unexplained infertility' the sperm of one in three men have severely defective fertilising ability tested by hamster egg penetration. Controlled trials of, for example, hormonal stimulation, artificial insemination or sperm prepared by intrauterine insemination (IUI) have failed to show any benefit. However, treatment to suppress production of seminal antisperm antibodies may be beneficial. Surgical excision of a varicoele does not necessarily improve fertility. The best treatment option in cases of sperm dysfunction is assisted conception.

Unexplained infertility

Most couples with unexplained infertility of less than three years' duration are normal and have simply been unlucky. Most will conceive within two years and no treatment is needed. There is no evidence of any benefit from simple treatment such as clomiphene. After more than three years the chance of natural conception is reduced to between 1 and 3 per cent (Fig 1.6). IVF should be offered to those with unexplained infertility of more than three years' duration. Such couples may expect a 40 per cent 'take home' baby rate per cycle (see Table 1.14).

In vitro fertilisation treatments (IVF, GIFT and superovulation/IUI)

Main indications
- Severe tubal disease
- Unexplained infertility of more than three years' duration
- Significant sperm dysfunction.

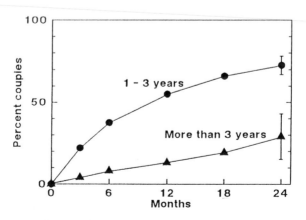

Fig. 1.6 Cumulative fertility in couples with unexplained infertility of less than 3 years and greater than 3 years. (Courtesy Professor M.G.R. Hull.)

Table 1.14 'Take-home baby' rates after IVF treatment.

82% after six cycles with a 'take home baby' rate of 70% (Hull *et al.*, 1992)
43–48% after five cycles (Tan *et al.*, 1992)
The cumulative 'take-home baby' rate can be up to 70% after six cycles and 90%
   after nine cycles in women under 40 years of age and men with normal
   spermatozoa

Pregnancy rates of 28–30 per cent per cycle can be expected as the norm now.

Age causes a decline in conception rates (see Table 1.15). For women up to the age of 34, IVF will result in 55 per cent becoming pregnant and 45 per cent having a livebirth within five cycles (see Fig. 1.5).

Table 1.15 Success of IVF in relation to maternal age. (Source Tan *et al.*, 1992.)

Age	Cumulative pregnancy rates (per cent) after 5 treatment cycles	
	Conception	Livebirth
20–34 years	54	45
35–39 years	39	29
40+ years	20	14

Ovulation induction

Ovulation induction regimens aim to restore the chance of conception to that in the normal fertile population which gives cumulative rates of conception at 6 and 12 months of about 75 per cent and 90 per cent respectively. After excluding women with primary ovulation failure, gonadotrophin therapy in amenorrhoeic women results in a conception rate per cycle of 15–18 per cent for 6 to 12 cycles. In women with oligomenorrhoea, the majority of whom have polycystic ovarian disease (PCOD), the conception rates with gonadotrophin therapy are reduced to about half those achieved in women without PCOD who are amenorrhoeic.

The appropriate method of ovulation induction depends on the type of ovulation disorder, which can be broadly classified into two groups:
▪ women who have amenorrhoea (oestrogen deficient), most of whom

have hypothalamic or pituitary causes accounting for their anovulation;
- women with oligomenorrhoea, mostly due to polycystic ovarian disease.

Before ovulation induction is attempted the underlying cause of a woman's amenorrhoea or oligomenorrhoea should be established. There are three possible causes:

1 Disorders of the hypothalamic/pituitary/ovarian axis
Primary failures
- Hypothalamic, e.g. Kalman syndrome;
- Pituitary, e.g. tumours such as non-secretory adenomas or craniopharyngiomas, or previous surgery.
- Ovarian, e.g. dysgenesis, premature menopause, destruction by radiation or chemotherapy and autoimmune failure.

2 Functional disorders
- Hypothalamic
- Psychological disorders
- Weight loss
- Exercise related
- Pituitary prolactinoma

3 Polycystic ovarian disease

Investigations

Primary ovarian failure

This is characterised by raised follicle-stimulating hormone (FSH) levels (> 50 IU/L) and luteinising hormone (LH) levels and hypoestrogenism (serum oestradiol < 100 picomol/L or negative response to a progestogen challenge test).

Secondary ovarian failure (hypothalamic or pituitary failure)

FSH and LH levels are normal or low (usually < 4 IU/L). On transvaginal ultrasonography the ovaries show as totally inactive with no evidence of any visible follicles, or they may have a multifollicular appearance during the recovery phase from secondary ovarian failure.

Polycystic ovarian disease

This is characterised by raised serum LH levels (usually > 10 IU/L), hyperinsulinaemia, increased androgen production by the ovarian theca and stromal cells, non-elevated FSH, oestrogenisation and usually hirsutism with androgenic alopecia. The diagnosis is usually made from the ovarian morphology at (preferably transvaginal) ultrasound scan. The appearance will be of an expanded echogenic stroma, and multiple (usually > 15), small (usually 2–10 mm diameter) follicles lying in the cortical margin which has been likened to a 'pearl necklace' effect. The ovary is usually enlarged, occasionally to a considerable degree. The diagnosis having been made ultrasonographically, the severity is usually determined endocrinologically.

Treatment

Treat specific underlying causes, e.g. hypothyroidism, before instituting any ovulation induction therapy.

Hyperprolactinaemia – bromocriptine

If the prolactin level is elevated (> 1000 units) ovulation will return with the following treatment with bromocriptine:

- Commence treatment using 2.5 mg nightly for seven days, then increase to 2.5 mg b.d. for seven days and then 2.5 mg t.d.s.
- Check serum prolactin after six weeks on 2.5 mg t.d.s. if patient remains amenorrhoeic and exclude pregnancy.
- Recheck serum prolactin concentration on this dosage.
- If gastrointestinal side effects are troublesome cut the starting dose to 1 mg/day, increasing by 1 mg increments in divided doses at seven day intervals until the maximum tolerated dose is achieved. It is also possible to use the oral tablets rectally. Absorption from the rectum usually gives higher serum bromocriptine levels and a lower dose may be required to control hyperprolactinaemia.

Hypothalamic disorders and failure

Initally attempt induction of ovulation with pulsatile LH-releasing hormone (LHRH) (see below). If unsuccessful the woman may need gonadotrophin therapy.

Amenorrhoeic women with PCOD

Amenorrhoeic women with PCOD who are oestrogenised may require either clomiphene or gonadotrophin therapy for ovulation induction. A positive progestogen challenge test is useful in predicting that a woman should respond to clomiphene citrate (Provera 5 mg/day

1

for five days followed by a withdrawal bleed within seven days). In women with no withdrawal bleeding it is best to use gonadotrophin therapy from the outset.

Avoid clomiphene or simple gonadotrophin therapy if the LH level is > 10 IU/L in the early follicular phase because of the potential increased risk of miscarriage.

Clomiphene citrate

Mechanism of action

Clomiphene citrate is predominantly antioestrogenic in action but also weakly oestrogenic. It competitively blocks the negative feedback effect of oestradiol and causes an increase in the release of pituitary gonadotrophins.

Indications

Useful in the treatment of anovulation in women with an intact and functional hypothalamic-pituitary-ovarian axis who are oestrogenised and, therefore, able to respond to its antioestrogenic actions.

Administration and management of clomiphene therapy

- Dose: 100 mg, given on days 2–6, inclusive, of the cycle.
- Lower doses are only appropriate for women who get side effects at 100 mg/day. Almost all women who are going to respond to clomiphene will do so at 100 mg dosage whereas only about 70 per cent of potential responders will do so on 50 mg doses.
- Clomiphene citrate also has antioestrogenic actions which adversely affect cervical mucus development in some patients, particularly if clomiphene is inappropriately used as an empirical treatment in women who are already ovulating.
- Fewer than 10 per cent of oestrogen deficient women will ovulate with clomiphene therapy. In oestrogenised women 62 per cent will ovulate in the first cycle and 86 per cent within three cycles. Therefore, clomiphene treatment should be pursued for at least three cycles in oestrogenised patients. If there is no evidence of ovulation (mid-luteal serum progesterone levels less than 30 nanomol/L) after three cycles of clomiphene, commence gonadotrophin therapy.
- There is no benefit from using more than 100 mg doses of clomiphene, other than perhaps in grossly obese women.
- Ovulation is determined by mid-luteal serum progesterone levels. In

stimulated cycles a higher mid-luteal progesterone level than usual may need to be taken as evidence of ovulation (60 nanomol/L rather than 30 nanomol/L) because of the contribution of smaller subsidiary follicles which may still become luteinised.

■ If conception does not occur within six cycles of clomiphene, despite mid-luteal progesterone levels suggestive of ovulation, gonadotrophin therapy should be considered.

Gonadotrophins

Choice of gonadotrophin

The choices are 'pure' FSH or a combination of LH and FSH (human menopausal gonadotrophin (hMG)). In cases of PCOD there are theoretical advantages of using 'pure' FSH, which avoids giving further exogenous LH when there is already an excess of endogenous LH in this condition. However, there is no specific clinical evidence for any advantage of using 'pure' FSH in women with PCOD, but there may be more advantage from using it or hMG with pituitary down regulation.

Regimen for managing women on gonadotrophin therapy for ovulation induction

■ The woman telephones with the date of her last menstrual period. If she is amenorrhoeic she should have a five day course of progestogen (5 mg/day) to induce shedding of any residual endometrium.

■ The woman then visits within three days for a baseline serum oestradiol level to be measured and a treatment schedule to be given (Fig. 1.7).

■ Start dose for injections – 1 ampoule of hMG or 'pure' FSH daily (75 IU) for women with PCOD, 150 IU for those without PCOD.

■ The woman returns on day five of treatment for repeat serum oestradiol measurement.

■ When results are available, the woman telephones for modification of the dosage regimen, i.e. the number of ampoules of hMG to be given. The serum oestradiol should have risen from the baseline level and, if not, the gonadotrophin dosage should be increased. In general the rise in oestradiol level should be exponential, doubling every 48–72 hours, and commensurate with 600–1000 picomol/L per mature follicle at the time of ovulation.

■ Continue daily injections. The woman attends at 2–3 day intervals

OVARIAN INDUCTION SCHEDULE

Special instructions   Name, No. or ID label:

History: PCOD/Hypothalamic/Other................
Pretreatment: LHRH/Norethisterone/Oestrogen
Treatment: None/Clom/FSH/LHRH   Starting dose:........amps.
Cycle No: ....
LMP: ..../..../.....   1st day   Rx:..../..../......   Previous cycles: Tel: Daytime:.............
Baseline   LH.........IU/L   FSH.........IU/L   Testosterone.......nmol/L   Evening:............

Date	Cycle day	Follicle diameters		Endometrium	Scan comments	Serum E₂	Serum LH	Treatment plan/comments	Dr
		L. ovary	R. ovary						

hCG 5000 units on:__/__/__   Day 5 hCG 2000 units on:__/__/__   Day 10 hCG 2000 units on:__/__/__
Mid luteal progesterone.........nmol/L   Period date:__/__/__

Fig. 1.7 Ovulation induction schedule.

for serum oestradiol measurement and ultrasound scans to check the number and size of developing follicles.

- The dosage may be increased if there is no evidence of a rise in serum oestradiol after eight days' treatment. (Dosage increment will depend on underlying indication for treatment.) If the diagnosis is PCOD, the increment should only be half an ampoule daily with no increase more frequent than every 10 days to avoid hyperstimulation. For women who do not have PCOD, the dosage increase should be 1 ampoule increments.

- When there are no more than three follicles >17 mm in size on ultrasound scan and a serum oestradiol commensurate with the number and size of the follicles, ovulation is induced with intramuscular hCG 5000 IU. Sexual intercourse should be advised at this stage; preferably daily for the subsequent three days. Seven days after the ovulatory dose of hCG take blood for a progesterone level measurement. A level of >30 nanomol/L is suggestive of ovulation.

- If the woman fails to conceive, she should expect a period 14–16 days after the hCG. Wait one week past the expected date of a period. If it has not arrived advise a pregnancy test to be done. Treatment may be given in consecutive cycles without any adverse effect on the chance of conception.

Ovulation induction with gonadotrophin (with pituitary down regulation)

GnRH (FSH- and LH-releasing hormone) agonists in combination with gonadotrophins for the induction of superovulation may overcome possible adverse effects of endogenous tonic raised LH or premature LH surges on the chances of pregnancy. There is some evidence that the viability of embryos derived from oocytes exposed to inappropriately raised LH levels may be adversely affected. If these embryos implant the pregnancy is more likely to result in an early miscarriage. If GnRH analogues are used with gonadotrophins, they eliminate the risk of premature luteinisation.

Ovulation induction with pituitary down regulation using a GnRH analogue

The following regimen is used for patients with PCOD (LH >10 micromol/L), in women who are responding unpredictably to gonadotrophins alone, and for patients who are getting a premature endogeneous LH rise with simple gonadotrophin therapy.

- The woman telephones in with the date of her last menstrual period.
- Start norethisterone 5 mg/day for seven days from day 17 of the cycle.
- Start intranasal buserelin 100 micrograms four times a day and 200 micrograms at night (600 micrograms/day in divided doses) from day 21.
- At least 14 days later take blood for baseline serum oestradiol and LH levels to confirm adequate pituitary suppression. If appropriate, commence gonadotrophin injections – 1 ampoule/day to start with if it is the first cycle of hMG or 'pure' FSH. Give the woman a treatment schedule.
- The woman returns on day 5 of gonadotrophin therapy for blood to be taken for 'same day' oestradiol estimation. She telephones in the evening for information on any dosage change and when to return for her next serum oestradiol estimation and scan. In general, an ultrasound scan for follicular size is not necessary until the serum oestradiol level is >500 picomol/L. Ultrasound scans and serum oestradiol monitoring should then be done on alternate days.
- Continue buserelin intranasally with daily gonadotrophins until there are not more than three follicles >17 mm in size with a serum oestradiol level of 600–1000 picomol/L for each mature follicule. At this stage, hCG 5000 IU is given and the woman can discontinue her intranasal buserelin. Ovulation occurs 36–42 hours after hCG so the couple should be advised to have intercourse for the next two or three days to optimise the chance of conception.
- If there are more than three mature follicles then there is a substantial risk of a high order multiple pregnancy; hCG should be witheld under these circumstances.
- Do not give the ovulatory dose of hCG if the serum oestradiol exceeds 8000 picomol/L as this is associated with an increased risk of ovarian hyperstimulation syndrome which has serious and potentially life-threatening implications.
- hCG 2000 IU should be given five and ten days after the ovulatory dose of hCG for luteal phase support.

Ovarian electro-cautery

There is some evidence that treatment with electrocoagulation (a 4 second pepper-pot burn to the surface of the ovary using a needle diathermy point at 20 Watt settings) results in ovulation rates of 80 per cent and pregnancy rates in 75 per cent of those women with PCOD within 6 months of surgery.

Superovulation for *in vitro* fertilisation

- The woman starts GnRH therapy in the midluteal phase of the cycle. In women with variable cycle lengths this is best identified as the length of her shortest normal menstrual cycle minus seven days.
- Commence on buserelin 100 micrograms four doses intranasally at 08.00, 12.00, 16.00, 20.00 hours and 200 micrograms at night at bedtime. An alternative is nafarelin 400 micrograms twice daily to give a total daily dose of 800 microgram/day.
- Anticipate a period within 14 days of starting GnRH. If the woman does not have a period, then a pregnancy test should be arranged as approximately 1 per cent of women without bilateral tubal occlusion will have conceived.
- Commence daily injections of FSH 150 IU after pituitary down regulation is complete (i.e. observe dormant ovaries on ultrasound scan, a serum oestradiol level <100 picomol/L or serum LH <2 IU/L).
- Serum oestradiol and ultrasound monitoring should commence from day 8 of gonadotrophin stimulation. If there is no rise of oestradiol from the baseline by day 8, consider increasing the dose of gonadotrophin. Anticipate a doubling of serum oestradiol concentration every 48–72 hours from day 8.
- The ovulatory dose of hCG 5000 IU is given when there are at least three follicles of 16 mm or more in diameter with commensurate oestrogen levels of 600–1000 picomol/L for each mature follicle. Oocyte retrieval is planned for 36 hours later.
- If the serum oestradiol is 10 000 picomol/L consider abandoning the cycle because of the risk of ovarian hyperstimulation syndrome.
- Stop FSH and buserelin after the ovulatory dose of hCG.
- Give hCG 2000 IU on the day of embryo transfer and on day 5 post embryo transfer, for luteal phase support. Reduce these dosages if there is considered to be a high risk of ovarian hyperstimulation such as when the pre-hCG serum oestradiol is greater than 8000 picomol/L or if the patient has abdominal pain, abdominal bloating, nausea and vomiting.

Setting up an LHRH pump

1

A Graseby Driver Type MS 27 pulsatile battery operated syringe pump or similar is required.

- The pulse rate should be set at 90 minute intervals.
- Press the 'start/test' button to check it is working.
- Use a microflex butterfly infusion set 1000 mm × 0.5 mm gauge 25.
- A Vecafix dressing is required.
- A 10 ml sabre syringe is required to fit the pump accurately and give an appropriate metred dose of 15 micrograms with each pulse.
- Fill the syringe with LHRH (Fertiral) diluted 50:50 with normal saline. Each ampoule contains 1000 micrograms in 2 mL (500 microgram/mL).
- Use two ampoules (4 mL) of LHRH and combine with 4 mL of normal saline (0.9 per cent). Fill the dead space in the giving set and butterfly needle completely after connection to the syringe.
- Break off one of the wings on the syringe to allow it to fit into the delivery apparatus snugly.
- Attach the protective shield. The syringe driver can comfortably be carried on a waist money bag or 'shoulder holster'. Test the driver with a pulse dose.
- Insert the butterfly needle subcutaneously between the lower ribs parallel to them and below the normal 'bra-line'.
- Expect a delivery rate at 1½ mL/day. Top up the syringe after five days.
- Refill the syringe with 50:50 mixture of LHRH and normal saline.
- After five days arrange an ultrasound scan to monitor follicular development and to give advice regarding appropriate timing of intercourse.
- If there is no follicular growth after 14 days, increase the solution to full strength by refilling the syringe with undiluted LHRH.
- Repeat scans at five day intervals when syringe is refilled.
- When a follicle of 17–18 mm is anticipated (assuming a growth rate of 1½–2 mm/day after a 12 mm diameter is achieved), advise sexual intercourse, assuming spontaneous ovulation. Scan 36 hours later when it is expected that the follicle will have disappeared.
- Once ovulation has occurred the pump can be taken down and hCG 5000 IU given. Alternatively, the pump may he left in place to provide 'luteal support'. A blood sample for serum progesterone seven days

after presumed ovulation will confirm whether this has occurred. The level should be above 30 nanomol/L.

LHRH test – for possible hypopituitarism

This test is most useful after pituitary surgery as a dynamic test of pituitary gonadotrophin function. It may be combined with dynamic testing of pituitary TSH production.

Combined LHRH and thyrotrophin-releasing hormone (TRH) test

- A blood sample is taken before the administration of LHRH – TRH to measure baseline concentration of LH/TSH and prolactin.
- LHRH 100 mg and TRH 200 mg are given intravenously as a bolus. The bolus injection should be given slowly, especially in patients with hypertension as there may be some elevation of blood pressure. In hypertensive patients the dose of TRH should be reduced to 100 mg.

Note. Patients may get a strong urge to micturate shortly after the LHRH and TRH have been given.

BIBLIOGRAPHY

Abdel Gadir Mowafi, R.S., Alnaser, H.M.I., Alfrashid, A.H., Alonezi, O.M. & Shaw, R.W. (1990) Ovarian electrocautery versus human menopausal gonadotrophins and pure follicle stimulating hormone therapy in the treatment of patients with polycystic ovarian disease. *Clinical Endocrinology*, **33**, 585–592.

Alberman, E. (1988) The epidemiology of repeated abortion. In *Early Pregnancy Loss: Mechanism and Treatment* (Ed. by R.W. Beard & S.N. Sharp), pp 9–17. Royal College of Obstetricians and Gynaecologists, London.

Berkowitz, R.L. Lynch, L., Lapinskki, R. & Bergh, P. (1993) First-trimester transabdominal multifetal pregnancy reduction: a report of two hundred completed cases. *American Journal of Obstetrics & Gynecology*, **169**, 17–21.

Bruhart, A., Manhes, H., Mage, C. & Pouly, J.L. (1980) Treatment of ectopic pregnancy by means of laparoscopy. *Fertility & Sterility*, **33**, 411–414.

DeCherney, A.H. & Kase, N. (1979) The conservative surgical management of unruptured ectopic pregnancy. *Obstetrics & Gynecology*, **54**, 451–454.

Fernandez, H., Lelaidier, C., Batson, C., Bourget, P. & Frydman, R. (1991) Return of reproductive performance after expectant management and local treatment for ectopic pregnancy. *Human Reproduction*, **6**, 1474–1477.

Fernandez, H., Lelaidier, C., Thouvenez, V. & Frydman, R. (1991) The use of a pretherapeutic, predictive score to determine inclusion criteria for the non-surgical treatment of ectopic pregnancy. *Human Reproduction*, **6**, 995–998.

Fernandez, H., Rainhorn, J.D., Papernik, E., Bellet, D. & Frydman, R. (1988) Spontaneous resolution of ectopic pregnancy. *Obstetrics & Gynecology*, **71**, 171–174.

Hallatt, J.G. (1986) Tubal conservation in ectopic pregnancy: a study of 200 cases. *American Journal of Obstetrics & Gynecology*, **154**, 1216–1221.

Harp, S.N. (1988) A prospective study of spontaneous abortion. In: *Early Pregnancy Loss: Mechanism and Treatment* (Ed. by R.W. Beard), pp 23–37. Royal College of Obstetricians and Gynaecologists, London.

Hull, M.G.R., Eddowes, H.A., Fahy, U., Abuzeid, M.I., Mills, M.S., Cahill, D.J., Fleming, C.F., Wardle, P.G., Ford, W.C.L. & McDermitt, A. (1992) Expectations of assisted conception for infertility. *British Medical Journal*, **304**, 1465–1469.

Hull, M.G.R., Glazener, C.M.A., Kelly, N.J., Conway, D.I., Foster, P.A., Hinton, R.A., Coulson, C., Lambert, P.A., Watt, E.M. & Desai, K.M. (1985) Population study of causes, treatment and outcome of infertility. *British Medical Journal*, **291**, 1693–1697.

Hull, M.G.R., Savage, P.E. & Jacobs, H.S. (1979) Investigation and treatment of amenorrhoea resulting in normal fertility. *British Medical Journal*, **1**, 1257–1261.

Newlands, E.S. (1983) Treatment of trophoblastic disease. In *Progress in Obstetrics* Vol. 3 (Ed. by J. Studd), p. 162, Churchill Livingstone, London.

Pouly, J.L., Mahnes, H., Canis, M., *et al.* (1986) Conservative laparoscopic treatment of 321 ectopic pregnancies. *Fertility & Sterility*, **46**, 1093–1097.

Regan, L., Braude, P.R. & Trembath, P.L. (1989) Influence of past reproductive performance on risk of spontaneous abortion. *British Medical Journal*, **299**, 541–545.

Regan, L. (1991) Recurrent miscarriage. *British Medical Journal* (Editorial) **302**, 543–544.

Stirrat, G.M. (1990a) Recurrent miscarriage I: definition and epidemiology. *The Lancet*, **366**, 673–675.

Stirrat, G.M. (1990b) Recurrent miscarriage II: clinical associations, causes and management. *The Lancet*, **336**, 728–733.

Tan, S.L., Royston, P., Campbell, S., Jacobs, H.S., Betts, J., Mason, B. & Edwards, R.G. (1992) Cumulative conception and live birth rates after in-vitro fertilisation. *The Lancet*, **339**, 1390–1394.

Tietze, C. (1986) Fertility after the discontinuation of intrauterine and oral contraception. *International Journal of Fertility*, **13**, 385–389.

Vermesh, M. (1989) Conservative management of ectopic gestation. *Fertility & Sterility*, **51**, 559–567.

Vessey, M.P., Wright, N.H., McPherson, K. & Wiggins, P. (1978) Fertility after stopping different methods of contraception. *British Medical Journal*, **i**, 265–267.

2 Antenatal Fetal Diagnosis

ULTRASOUND MEASUREMENTS OF THE FETUS

Clinical estimation of gestational age

Naegele's formula is used to estimate gestational age.

- Add seven days to the last menstrual period, subtract three from the month and add one to the year.

This formula assumes a pregnancy length of 40 weeks (280 days) and that conception occurred two weeks after the LMP. Postmaturity is defined as a pregnancy longer than 42 weeks (294 days) of gestation.

Ultrasound imaging provides verification of the 'dates' and establishes viability of the pregnancy.

Gestation sac

The first evidence of an intrauterine pregnancy is the presence of an intrauterine sac.

The gestation sac is first measurable by vaginal ultrasonography at just over 4 weeks from the last menstrual period (see Table 2.1).

Table 2.1 Gestation sac size (mm) and weeks of gestation.

Gestation sac size (mm)	Weeks of gestation
2	4
5	5
10	6
20	7
25	8

Crown–rump length (CRL)

CRL is used to identify gestational age in the first trimester of pregnancy (Fig. 2.1). It measures a straight line from one fetal pole to the other along its longitudinal axis. Between 12 and 14 weeks accurate assessment of gestational age is difficult by measuring CRL due to fetal flexion.

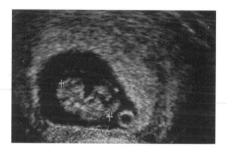

Fig. 2.1 Crown–rump length. Yolk sac is visible on the right.

Bi-parietal diameter (BPD)

BPD is measured to assess gestational age from 14 weeks onwards. The ultrasound probe images the fetus longitudinally and then it is rotated 90° to obtain the transverse plane through the fetal head (Fig. 2.2).

- The head should be oval. Exclude any defects of the bony outline or soft tissue excrescences.
- Check the midline echo and presence of the cavum septum pellucidum which looks like an = sign between the anterior $\frac{1}{3}$ and posterior $\frac{2}{3}$ interrupting the midline.

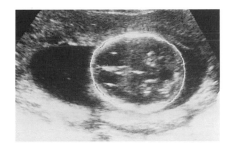

2

Fig. 2.2 Biparietal diameter (BPD).

- The BPD is measured between the leading edge of the echoes from the proximal and distal skull bones.
- It increases by **3–4 mm per week** in the early second trimester but only by **1–2 mm per week** in the late third trimester.
- The lateral ventricles are recognised as echopoor structures, the anterior horns lying medially and the posterior horns more laterally.

Head circumference (HC)

- The same section is taken as that which derives the BPD. It is obtained by measuring around the circumference of the head with electronic calipers or by taking the occipito-frontal diameter (OFD), adding it to the BPD and dividing by two.
- The dumbell shape of the cerebellum and fluid filled cisterna magna can be seen on the suboccipto-bregmatic view.
- Transcerebellar diameter in millimetres gives the gestational age in weeks. It remains constant in growth retardation.

Abdominal circumference (AC) (Fig. 2.3)

- The fetus is imaged by identifying a longitudinal section through the fetal aorta. The transducer is rotated through 90° at the level of the umbilical vein. The correct cross section across the fetal abdomen is identified by a circular outline of the spine. The aorta should also be circular and the stomach bubble visualised. The umbilical vein is visualised approximately a third of the distance from the edge of the abdomen in cross section.

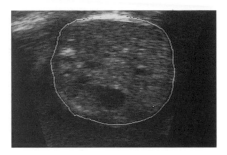

Fig. 2.3 Abdominal circumference.

▪ The abdominal circumference is determined by tracing around the outline or by adding together two cross sectional measurements at right angles, dividing them by two, and multiplying by 22/7.

The head circumference/abdominal circumference should approximate to one near term.

Intrauterine growth retardation (IUGR)

IUGR is detected by serial measurement of both HC and AC. It can be **symmetrical** (i.e. the growth of all organs and structures is equally impaired) or **asymmetrical** (in which there is relative sparing of head growth).

Femur length (FL)

The fetal thigh is identified and the femur measured in the plane where the buttocks and knee are included in the view (Fig. 2.4). The femur should be imaged parallel to the transducer. FL can be underestimated if the incorrect plane is obtained; it cannot be overestimated.

Note: The femoral capital epiphysis does not ossify until 6 months after birth.

Ultrasound assessment of gestational age

BPD and FL give the same assessment of gestational age. If this differs from the menstrual dates by more than one week at an early scan

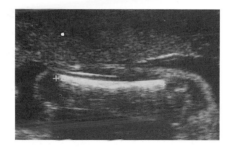

Fig. 2.4 Femur length.

(<20 weeks), the ultrasonic measurements should be taken as indicating the gestational age and the expected date of delivery adjusted accordingly.

A discrepancy in the estimate of gestational age between the BPD and FL may be due to dolicocephaly i.e. the breadth of the skull is less than 4/5 of the length. In this case the head circumference should be measured.

During the third trimester, sonographic detection of lower limb epiphyseal ossification centres is an accurate indicator of gestational age.

Tables and graphs for plotting ultrasonically determined measurements may be found in Chapter 11.

Ultrasound equipment

Antenatal diagnosis by abdominal sonography uses a 3.5 or 5 MHz probe. Higher frequency probes give improved resolution with decreased tissue penetration. With term pregnancies or obese patients in the second trimester a 3 or 3.5 MHz probe may enhance tissue penetration but decreases resolution.

Knowledge of the use of the following controls is essential:

- **Focal depth** should be set at a level appropriate for the structures being imaged, i.e. 2 cm or 10 cm.
- **Gain** (intensity). Increasing the gain amplifies all information – both the true signal and random noise. It must be set for optimum imaging.

Safety of ultrasound

There is no confirmed scientific evidence for adverse effects on humans at levels of intensity used for diagnostic purposes although, on grounds of caution, it may be best to avoid pulsed Doppler in the first trimester.

2

Biological effects of ultrasound

At higher intensities than those used clinically ultrasound may have adverse effects by causing thermal changes and induction of microcavitation.

- Significant heating (>1°C) is not caused by the levels of intensity to which the tissue is exposed with diagnostic ultrasound – less than 20 milliwatts per square centimetre (20 mW/cm^2). Mammals tolerate increases in heating of up to 4°C.
- Microcavitation is the interaction of sound with the microscopic gas bubbles that occur in tissues, causing the bubbles to increase and decrease rapidly in size. It must be noted that diagnostic ultrasound involves short pulses with long intervals between adjacent pulses, i.e. if the mean examination time was 10 minutes, fetal exposure would be less than 2 minutes. Calculations of exposure time depend on the particular instrument, the transducer characteristics and the size and orientation of the fetus.

Psychological effects of ultrasound

Many women are reassured by routine ultrasound examination and enjoy seeing 'their baby'. A small number are caused great (and often unnecessary) anxiety by uncertain findings, the real significance of which is not known.

INVASIVE PROCEDURES FOR IDENTIFICATION OF THE FETAL KARYOTYPE

Karyotyping

Karyotyping is usually offered when the risk of a chromosomal abnormality is at least 1 per cent. This is an empirical approach based on the approximate risks of miscarriage as a result of invasive fetal sampling procedures (amniocentesis, chorionic villus sampling or cordocentesis – see below).

Indications for karyotype analysis

- The risk of a fetus at 16 weeks being karyotypically abnormal is greater than the risk at birth (see Tables 2.2, 2.3 and 2.4).
- A Down's syndrome screening programme suggests an unacceptably high risk of Down's syndrome. Risk assessment is based on maternal age, and serum alphafetoprotein (AFP), hCG and, in some centres, oestriol levels measured at 16 to 18 weeks. Each centre must set its own definition of 'unacceptably high risk'. An estimated risk of worse than one in three hundred will identify 60 per cent of Down's syndrome fetuses if karyotyping is done (usually by amniocentesis).

This screening can cause serious anxiety to a small but increasing number of women who are thought to be at higher than average risk. The rationale behind screening is often not fully understood. Women at 'low risk' often wrongly consider this is a total reassurance about the baby not having Down's syndrome.

- Structural abnormalities are found by ultrasound on routine scanning at 18 weeks (Tables 2.5 and 2.6). The commonest associated

Table 2.2 Overall incidence of chromosomal abnormalities.

Sex chromosome abnormalities In males	
XXY (Klinefelter's syndrome)	1/1000
XYY	1/1100
Other	1/1700
Total	1/400
Sex chromosome abnormalities in females	
45,X (Turner's syndrome)	1/7500
XXX	1/1200
Other	1/300
Total	1/750
Autosomal trisomies	
Trisomy 13	1/15 000
Trisomy 18	1/11 000
Trisomy 21	1/900
Other trisomies	1/22 000
Overall incidence	1/800

Table 2.3 Maternal age associated specific risks of all chromosome anomalies derived from amniocenteses at 16 weeks' gestation. (Source: Ferguson-Smith M.A. & Yates J.R.W. (1984) Maternal age specific rates for chromosome aberrations and factors influencing them; a report of a collaborative European study on 52,965 amniocenteses. *Prenatal Diagnosis*, **4**, 5–44.)

Age (years)	Incidence	Percentage risk
35	1/250	0.4
36	1/143	0.7
37	1/125	0.8
38	1/111	0.9
39	1/83	1.2
40	1/71	1.4
41	1/63	1.6
42	1/30	3.3
43	1/43	2.3
44	1/22	4.6
45	1/12	8.2

chromosome anomalies (especially if more than one structural abnormality is found) are:

> Trisomy 13
> Trisomy 18
> Trisomy 21
> Turner's
> Unbalanced chromosomal rearrangements

(See Table 2.2.)

Amniocentesis technique

- The maternal skin is swabbed with povidine iodine.
- A 20–22 gauge spinal needle, 7–10 cm in length is used.
- It is inserted with or without local anaesthetic under continual ultrasound imaging.
- The stylet is removed and 1–2 mL of amniotic fluid is aspirated and discarded to minimise maternal cell contamination.
- A second syringe is attached to the hub of the needle and 10–15 mL of amniotic fluid withdrawn.
- The needle is withdrawn.

Table 2.4 Age specific risk of chromosome abnormality derived from livebirths. (Source: Hook E.B. (1981) Rates of chromosome abnormalities at different maternal ages. *Obstetrics & Gynecology*, **58**, 282–285.)

Maternal age (years)	Risk of Down's syndrome	Risk of all abnormalities
20	1/1667	1/526
21	1/1667	1/526
22	1/1429	1/500
23	1/1429	1/500
24	1/1250	1/476
25	1/1250	1/476
26	1/1176	1/476
27	1/1111	1/455
28	1/1053	1/435
29	1/1000	1/384
30	1/952	1/385
31	1/909	1/322
32	1/769	1/317
33	1/625	1/260
34	1/500	1/204
35	1/385	1/164
36	1/294	1/130
37	1/227	1/103
38	1/175	1/82
39	1/137	1/65
40	1/106	1/51
41	1/82	1/40
42	1/64	1/32
43	1/50	1/25
44	1/38	1/20
45	1/30	1/15
46	1/23	1/12
47	1/18	1/10
48	1/14	1/7
49	1/11	

Risks of amniocentesis

Two studies have failed to detect any excess risk (National Institute of Child Health and Human Development, 1976; Simpson *et al.*, 1976) but others (MRC, 1978; Tabor, 1986) have suggested the following additional risks:

■ **Miscarriage** (1 per cent) particularly if maternal serum AFP is elevated beforehand, the placenta has been perforated or discoloured amniotic fluid is withdrawn

Table 2.5 Ultrasonic structural appearances of fetuses with common chromosomal defects.

Trisomy 21 (Down's syndrome)	Trisomy 18 (Edwards' syndrome)	Trisomy 13 (Patau's syndrome)
Nuchal oedema	Strawberry-shaped head	Holoprosencephaly
Macroglossia	Choroid plexus cysts	Facial cleft
Atrioventricular septal defects	Facial cleft	Cardiac defects
Mild hydronephrosis	Micrognathia	Hydronephrosis
Clinodactyly	Heart defects	Polydactyly
Sandal gap	Exomphalos	Overlapping fingers
	Malformations of the hands and feet	Clubfoot
	Growth retardation	

Turner's syndrome	Triploidy	
Nuchal cystic hygromata	Early-onset severe asymmetrical growth retardation	
General oedema	Ventriculomegaly	
Brachycephaly	Syndactyly	
Cardiac defects	Molar pregnancy (6/42) cases	

Table 2.6 Frequency of chromosomal anomalies associated with fetal structural defect. (Adapted from Nicolaides *et al.* (1992))

Chromosomal anomaly	Incidence (per cent)
Isolated defect detected	2
More than 1 defect detected	29
Overall	14

- **Leakage of liquor** within six weeks of test
- **Respiratory distress syndrome**
- **Talipes**.

In the MRC study the incidence of perinatal death was higher in the amniocentesis group but the inherent risk may have been greater in those having the test.

Chorionic villus sampling (CVS)

Chorionic villus sampling is done after ten weeks' gestation (CRL

35 mm). This not only excludes those pregancies that miscarry early in gestation but also minimises the risk to the fetus.

▪ A single (18–20 gauge) or double (17–18 outer and 19–20 inner) gauge needle may be used. The latter allows multiple samples to be aspirated.

▪ The point of entry in the skin is infiltrated with a local anaesthetic agent and the needle passed into the placenta under ultrasound guidance.

▪ Villi are identified as pale pink lace-like fronds. Between 5 and 30 mg of villi are usually required. (Maternal decidua is white, more solid and homogenous.)

Risks of CVS

In the Medical Research Council European Trial of CVS (MRC Working Party, 1991) (3248 women) 86 per cent and 91 per cent had a liveborn infant in those who had CVS and amniocentesis respectively. The excess risks among those having CVS were:

▪ more spontaneous fetal deaths before 28 weeks' gestation (2.9 per cent (0.6–5.3 per cent));

▪ more terminations of pregnancy for chromosomal anomalies (1 per cent (0.0–2.1 per cent));

▪ more neonatal deaths (0.3 pcr cent (0.1–0.7 per cent)) in those who had CVS, due to a preponderance of very immature liveborn infants in that group;

▪ more abnormal diagnoses followed chorion villus than amniotic fluid analyses (5.6 per cent versus 3.9 per cent). (This difference was largely due to diagnoses of trisomy 18 and or (usually mosaic) abnormalities known to be confined to the placenta.)

Three terminated pregnancies wcre false positives (one tested by CVS and two by amniocentesis) and two other mosaic cases diagnosed by CVS may have been false positives. There was one false negative result in the chorion villus sampling group.

Cell analysis with CVS

There are two methods:

1 **Direct analysis** gives a cytogenetic analysis carried out on metaphase spread of chromosomes, usually within 48 hours. Abnormalities confined to the placenta are found most frequently in the cytotrophoblastic cells studied in the **direct** preparations (see below).

Chromosome banding is more difficult with this method but avoids maternal cell contamination (see below).

2 **Long-term culture** utilises mesenchymal cells which have the same karyotype as the fetus, takes longer, but produces better metaphase spreads. Long-term culture (about 10 days for a result) allows the identification of small chromosomal deletions and duplications (thus avoiding some false negative results), has lower rates of confined placental abnormalities, but has higher rates of maternal cell contamination.

Therefore proper CVS examination involves both a direct and indirect karyotype analysis.

Diagnostic accuracy of karyotyping process

Occasionally there is discrepancy between the result of the amniocentesis or the placental biopsy at CVS and the true fetal karyotype. Among the possible reasons are maternal cell contamination, placental mosaicism and death of an abnormal twin.

Maternal cell contamination

The incidence may be as high as 0.5 per cent. The following will minimise the risk at **amniocentesis**:

- discard the first 1–2 mL of amniotic fluid
- use a 20 gauge needle (or smaller)
- always keep the stylet in the needle during insertion
- strive to avoid a bloody tap.

Placental mosaicism

Mosaicism is the presence of two or more cell lines with different karyotypes in a prenatal diagnostic sample or an individual. Most cases of true mosaicism arise as a result of an error in an early division in the zygote rather than a parental non-disjunctional error. Although mosaicism in CVS may be associated with true mosaicism in the fetus, it is more often due to **placental mosaicism** which arose as a result of the expression of genes in the trophoblast which are not expressed in the fetus. It occurs in between 0.4 and 4 per cent of CVS samples.

Long term culture reduces the risk but occasionally further investigation (e.g. cordocentesis) is required with additional procedure-related fetal risks.

Death of an abnormal twin

Very rarely a discrepancy may arise from the death of an abnormal twin but survival of that twin's trophoblast which happens to have been sampled.

TYPES OF CHROMOSOMAL ABNORMALITY

2

The four most important are:

- autosomal trisomies
- sex chromosome abnormalities
- chromosomal rearrangements
- polyploidy.

Autosomal trisomies

Autosomal trisomies are either associated with recognisable clinical syndromes, e.g. trisomies 8, 9, 13, 18, 21 and 22, or are not associated with clinically recognisable syndromes (e.g. trisomies 3, 6, 7, 14, 15, 16 and 20). The latter are usually confined to the placenta but may indicate a risk of adverse pregnancy outcome.

No case of false positive diagnosis for pure trisomy 21 has yet been reported, although there are false positive results for trisomy 21 mosaicism. False positive results for other trisomies (usually trisomy 18) are frequent.

Sex chromosome abnormalities

These include two major problem groups, 45X cell lines (often not real in the fetus) and 46XX/46XY mosaicism which usually involves maternal cell contamination but may indicate true hermaphroditism. Other forms of mosaicism involve 47XXX, 47XXY and 47XYY.

Chromosomal rearrangements

Chromosomal rearrangements are a very heterogeneous group of abnormalities including de novo translocations, inversions, deletions and duplications as well as 'supernumerary marker' chromosomes. The risks depend on the type of rearrangement (whether balanced or unbalanced) and the chromosome regions involved. Even if they are real, the prognosis is difficult to predict.

Polyploidy

This includes triploidy and tetraploidy, which have entirely different origins and implications. Tetraploidy occurs frequently in CVS and is one of the leading causes of false positive results in CVS. Triploidy occurs less frequently and in some cases involves twin pregnancy with death of the triploid twin but survival of its trophoblast.

Anomalous test results

The highest risks for false positive results occur for trisomies 3, 7, 8, 9, 12, 13, 15, 16, 18, 20, 23, 22, 45, X, polyploidy especially tetraploidy, 47XXY and supernumerary markers.

46/47,+20 mosaics are almost always extra-embryonic and therefore not representatitive of the fetus. Ninety per cent of cases with 45X/XY are associated with normal male phenotype.

MID TRIMESTER ULTRASOUND SCANNING FOR STRUCTURAL ANOMALIES

Detailed ultrasound scanning is done at 18 weeks gestation to assess structural normality of the fetus.

Intracranial abnormalities (see Table 2.7)

Ventriculomegaly (associated with hydrocephalus)

This is the most common intracranial abnormality, with an incidence of 0.3–1.5/1000 births. It may be isolated or associated with neural tube defects which occur in 1–2/1000 births.

On ultrasound examination the biparietal view includes the lateral

Table 2.7 Types of CNS abnormalities and their incidence.

Spina bifida	1/1000
Anencephaly	1/1000
Encephalocoele	1/10 000
Hydrocephalus	1–2.5/1000
Agenesis of the corpus callosum	1/100–1/19 000
Holoprosencephaly	1/1660–1/16 000
Iniencephaly	1/1000–1/100 000

ventricles (which are echo-poor structures) with anterior horns lying medially and the posterior horns lateral to the midline echo.

Ventricular dilatation should be assessed. Ventriculomegaly is diagnosed if either or both ventricles measures 10 mm or more or the width of the anterior or posterior horn compared to the width of the hemisphere (V/H ratio) is greater than 0.5 from 16 weeks onwards.

If hydrocephalus is identified, the site of the obstruction may be inferred by identifying the enlarged portion of the ventricular system. Marked dilatation of the lateral and third ventricle suggests aquaduct stenosis. Enlargement of all ventricles and the presence of a normal cerebellar vermis associated with distension of the sub-arachnoid system suggests communicating hydrocephalus.

Congenital hydrocephalus

Congenital hydrocephalus has various causes:

- It may be due to aquaductal stenosis possibly as a result of intrauterine infections such as toxoplasmosis, syphilis, cytomegalovirus, mumps or influenza.
- Familial cases due to X-linked pattern of transmission causes up to 25 per cent of lesions in males.
- 'Dandy Walker' malformation is a defect in the cerebellar vermis through which the posterior fossa communicates with the fourth ventricle which causes hydrocephalus. It is frequently associated with another nervous system abnormality.

Each of these forms of anatomical hydrocephalus has a different prognosis.

- All cases of ventriculomegaly should be karyotyped.
- Aquaductal stenosis has a mortality of between 10 and 30 per cent; of those surviving the mean IQ is 71.
- Isolated communicating hydrocephalus carries a good prognosis with those treated having no excess mortality and normal intelligence.
- 'Dandy Walker' malformation has an overall mortality rate of 12–26 per cent and an IQ below 80 in 60–70 per cent of cases.

Neural tube defects

In addition to the visualisation of the actual defect the following can be helpful:

- **Lemon sign** This is the scalloped appearance of the fronto-parietal bones due to an Arnold–Chiari malformation at the foramen magnum. It is not present in late pregnancy (i.e. it is only observed in the second trimester).

▪ **Banana sign** Instead of the normal dumb-bell shape of the cerebellum imaged on the sub-occipito-bregmatic view (Fig. 2.5) the Arnold–Chiari malformation causes the cerebellum to be pulled caudally producing the banana shape on imaging. If severe, the cerebellum may not be seen intracerebally because it has been pulled into the upper cervical spinal canal.

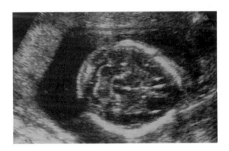

Fig. 2.5 Normal cerebellum.

Choroid plexus cysts

The chorid plexus is a vascular structure located within the lateral, third and fourth ventricles that produces cerebro spinal fluid (CSF). It is particularly prominent between late first and second trimesters (16–21 weeks) where they occupy most of the cerebral ventricle.

Choroid plexus cysts are generally bilateral and can be seen in 0.1–0.8 per cent (one in 120–400) of fetuses. They are well defined round cystic structures within the choroid plexus, thought to be due to neuro-epithelial folds that fill with CSF and cellular debris. Most resolve spontaneously by 24 weeks but they can be associated with trisomies (particularly trisomy 18).

If other markers for chromosome abnormalities are present or there are other structural abnormalities, karyotyping is indicated.

CARDIAC ULTRASOUND SCANNING

Congenital heart defects (CHD) occur in 8–9/1000 livebirths, with a higher frequency in spontaneous abortions.

Chromosomal aberrations are found in 4–5 per cent of cases of CHD. There is a higher incidence in children of mothers with CHD. Cardiac scans are best done at 20 weeks gestation (see Table 2.8).

Table 2.8 Echocardiography: indications for fetal echocardiography.

	Recurrence risk
A family history of CHD	
One previous child has had CHD	1/50
Two affected children	1/10
Affected parent: risk of a child being affected	1/10
Maternal history/medical conditions	
Alcoholism	
Diabetes	
Drug exposure during pregnancy	
Infections during pregnancy	
Phenylketonuria	
Systemic lupus erythematosus	
Fetal indications	
Chromosomal abnormalities	
Dysrhythmias – especially complete heart block which produces a sustained bradycardia of less than 100 beats per minute	
Extracardiac abnormalities	
Non-immune hydrops	
Polyhydramnios	
Symmetrical growth retardation	
Structural abnormality of the fetus on ulrasound	
Teratogens, e.g. lithium, phenytoin or steroids	

Cardiac malformations

Those that may be diagnosed by ultrasound in utero include:

- aortic, mitral, pulmonary, or tricuspid atresia
- aortic over-ride
- atrioventricular septal defect
- double inlet ventricle
- Fallot's tetralogy
- mitral atresia
- severe coarctation or interruption of the aorta
- severe Ebstein's anomaly or tricuspid dysplasis

- total anomalous pulmonary venous drainage
- transposition of the great arteries
- ventricular septal defect.

Four chamber view of the heart

Detects 2/1000 cardiac defects (Fig. 2.6). A complete fetal echo-cardiogram identifies all the cardiac connections and should detect about four to five forms of heart disease per 1000 fetuses scanned.

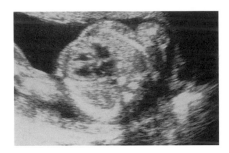

Fig. 2.6 Normal four-chamber view of the heart.

It is obtained by imaging a transverse section of the thorax just above the diaphragm. The heart lies mainly in the left chest.

The heart occupies about a third of the thorax. The two atria are approximately equal in size. There are two ventricles of approximately equal size and thickness. Both contract equally. The atria and ventricular septa meet the two atrioventricular valves at the crux of the heart in an offset cross. The apex points towards the left anterior chest wall. The ventricular and atrial septums may be observed and the atrioventricular valves can be demonstrated. The right ventricle is below the sternum.

The descending aorta is seen as a circle in the mediastinum. It lies anterior to the spine. The left atrium lies anterior to the aorta (Fig. 2.7).

Imaging the heart for connection abnormalities

- **Six connections**: Atria, ventricles and great arteries.
- **Four chamber view**: Demonstrates the pulmonary veins, and atria, the atrioventricular connections and the two ventricles.

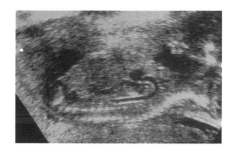

Fig. 2.7 A normal longitudinal view of the chest showing the arch of the aorta.

- **Right side of the heart**: The inferior and superior vena cavae drain to the right atrium, which connects through the tricuspid valve to the right ventricle. The pulmonary artery arises from the right ventricle.
- **Left side of the heart**: The left atrium receives the pulmonary veins. The left atrium connects via the mitral valve to the left ventricle which gives rise to the aorta.

Prognosis for ultrasonically antenatally diagnosed cardiac disease
(see Table 2.9)

Up to 25 per cent of continuing pregnancies with CHD result in spontaneous fetal loss. Up to 75 per cent of women elect to have a termination of pregnancy at the time of diagnosis. Twenty per cent of detected cardiac abnormalities have associated chromosome defects. Of these cardiac disorders diagnosed antenatally, only 10 per cent will be born alive and a substantial proportion of those will not survive infancy.

Heart defects which do not involve a connection abnormality are

Table 2.9 The outcome of structural abnormalities of the heart diagnosed in utero (at gestation of referral) for 613 cases of fetal cardiac anomaly detected at the end of 1991.

Outcome	Number	Per cent
Termination of pregnancy	315	51
Intrauterine death	66	11
Neonatal death	102	17
Born alive	92	15
Survived into infancy	28	6

usually relatively minor defects with a good chance of successful correction.

THORACIC ABNORMALITIES

During ultrasound examination the relationship of the heart to the lungs is assessed with regard to the size and position. In a normal view the thorax is at the level of the four chamber view of the heart. The cross sectional area of the heart is $\frac{1}{3}$ of the total area of the thorax. The heart lies slightly to the left of the midline. The smaller left lung lies posterior.

An intrapulmonary lesion will lead to mediastinal shift causing displacement of the heart away from the lesion. This may result in pulmonary hypoplasia, the degree of which may only be assessed post-natally. There may be associated pleural effusions and obstruction of the inferior vena cava may cause ascites.

Fetal breathing is observed as rhythmic bursts of activity with movement of the diaphragm downwards, rather than chest expansion outwards.

Primary lung abnormalities are rare. The most important are cystic adenomatoid malformations.

Cystic adenomatoid malformations

These are usually unilateral with a wide spectrum of appearances and prognosis.

Type I   A single or multiple large cysts of > 2 cm diameter
Type II   Multiple small cysts of <1 cm diameter
Type III   Echogenic due to the presence of multiple tiny cysts which often produce mediastinal shift.

In most of cases of Type III there is accompanying polyhydramnios and fetal hydrops giving a poor prognosis.

Severe mediastinal shift is not necessarily associated with a bad outcome.

The rare mediastinal teratoma and rhabdomyoma may also be detected at ultrasound examination.

Congenital diaphragmatic hernia

- Incidence 1:2000 births.

- 75 per cent are left sided with 3 per cent bilateral.
- The severity of lung hypoplasia depends on the stage of pulmonary development when herniation took place and the size.
- Associated abnormalities: congenital heart lesions, chromosome – trisomy 13, 18 and 21 neural tube defects, other central nervous system abnormalities, renal and skeletal.
- Ultrasound diagnosis depends upon visualision of the abdominal organs in the thorax. Most commonly the stomach will be noted in the left hemithorax lying adjacent to the heart which is displaced to the right. This may be seen even at the 18 week scan.
- Bowel loops are differentiated from other cystic lesions of the thorax by observing the paradoxical movement of the viscera with fetal respiration and peristalsis of the bowel. These signs may not be seen until the third trimester.
- Prenatal diagnosis enables delivery in a centre with paediatric facilities which significantly improves the prognosis.
- Overall survival rate in the neonatal period can be as high as 60 to 70 per cent.
- The recurrence rate is about 2 per cent (except when it occurs as part of a syndrome, when the recurrence risk is that of the syndrome).

HEAD AND NECK LESIONS

Cleft lip and palate

- The fetal face is examined in the sagittal and coronal views.
- A normal fetal profile is seen in Fig. 2.8 and normal lips in Fig. 2.9.
- Facial clefts occur in one in 700 live births and account for just over 10 per cent of congenital anomalies.
- Cleft lips are easily visualised but cleft palate is a difficult diagnosis and often missed. Scan in the axial plane. Lateral clefts of the lip and palate are common and may be unilateral or bilateral.
- The development of the midline structure of the face is closely linked with the differentiation of the forebrain. A midline cleft is rare and indicates the need to carefully examine for holoprosencephaly and exclude an abnormal karyotype.

Cystic hygroma

This is the most common fetal tumour with an incidence of 1:200 pregnancies.

2

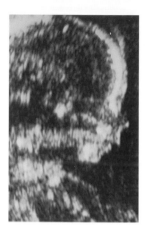

Fig. 2.8 A normal fetal profile.

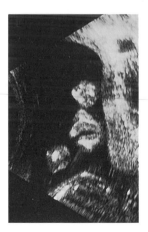

Fig. 2.9 Normal fetal lips.

▪ It is a pathological dilatation of the jugular lymphatic sac which is a primitive structure draining the embryological lymphatic system. It connects to the jugular vein at 9 weeks of gestation. If this link does not occur then peripheral oedema accumulates that will eventually cause heart failure.

- It may involve the posterior neck. It is symmetrical with a midline septum, may be huge and associated with fetal hydrops. Cystic hygromas should always be karotyped because more than 70 per cent may be associated with Turner's syndrome (XO).
- Cystic hygromas may also affect the axillae, the mediastinum and groin when they are less likely to be associated with karyotype abnormalities.

GASTROINTESTINAL ABNORMALITIES

The normal stomach is invariably visualised as a cystic structure in the left upper quadrant. Normal small and large bowel cannot be distinguished at 18 weeks, but by the thrid trimester the meconium filled large intestine is easily seen. However, the small intestine is not clearly defined.

Oesophageal atresia

- Incidence 1/3000–3500 livebirths.
- Rarely diagnosed prenatally as 85 per cent are associated with tracheoesophageal fistula. If no fistula is present, then it may present as polyhydramnios and non-visualisation of the fetal stomach.
- A proximal obstruction can be seen with approximately 1/15 pregnancies with polyhydramnios.

Duodenal obstruction

- Incidence 1/7500–10 000 live births.
- Thirty per cent of affected fetuses have trisomy 21.
- Other common anomalies include structural cardiac anomalies (20 per cent) malrotation of the colon (22 per cent), tracheo-oesophageal fistula and renal malformations.
- Ultrasound reveals polyhydramnios and a double bubble sign of the dilatation of the proximal and distal duodenum. It rarely presents before 26 weeks' gestation.

Small intestine obstruction

May affect the jejunum or ileum at one or more levels. It may present with hydramnios depending on the level of obstruction. It is less likely if the obstruction is low as the proximal fluid is absorbed. Peristalsis in multiple dilated fluid filled loops of bowel are seen on ultrasound.

Aetiology

Bands, atresias, stenosis, and associated with gastroschisis or cystic fibrosis.

Large intestine obstruction

Usually distal and related recto-anal atresia or Hirschsprung's disease. Dilated meconium filled large bowel may be seen but no hydramnios is present. Abnormalities involving other systems are common e.g. VATER syndrome, in which there are **V**ertebral, **A**nal, **T**racheo- or **E**sophageal and **R**enal lesions.

Gastroschisis

▪ The herniation generally of small intestine through a right sided umbilical defect of the anterior abdominal wall. The umbilical cord is normally inserted (Fig. 2.10).

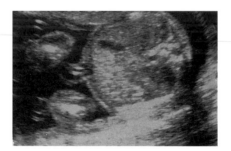

Fig. 2.10 Normal umbilical cord insertion.

Ultrasound diagnosis at 18 weeks' gestation in the presence of a gastroschisis shows an irregular, echogenic cauliflower like shaped mass related to the anterior abdominal wall. There is no membraneous covering and loops of bowel may be seen floating in the amniotic fluid. (This is important in differentiating it from omphalocoele.)

- By the late second trimester, fluid will be observed within the loops of small intestine.
- Incidence 1:12 000 live births. It is usually an isolated lesion but congenital heart defects have been noted in up to 8.5 per cent of cases.
- Neonatal surgery – survival rates up to 95 per cent. Other causes of death are usually associated with other abnormalities or sepsis.
- Karyotype abnormality with gastroschisis is rare. However, in up to 25 per cent of cases there may be gastrointestinal problems due to vascular impairment and adhesions. Malrotation and intestinal atresia and stenosis also occur.
- There is no clear advantage of delivery by caesarean section.
- Recurrence risk <1 per cent.

Omphalocoele (exomphalos)

- An anterior abdominal wall defect resulting from herniation of the intra-abdominal contents into the base of the umbilical cord. The size and contents of the defects are very variable, most commonly bowel and liver. The incidence is about 1:10 000 live births.
- Ultrasonographically, the midline hernia is covered with membrane and the umbilical cord is inserted into the apex.
- The differential diagnosis from gastroschisis is very important because omphalocoele is associated in 45 per cent of cases with other congenital abnormalites (unlike gastroschisis where the incidence of other abnormalities is probably much less than 5 per cent) and has a high risk of other structural and chromosomal abnormalities. Karyotyping is therefore indicated.
- Large defects which include the liver and heart have a worse prognosis than small defects in which only bowel loops are extruded.

Intra-abdominal cysts

Ovarian cysts

These may be single, bilateral, unilocular or multilocular. Most resolve postnatally and do not require surgery.

Other cysts

Among other cysts which can be detected are mesenteric (generally single and unilocular), omental and choledochal. Ultrasound diagnosis of the last depends on visualisation of an echo-free, non-pulsatile area in the right side of the fetal abdomen near the portal vein. It is an important diagnosis to make as it requires postnatal surgery to avoid portal hypertension and biliary sclerosis. There is a 10 per cent operative mortality.

RENAL ABNORMALITIES

Renal anomalies are very common and range from minor renal pelvis dilatation to bilateral obstruction. Most are incidental findings, but must be carefully sought, particularly in the presence of oligohydramnios.

Severe urinary tract abnormalities are often associated with oligohydramnios either due to bilateral absence of kidneys, cystic renal dysplasia or to bilateral obstructive uropathy.

Ultrasound findings

- Normal amniotic fluid volume implies the presence of at least one functioning kidney.
- The ratio of the area of both kidneys to abdominal area is 1/3.
- The fetal bladder should always be seen by 15 weeks (Fig. 2.11). It fills and empties every 30 to 45 minutes.

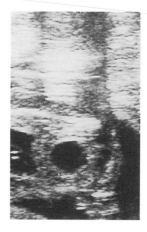

Fig. 2.11 Fetal bladder.

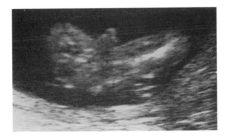

Fig. 2.12 Male genitalia.

- The external genitalia may be identified from 15 weeks onwards with careful scanning (Fig. 2.12 and Fig. 2.13).

Among the implications to be considered in the presence of **oligohydramnios** is Potter's syndrome (pulmonary hypoplasia, skeletal deformities e.g. club feet, typical facies, characterised by low-set ears).

Absence of urine within the fetal bladder over a long period suggests renal agenesis rather than the differential diagnosis of intrauterine growth retardation or prolonged rupture of the membranes.

Doppler ultrasound may be of value to show normal umbilical arterial flow and therefore exclude intrauterine growth retardation and absence of renal arteries.

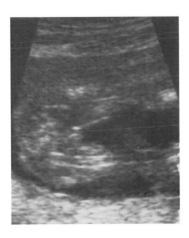

Fig. 2.13 Female genitalia.

Renal agenesis

- It is bilateral with an incidence of 1/4000 births. It is more common in male than female fetuses.
- At ultrasound examination neither amniotic fluid nor the kidneys and bladder can be seen.
- The recurrence risk is about 2 to 3 per cent.

Polycystic kidney disease

Appearances are variable depending on the pathology and severity. Although severe cases may have oligohydramnios from 16 weeks' gestation, in less severe cases, the kidney may appear relatively normal with good normal function as evidenced by normal filling and emptying of the fetal bladder and normal liquor volume.

(1) Infantile polycystic kidney

- It is due to a defect of the collecting system. Both kidneys are symmetrically enlarged and contain multiple minute cysts.
- Ultrasound appearance reveals extreme enlargement of both kidneys which are hyperechogenic, due to the multiple minute cysts. The bladder may or may not be seen, depending on the severity. Oligohydramnios is present.
- In severe cases, compromised renal function leads to a marked oligohydramnios, which leads to pulmonary hypoplasia and skeletal deformities, resembling Potter's syndrome.
- It is an autosomal recessive disease with a recurrence risk of 25 per cent.

(2) Adult polycystic kidney disease (APCK)

- Bilateral and symmetrical enlargement of kidneys. Small cysts may be visualised.
- Inherited as an autosomal dominant (1:2).
- It may be associated with Meckel–Gruber syndrome (occipital encephalocoele) a lethal autosomal recessive condition.
- It usually leads to hypertension and renal failure in adulthood.
- There is overlap in appearances and prognosis APCK and MCKD (see below).

(3) *Multicystic dysplastic kidney disease (MCKD)*

- Renal dysplasia involves the replacement of renal parenchyma by cysts of variable size, thought to be due to long standing obstruction. Usually one kidney is affected. The dysplastic process is usually limited to the medulla.
- Incidence 1/1000 live births.
- The diagnosis must be differentiated from hydronephrosis: in multicystic kidney disease, the cysts do not communicate unlike the calyces and pelvis with hydronephrosis.
- In cases of unilateral MCKD with no sign of renal failure, and no associated anomalies, the prognosis is good. In many cases the affected kidney will shrink and may not be visualised postnatally. The prognosis depends on the type and severity of associated abnormalities.
- Bilateral MCKD is lethal.

DILATATION OF RENAL TRACT

- It is common but the true incidence is unknown. No dilatation does not imply no obstruction.
- Prenatal ultrasound diagnosis is based on the finding of a dilated renal pelvis. An antero-posterior (AP) diameter >10 mm is abnormal. Less than 5 mm is normal and the significance of a diameter between 5 and 10 mm is uncertain.
- Follow up all cases with an AP diameter of more than 5 mm, because it may result from vesico-ureteric reflux with increased risk of urinary tract infections in infancy.
- Ultrasound appearances of renal tract dilatation are very variable depending on the level of the obstruction of the urinary tract.

    High   Pelvi-ureteric junction obstruction
    Mid   Ureter/uretero-vesical junction
    Low   Bladder outflow

    High obstruction results in a variable degree of unilateral/bilateral pelvi-calyceal dilatation.

    Mid level obstruction is rare due to congenital megaureter and vesico-ureteric reflux.

    Low level obstruction usually occurs in the urethra and is generally due to posterior urethral valves. It occurs mostly in a male fetus, although it may occur in the female due to stenosis or atresia.

- The appearances are variable depending on severity with or without associated oligohydramnios; dilatation of the bladder; dilatation of the ureter and pelvi-calyceal collecting system; urinary ascites or renal cystic dysplasia.

Assessment of impaired renal function

In the fetus this is problematic. Biochemistry of fetal urine from aspiration may be of some value. A high urinary sodium is usually associated with a poor prognosis. In very carefully selected cases, shunting has been shown to be of some value.

LIMBS AND SKELETON

Generalised skeletal bone dysplasias (see Table 2.10)

The commonest skeletal dysplasia is achondroplasia which is not lethal and generally not diagnosed pre-natally as limb shortening is not apparent until after 22 weeks' gestation. (Normal limbs are shown in Fig. 2.14a and 2.14b.)

Table 2.10 Approximate incidence of 'common' lethal skeletal dysplasia. (Reproduced with permission from Griffin, D.R. & Chitty, L.S. The skeleton. In *Ultrasound in Obstetrics and Gynaecology* (Ed. by K. Dewbury, H. Meire & D. Cosgrove), p. 383. Churchill Livingstone, London.)

Thanatophoric dysplasia	1 in	30 000
Osteogenesis imperfecta (type II)	1 in	55 000
Achondrogenesis (all types)	1 in	75 000
Chondrodysplasia punctata	1 in	85 000
Hypophosphatasia (severe form)	1 in	110 000
Campomelic dysplasia	1 in	150 000

Focal skeletal abnormalities

- Absence of limbs
  Amelia (complete absence of a limb)
  Meromelia (partial absence of a limb or limb segment)
  Phocomelia (absence of long bones with hands or feet attached to the body).
- Micromelia (small limbs).

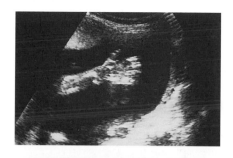

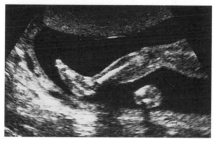

Fig. 2.14 (a) Normal hand. (b) Normal leg.

- Club foot – diagnosed when the foot is not observed in the usual position of almost at right angles to the lower leg, but it seen continous with the length of the tibia and fibula.
- Shortening of the long bones. Check all long bone lengths. Several scans may be needed. Check for extra digits, skeletal deformities of the spine, rib cage and extremities (see Table 2.11).
- Defective mineralisation and fracture (see Table 2.12).

Table 2.11 Skeletal dysplasia characterised by short ribs. (Reproduced with permission from Griffin D.R. & Chitty L.S. (1993) The skeleton. In *Ultrasound in Obstetrics & Gynaecology* [Ed. by K. Dewbury, H. Meire & D. Cosgrove], p. 386. Churchill Livingstone, London.)

Type and inheritance	Long bones	Spine	Other features	Prognosis
Thanatophoric (sporadic) dysplasia	Severe micromelia Thick diaphysis +/- bowing	Flat vertebral bodies	Polyhydramnios Megalocephaly Ventriculomegaly +/- Cloverleaf skull Renal & cardiac anomalies Trident hand	Lethal
Campomelic dysplasia (AR)	Moderate shortening Bowed femur/tibia Hypo/asplastic fibula	Flat vertebrae	Short clavicles Micrognathia, Talipes eq. varus Sex reversal	Usually lethal

Table 2.12 Skeletal dysplasia characterised by poor mineralisation. (Reproduced with permission from Griffin, D.R. & Chitty, L.S. (1993) The skeleton. In *Ultrasound in Obstetrics & Gynaecology* [Ed. by K. Dewbury, H. Meire & D. Cosgrove], p. 385. Churchill Livingstone, London.)

Type and inheritance		Long bones	Spine	Ribs	Other features	Prognosis
Achondrogenesis (type I)	(AR)	Extreme micromelia	Poorly mineralised Short	Short	Polyhydramnios Hydrops Very poor cranial ossification	Lethal
Achondrogenesis (type II)	(AR)	Severe micromelia	Unossified spine and sacrum	Short	Polyhydramnios Micrognathia Good cranial ossification	Lethal
Osteogenesis (type II)	(VAR)	V. short, crumpled multiple fractures	Vertebrae may be flattened	Beaded +/– short	Polyhydramnios Unossified skull Brachycephaly	Lethal
Hypophosphatasia (lethal form)	(AR)	Short, bowed	May show deformity	Thin +/– short +/– beaded	Poorly ossified skull	Lethal

Table 2.13 Clues to the differential ultrasound diagnosis of skeletal dysplasias. (Reproduced with permission from Griffin, D.R. & Chitty, L.S. (1993) The skeleton. In *Ultrasound in Obstetrics & Gynaecology* (Ed. by K. Dewbury, H. Meire & D. Cosgrove), p. 384. Churchill Livingstone, London.)

Polyhydramnios	Achondrogenesis type I or II
	Thanatophoric dysplasia
	Short rib–polydactyly (SRP) syndrome
Fetal hydrops	Achondrogenesis type I
	SRP syndromes
Undermineralised skull	Osteogenesis imperfecta (IIa)
	Achondrogenesis type I
	Hypophosphatasia
Clover leaf skull	Thanatophoric dysplasia
Small thorax	Achondrogenesis
	Hypochondrogenesis
	Thanatophoric dysplasia
	SRP syndromes
	Chondroectodermal dysplasia
	Campomelic dysplasia
Marked femoral bowing	Campomelic dysplasia
	Osteogenesis imperfecta
	Hypophosphatasia
Talipes equinovarus	Campomelic dysplasia
	Diastrophic dysplasia
Polydactyly	Chondroectodermal dysplasia
	SRP syndromes
	Grebe syndrome
	Jejune thoracic dystrophy
Short clavicles	Campomelic dysplasia
	Cleidocranial dysostosis
	Kniest syndrome

BIBLIOGRAPHY

Allan, L.D., Crawford, D.C., Chita, S.K. & Tynan, M J. (1986) Prenatal screening for congenital heart disease. *British Medical Journal*, **292**, 1717–1719.

The British Medical Ultrasound Society Fetal Measurements Working Party. (1990) *Report*. British Institute of Radiology, London.

Cuckle, H.S., Nanchahal, K. & Wald, N.J. (1991) Birth prevalence of Down's syndrome in England and Wales. *Prenatal Diagnosis*, **11**, 29–34.

Dewbury, K., Meire, H. & Cosgrove, D. (1993) *Ultrasound in Obstetrics and Gynaecology*, Churchill Livingstone, London.

Ferguson-Smith, M.A. & Yates, J.R.W. (1984) Maternal age specific rates for chromosome aberrations and factors influencing them: report of a collaborative European study on 52,965 amniocenteses. *Prenatal Diagnosis*, **4**, 5–44.

Gilbert, W.M. & Nicolaides, K.H. (1987) Fetal omphalocele, associated malformations and chromosomal defects. *Obstetrics & Gynecology*, **70**, 633–635.

Griffin, D.R. & Chitty, L.S. (1993) The skeleton. In *Ultrasound in Obstetrics and Gynaecology* (Ed. by K. Dewbury, H. Meire & D. Cosgrove) pp. 383–386, Churchill Livingstone, London.

Hook, E.B. (1981) Rates of chromosome abnormalities at different maternal ages. *Obstetrics & Gynecology*, **58**, 282–285.

Medical Research Council Working Party. (1978) An assessment of the hazards of amniocentesis. *British Journal of Obstetrics & Gynaecology*, **85** (suppl.).

Medical Research Council Working Party. (1991) Medical Research Council European Trial of chorionic villus sampling. *The Lancet*, **337**, 1491–1499.

National Institute of Child Health and Human Development (1976) Mid trimester amniocentesis for prenatal diagnosis. Safety and Accuracy. *Journal of American Medical Association*, **236**, 1471–1476.

Nicolaides, K.H., Snijders, R.J.M., Gosden, C.M., Berry, C. & Campbell, S. (1992) Ultrasonically detectable markers of fetal chromosomal abnormalities. *The Lancet*, **340**, 704–707.

Simpson, N.E., Dallaire, L. Miller, J.R., Siminovicah, L., Hamerton, J.L., Miller, J. & McKeen, C. (1976) Prenatal diagnosis of genetic disease in Canada; report of a collaborative study. *Canadian Medical Association Journal*, **115**, 739–746.

Tabor, A., Madsen, M., Obel, E.B., Philip, J., Bang, J. & Norgaard-Pedersen, B.N. (1986) Randomised controlled trial of genetic amniocentesis in 4606 low-risk women. *The Lancet*, **i**, 1287–1293.

3 Genetics

Peter Lunt

INTRODUCTION

Genetics and antenatal care

Genetic aspects are important both for the individual family and at a population level. Counselling is required for the individual couple concerned that their offspring may be at risk of a specific genetic problem which has already presented in their family, or following unexpected detection of a genetic abnormality in a population screening test.

Advances in molecular genetics and gene mapping now enable specific genetic advice, including risk assessment and prenatal testing, to be offered in many cases. Counselling should not be directive, but rather should help support the couple to come to whatever decision they feel to be right for them. Therefore, advice as to diagnostic techniques depends on the couple's consent.

Genetic assessment of risk should where possible commence prior to onset of a pregnancy, to allow sufficient time for laboratory investigation of appropriate family members, and in many cases to be able to offer couples the confidence of knowing that they are not at risk.

Members of the wider family may also unknowingly be at risk (especially in dominant or X-linked conditions or chromosome rearrangements) and should be contacted where applicable, usually through involvement of the Clinical Genetic Service.

Prenatal diagnostic options

The method chosen depends on feasibility and availability of test, prior risk of abnormal result, iatrogenic risk to fetus, time to obtain result, gestation at presentation, past obstetric history, future reproductive potential, and parental anxiety level. In general, amniocentesis is applicable where reassurance is being sought (prior risk ≤5 per cent): chorionic villus biopsy is more applicable where the genetic risk is high (≥10 per cent).

■ Amniocentesis (16–17 weeks) provides amniotic fluid and amnion cells. In amniotic fluid the following can be measured: bilirubin (Rhesus disease), alkaline phosphatase (cystic fibrosis) and alphafetoprotein. Amniotic cells require culture (for 2–3 weeks) for chromosome and metabolic enzyme activity analysis. Increasingly, direct trisomy screening on uncultured cells is becoming possible using fluorescent *in situ* hybridisation (FISH). Cultured amnion cells are a poor source of DNA.

The miscarriage risk from amniocentesis is 0.5–1 per cent.

■ Chorionic villus sampling (CVS) can be performed from about 10 weeks onwards (CRL = 35 mm). The miscarriage risk is about 2–3 per cent.

CVS is particularly valuable for DNA based diagnosis and for metabolic enzyme studies. Direct trisomy screening using FISH and 48-hour chromosome-count analysis is possible on uncultured cells, but a one-week culture is required for accurate full karyotyping. Localised placental chromosome mosaicism can complicate a result and apparent mosaicism requires subsequent amniocentesis for clarification.

■ Fetal anomaly ultrasound scanning is usually performed at 18 weeks' gestation: fetal cardiac Doppler scanning can be performed at 20 weeks. Transvaginal fetal scans at 12 weeks may detect anencephaly or other major cerebral abnormality.

■ Cordocentesis (fetal blood sampling) is performed at 18 weeks' gestation onwards. It may be used, (i) in families with a haemoglobinopathy not elucidated by DNA analysis, (ii) to help clarify possibly fetal chromosome mosaicism, or (iii) for late fetal karyotyping if there are anomalies on ultrasound scan.

Population screening for genetic disorders

Spina bifida

Raised maternal serum alphafetoprotein (AFP) at 17 weeks' gestation can enable detection of nearly all babies with open spina bifida, but the test has poor specificity, and must be combined with ultrasound scan for accurate pregnancy dating in order to interpret the AFP level against the norm for gestation. In true positives scanning will confirm the diagnosis, and in many cases now is the primary method of diagnosis.

Amniotic fluid AFP and acetylcholinesterase are now rarely required.

Raised AFP is also seen in twin pregnancies, and in other open fetal malformations.

Prediction of a mitochondrial disorder in offspring

Several disorders affecting mitochondrial function arise from mutations in mitochondrial DNA (see Table 3.1). These pose a particular problem in antenatal counselling. Mitochondria of the embryo and fetus are inherited in large numbers in the egg from the mother, but not from sperm. Inheritance is therefore matrolinear.

All offspring may inherit faulty mitochondria from the mother, but the likelihood of symptoms in each offspring depends on the proportion of mitochondria which are faulty, and on their organ/tissue distribution. This cannot easily be determined. Therefore prenatal testing from CVS, amniocentesis, or cordocentesis would be unreliable in most cases.

Some mitochondrial disorders are determined by mutations in nuclear genes coding for other intro-mitochondrial proteins, and follow dominant recessive or X-linked inheritance patterns. Few if any are yet characterised.

Down's syndrome

An association between a lower mean AFP and raised hCG in pregnancies, giving rise to babies with t21 has led to the introduction of maternal serum screening for risk of Down's syndrome.

The serum levels of the biochemical markers (which may also include unconjugated oestriol) are expressed as multiples of the median (MoM) for the gestational age. The MoMs are combined with maternal age to give a composite risk figure. This may be higher or lower than the age-dependent risk alone, but can be used as a guide by staff and patient as to whether or not to request/offer amniocentesis. A risk figure of 1/250 is usually used as a threshold level.

The result of serum screening does not indicate that the fetus has a trisomy: it merely adjusts the risk estimate for this.

Accuracy of gestational assessment is essential as the MoM value is valid only for the specified gestational age. Usually serum screening is performed at 16–17 weeks to allow maximum time for cell culture from amniocentesis: other units take serum at 18 weeks as the MoM error for a given gestational inaccuracy is minimised.

Phenylketonuria (PKU)

From around 1960, newborns have been screened from heelprick Guthrie test for PKU. Maternal hyperphenylalaninaemia affects the developing fetal brain resulting in microcephaly and mental retardation. Some obstetric units offer routine screening of maternal blood at booking for phenylalanine levels, since hyperphenylalaninaemia does not usually give rise to symptoms in the mother.

COUNSELLING PROSPECTIVELY FOR IDENTIFIED FETAL CHROMOSOME ABNORMALITY

One in 20 women will have placental or amniotic cell karyotype during pregnancy. Counselling of parents whose fetus is found unexpectedly to have a chromosome anomaly can be difficult, but must be based on an unbiased overview of the possible problems and their range of severity.

Simple trisomy

t21 (Down's syndrome)

65–80 per cent of t21 fetuses are lost as spontaneous miscarriage or as stillbirth, a proportion therefore occuring after 18 weeks. Newborns are often small for dates and hypotonic. IQ in children ranges from 20 to 70, mean IQ = 50. Walking, language and self-care skills are attained, but rarely completely independent living. Complications may include hypotonia, congenital heart disease in 40 per cent (ventricular septal defect (VSD), atrioventricular (AV) canal, Fallot tetralogy, hypoplastic left heart, duodenal atresia (<10 per cent), leukemia (1 per cent) or other malformations.

Table 3.1 Availability and type of prenatal DNA test in some genetic disorders.

Disorder/Inheritance	Chromosome location	Gene cloned	Prenatal test	
			Direct	Indirect
Autosomal dominant				
Adenomatous polyposis cell	5q	FAP gene	+	+
Adult polycystic kidney disease	16p	–	–	+
Alzheimer's disease (early-onset)	21q	pre-Amyloid	+	+ (Some)
FSH muscular dystrophy	4p	–	(Some)	+
Huntington chorea	4p	Huntington	+	+
Hypertrophic cardiomyopathy	14q	ß-Myosin H chain	(Some)	+
Marfan syndrome	15q	Fibrillin	(V. few)	+
Myotonic dystrophy	19q	Myotonin	+	Redundant
Neurofibromatosis	17q	NF gene	(V. few)	+
Osteogenesis imperfecta (type 1)	7q/17q	Collagen 1	(Some)	+
Peroneal muscular atrophy (HMSN1)	17q		+	+
Retinitis pigmentosa (some)	3q	Rhodopsin	+	+
Retinoblastoma	13q	RB gene	(Some)	+
Tuberous sclerosis	9q/16p	Tinerom (16p)	(V. few)	Rarely
Autosomal recessive				
Albinism (tyrosinase negative)	11q	Tyrosinase	+	+
α-1-antitrypsin deficiency	14q	α-1-Antitrypsin	+	+
α-thalassemia	16p	α-Globin	+	+
β-thalassaemia/sickle cell	11p	β-Globin	+	+
Cystic fibrosis	7p	CFTR gene	+	+
Friedrich's ataxia	9q	–	–	+

Autoscmal recessive *continued*

Infantile polycystic kidneys	–	–	–	–
Phenylketonuria	12q	Phe hydroxylase	+	+
Spinal muscular atrophy	5q	–	–	+
X-linked recessive				
Christmas disease (factor IX)	Xq26	Factor IX	+	+
Duchenne/Becker muscular dystrophy	Xp21	Dystrophin	+	+
Fragile-X syndrome	Xq27	FraX gene	+	Redundant
Haemophilia A (factor VIII)	Xq28	Factor VIII	+	+
Retinitis pigmentosa (some)	Xp11	–	–	+
Mitochondrial				
Leber's optic atrophy	MT	NADH dehydrogenase	Difficult	
Leigh's disease	MT	PDH or cyt. oxidase	Difficult	
Mitochondrial cytopathy	MT	Mitochondrial genes	Difficult	

3

t18 (Edwards' syndrome) or t13 (Patau's syndrome)

Both are universally lethal, usually in the neonatal period. Survival to early childhood is recorded, but invariably associated with severe retardation and failure to thrive. Some of the longer survivors may be mosaics. In t18 and t13 cleft lip, cardiac, renal and other malformation is usual. Malformation in t13 is often more severe with holoprosencephaly, scalp defects, and polydactyly.

Triploidy

Rarely survives to live birth and then usually dies as neonate. Severe growth retardation and multiple malformation is the rule. Characteristic elongation of second digit and syndactyly of third/fourth digits may be seen. A few diploid/triploid mosaics have survived longer but show severe retardation.

Other autosomal anomalies

Unbalanced structural anomalies

Although many of the commoner deletions or duplications are well characterised, specific prediction is often not possible for unbalanced translocations involving simultaneous gain and loss of genetic material, as each rearrangement combination is often unique.

If an unbalanced anomaly can be observed in the chromosome preparation down the microscope, it involves sufficient genetic material to cause major problems, usually including malformation but invariably associated with some degree of mental retardation.

In general it is the origin of translocated chromosomal material which is of prime importance rather than the site to which it has been relocated.

Parental karyotyping should always be requested to identify a parental balanced rearrangement. This helps clarify the nature of a structural anomaly, determines recurrence risk and identifies the need for a wider family study.

Apparently balanced rearrangements (translocations or inversions)

In contrast to unbalanced structural anomalies the following points apply:
- Parental karyotyping is essential.

- Reassure if familial, and parent is clinically normal: a wider family study is indicated.
- If the lesion is de novo (i.e. parents' karyotypes are normal) there is an empirical 10 per cent risk of retardation or malformation; counselling and detailed scanning are required.

Chromosome mosaicism

The abnormal karyotype may be present in only a proportion of cells from CVS or amniocentesis. However, mosaicism found at CVS may be confined to the placenta and should be confirmed by amniocentesis and/or fetal blood sampling.

Mosaicism at amniocentesis is more reliable. Fetal blood sampling may be required to assess the likely extent of fetal tissues and proportion of cells involved.

Clinical effects in a mosaic are, in general, less severe than in the respective full abnormality.

Sex chromosome anomalies

XO (Turner's syndrome)

98 per cent of conceptuses abort spontaneously; the loss rate from 18 weeks onward is significant. Many fetuses have nuchal cyst or generalised oedema. Intelligence is in the normal range, but on average 10–15 IQ points below the mean for siblings. Infertility due to gonadal dysgenesis is expected. Most girls are diagnosed by short stature and primary amenorrhea at puberty. Neck webbing, coarctation of aorta and horseshoe kidney may be present. Mosaicism is common.

XXY (Klinefelter's syndrome)

Most men are diagnosed in life through adult presentation with a female partner at an infertility clinic. Secondary sexual changes occur but testes remain small. Mean adult height is 177.4 cm (5 ft 10 in). Intelligence is in the normal range, but on average 10–15 IQ points below the mean for siblings. Personality may tend to timidity and passivity. Homosexual orientation is not increased. Malformation is rarely a feature.

XYY

Most men are unaware of any problem. Normal intelligence (but an average 10 IQ points below siblings) and tall stature (mean height

184 cm) are the rule. Personality may tend to be immature with increased impulsive behaviour. A small proportion, but increased to five times normal, exhibit criminality; however, any tendency to this will be subject to upbringing. There is no associated major malformation.

XXX

Most affected women are unaware of any problem. The mean IQ is 20 points below the mean for siblings. Growth and fertility are normal. Mild facial dysmorphism may be recognised. Malformation is rare.

XXXY or XXXX

Rare. Significant retardation (IQ 30–80) and facial dysmorphism is expected. Usually infertile with short stature. Significant malformation is unusual.

Sex chromosome mosaics

These are not uncommon. Counselling is given as for the full abnormality, but with a likelihood of a lesser effect. Mixed sex mosaics may present with ambiguous genitalia.

INVESTIGATING AND MANAGING THE INDIVIDUAL FAMILY

Questions asked at antenatal/preconception clinic

- Is the baby/child at risk of inheriting a particular condition?
- If so, what is the expected range of severity or age at onset?
- Can the risk be excluded?
- If not, is there a prenatal test available?
- Can the severity be ascertained prenatally?
- Is the parent at risk of a fatal or disabling condition?
- What are the risks to a baby if parents are related (consanguinous)?

Family situations giving rise to these questions

- Parent with a disorder
- Family history of a disorder
- Parents with previous child/fetus with a disorder
- Parent at-risk of a late-onset disorder

- Cousin-marriage or other consanguinous partnership
- Previous recurrent miscarriages.

Answering the questions

- Take a full family history, including consanguinous relationships.
- Check for accuracy of diagnosis in index cases.
- Determine the result of any specific genetic test of index case.
- Are genetic tests now possible for determining carrier or presymptomatic status?
- Determine the result of previous genetic testing in the family.
- Examine at-risk parent for any relevant clinical feature.
- Genetic testing may require a family study using indirect DNA markers, but increasingly direct mutation testing may be possible.
- Beware that a direct prenatal test could be a predictive test for the parent.
- Discuss with parent whether they would wish to terminate the pregnancy according to a test result.

Type of disorder

Specific detailed genetic tests are only applicable for single gene or chromosomal disorders.

In many cases the concern will relate to more common disorders which follow a multifactorial inheritance pattern for which only empirical recurrence risks can be given (e.g. psoriasis, eczema or asthma, schizophrenia, cleft lip or palate, congenital heart disease, or cancer).

DIRECT AND INDIRECT DNA TESTING IN SINGLE GENE DISORDERS

Direct DNA testing

- Disease gene DNA sequence must be characterised or mutation pattern known.
- The specific mutation in the index case in the family must be identified,

or

the mutation must always be of one type (e.g. expansion of tandem triplet base repeat sequence).

- The result is absolute.
- Beware that a direct prenatal test could be a predictive test for the parent.
- Direct DNA testing is often possible in the following: fragile-X, myotonic dystrophy, Huntington disease (only if the parent is previously known to carry the mutation), Duchenne–Becker muscular dystrophy, cystic fibrosis, PKU, peroneal muscular atrophy (see Table 3.1).

3

Indirect DNA testing

- The chromosomal regional location of the disease gene must be known.
- DNA markers (probes) which can detect DNA sequence polymorphism (restriction fragment length polymorphism) closely linked to the disease gene must be available.
- An extended family study is often required. DNA samples from appropriate members of the nuclear and extended family must be available to determine which marker allele or haplotype is tracking with the faulty disease gene in that family (i.e. to determine the linkage phase).
- The family DNA study must be completed prior to offering a prenatal test, since not all families will be 'informative'.
- Possible genetic recombination limits the accuracy of a result.
- The accuracy of an indirect DNA test is also dependent on the accuracy of clinical diagnosis, since only in very large families can diagnosis be confirmed from the overall DNA study in the family.
- Similarly, the likelihood of genetic locus heterogeneity must be incorporated in the final risk estimate.
- Likely alternative risk figure outcomes should be discussed with the couple prior to offering the prenatal test.
- Indirect testing is still required for polycystic kidney disease, spinal muscular atrophy, and many other rarer conditions, including many cases of Duchenne muscular dystrophy (see Table 3.1).

Multifactorial/polygenic inheritance

Many common conditions follow multifactorial inheritance. The condition arises either from a combined pattern of polymorphic variation at several genes (polygenic cause), or from a combination of a susceptible genotype with an environmental 'trigger' factor. Specific genetic testing is rarely, if ever, possible.

Genetic risk

This increases with:
- closer pedigree relationship to the index case;
- increased number of affected cases in a family;
- increased severity of the index case;
- less frequently affected sex as index case (see Table 3.2).

3

Twinning (Table 3.3)

- The incidence is 1 in 90 pregnancies.
- The incidence of monozygous (MZ) 'identical' twins is constant in all racial groups at 4/1000 maternities.
- The incidence of dizygous (DZ) 'non-identical' twins varies between races (following the mother's ethnic risk in inter-racial partnerships);

Table 3.2 Examples of typical recurrence risks (per cent) in offspring.

Disorder	Prevalence (per cent)	Relative(s) affected				Caution
		Older child	Parent	Parent & child	Both parents	
Asthma	4	10	26		34	
Eczma	3	14	34		57	
Psoriasis		17	25	30	65	
Arthritis (RA/OA)		x2	x2			
Insulin dependent diabetes	0.2	7	3		20–50	
Epilepsy (child)	1	6	4	10	15	
Schizophrenia	1	9	13	15	40	
Affective psychosis (+ suicide)	1	13	15			
Cleft lip/palate	0.1	4	4	10		Beware syndrome
Congenital heart disorder	1	2	3	10		Deware Chr22del
Neural tube defect	0.2	5	4	10		

is greater with increased maternal age; and has tended to fall over recent years. The racial risks are: 3/1000 maternities in Orientals; 7/1000 maternities in Caucasians; 10/1000 maternities in some Black populations.

▪ Currently for Caucasians 36 per cent of twins are MZ and 64 per cent are DZ.

▪ Contrary to popular impression, familial recurrence risks are increased for both MZ and DZ twins, and are not restricted to one type in a family.

▪ The increased risk follows the maternal line in both types, but also the paternal line in DZ twins.

Table 3.3 Risk of twinning with positive family history.

Index case	Combined twin risk (Caucasians)
General population	1/90 (DZ 1/140; MZ 1/250)
Parents of DZ twins	Gen. pop. risk

Mother: one of DZ twins
    or has siblings who are DZ twins
    or has brother with DZ twin offspring
    or has sister with MZ twin offspring
	1/60

if has sister with DZ twin offspring **if** has brother with MZ twin offspring	1/40 Gen. pop. risk

Father: one of DZ twins
    has siblings who are DZ twins
    has siblings with twin offspring (MZ or DZ)
	Gen. pop. risk
	1/75
	1/60–1/75

Prenatal testing in a twin pregnancy

Selective CVS or selective amniocentesis are possible. Selective termination is possible but increases other risks to the remaining fetus. Careful counselling is needed.

COMMON SINGLE GENE DISORDERS THAT REQUIRE COUNSELLING

1 Autosomal recessive

Cystic fibrosis (CF)

CF is the commonest recessive condition in the UK population. **1/22 persons are carriers** (heterozygotes) for a faulty CF gene: approximately **1/500 couples are at 1/4 risk** of having an affected child.

Typically CF manifests as failure to thrive in childhood with malabsorption and recurrent chest infection. Routine treatment requires oral pancreatic enzyme replacement, prophylactic oral antibiotics and twice daily chest physiotherapy. Bronchiectasis, pneumothorax, haemoptysis, heart failure and cirrhosis can supervene. Survival beyond 25 years following childhood presentation is unusual.

Fetal or congenital presentation with meconium ileus and/or peritoneal calcification is not rare. Some 'milder' mutations are associated with longer survival including adult presentation. Anticipated future gene therapy may dramatically alter prognosis.

The CF gene is located on chromosome 7 (region 7q32). One mutation (δF508) accounts for 70 per cent of all faulty CF genes in the UK: a further five mutations (δ1507, G542X, G551D, R553X, 621+IG>T) account for a further 10 per cent. Routine CF mutation studies screen for the six most common mutations, thereby identifying 80 per cent of carriers.

Pre-pregnancy or antenatal situations

Risk to offspring of 'same couple' parents with an affected child is 1/4, but is low in all other situations, unless both parents are known to be carriers, or both have family history of CF. Investigation of parents will usually obviate the need for a prenatal test.

One parent affected with CF

Males with CF are usually subfertile or sterile. Females have reduced fertility but several pregnancies have been achieved. Genetic risk of CF in offspring is low (1/44 = 2.3 per cent).

DNA from the affected parent should be screened for CF mutations. DNA from the unaffected partner should be screened for the routine six mutations. If none is found their carrier risk falls to 1/106, and the risk of CF in the baby is 1/212. Prenatal testing would not provide any additional information. Prenatal testing is only offered if the partner has a CF mutation, giving 1/2 risk to fetus.

For affected mothers there is the risk of potentially fatal cardio-respiratory decompensation during pregnancy or in the postpartum period. Cardiorespiratory assessment is essential pre-pregnancy or in early pregnancy, with regular continued monitoring.

Couples with previous child with CF

The recurrence risk is 1/4 (25 per cent).

DNA should be studied from the affected child and from both parents for CF mutations **prior to pregnancy**. From a six-mutation screen, both mutations are identified for 64 per cent of CF children, one mutation is identified and one is unknown for 32 per cent of CF children, and in 4 per cent of CF children neither mutation is identified.

Prenatal testing can be offered easily (from 11-week CVS) only where both mutations are identified. The result takes seven days maximum (less with polymerase chain reaction (PCR) techniques) with an accuracy of 100 per cent.

For the 36 per cent where both mutations are not identified from routine screening, further mutation study is required. This cannot be offered as an urgent investigation during a pregnancy. However, prenatal diagnosis based on indirect DNA polymorphic marker analysis will be possible in over 95 per cent of these cases. Sufficient time (weeks) is required prior to CVS to determine which markers would be informative. Indirect testing for CF includes a recombination error risk of 1–2 per cent.

Alkaline phosphatase (ALP) assay on a 17-week amniotic fluid sample could be considered if DNA testing remains uninformative, but the false positive rate of 8 per cent limits applicability to the 1/4 risk situation.

Fetus identified on scan as having meconium ileus or peritoneal calcification

DNA should be obtained from CVS and analysed for CF mutations; or both parents should be tested. Detection of two mutations confirms the diagnosis: detection of only one mutation still makes CF extremely likely, especially if this is other than δF508.

If only one or no mutation is identified, offer amniocentesis for ALP assay if at 16–19 weeks.

Family history of CF or one partner has a CF child by a previous (different) partner

Carrier risk of the index parent depends on relationship to the affected child/adult. Assuming the partner has no family history of CF, the risks are as shown in Table 3.4. These risks are low and reassurance may be all that is needed.

The recommended course of action is as follows:

■ Ascertain whether mutations have been identified in the affected relative, and which one came from which parent.

■ Take blood for DNA from the index parent and their partner: run six-mutation screen on the partner, and as appropriate on the index parent.

■ If none of the six mutations is detected in the partner, his/her carrier risk (if of N European origin) falls to around 1/106, and the risk to the fetus is 1/424 at most. Reassure: prenatal testing could not provide additional information and is not indicated.

■ If the partner does carry a recognised mutation, but the carrier status of the index parent cannot be determined by specific or routine mutation study, extended mutation analysis of the affected relative, and/or a family study using indirect DNA markers is required. CVS for prenatal exclusion testing combined with ALP assay on 17 week amniocentesis can be offered.

■ If both parents carry a recognised mutation, offer CVS on 1/4 risk.

Other recessive disorders

For parents (same couple) with a previous affected child the recurrence risk is 1/4. Prenatal diagnosis is then possible from CVS in most

Table 3.4 Dependence of CF risk to child on familial CF incidence.

Affected relative	Carrier risk	CF risk to baby
Son/daughter by previous partner	Certain	1/88
Brother/sister	2/3	1/132
Half-sibling	1/2	1/176
Nephew/niece	1/2	1/176
Cousin	1/4	1/352
Cousin's child	1/8	1/704
Second cousin	1/16	$\approx$ 1/1400
None known	1/22	$\approx$ 1/2000

metabolic conditions by biochemical analysis, and in several others by DNA analysis provided that DNA is available from the affected child.

Conditions diagnosable by DNA tests require prior DNA investigation of the parents and the affected child, and can only be offered where a tissue or blood sample is available from the affected child.

Individually most serious recessive disorders are very rare (birth incidence <1/40 000) and the frequency of carriers in the general population is therefore <1/100.

For parents with a new partner, and for other family members, despite anxiety, reassurance should be given that the genetic risks are very low (mostly <1/400) except in cases of consanguinity.

In metabolic conditions, tests for heterozygote carrier status based on enzyme assay may be possible, but often show overlap with the normal range, and in general should be offered only according to individual special circumstances.

Prenatal testing in this low risk situation is not possible for tests which rely on DNA analysis using linked polymorphic markers, as there is no way of determining whether the gene copy from the population-risk partner is normal or faulty. Even where a diagnosis could be established in a fetus with certainty from biochemical analysis, the use of invasive (and perhaps expensive) prenatal diagnosis in a very low risk situation is questionable.

In different racial groups certain recessive conditions are more frequent and the approach to antenatal diagnosis is similar to that for CF in Caucasians. These conditions include thalassaemias in Asian, African and Mediterranean populations, sickle cell disease and other haemoglobinopathies in African and Negro populations, and Tay–Sachs disease in Ashkenazi Jews.

Thalassaemias (α or ß)
Following a previous affected child, DNA-based prenatal diagnosis is possible from CVS if DNA samples are available from both parents and the child. The procedure is to:
- screen for carrier status by routine full blood count, blood film, and haemoglobin electrophoresis;
- take blood from both parents for DNA mutation study, if both are carriers of the same type of thalassaemia (α and ß globin chains are coded for by different gene loci);
- if both mutations are identified offer CVS for DNA based prenatal

diagnosis; otherwise a fetal blood sample is required to study globin chain synthesis.

Sickle-cell disease

Direct DNA testing on CVS is available because the sickle-cell mutation alters a restriction enzyme chopping site in the ß-globin gene.

▪ Screen for carrier status by the sickle test in members of the Afro-Caribbean population.

Consanguinity

All consanguinous couples have an increased risk of having a child with a serious recessive condition.

▪ Take a detailed family history to identify any possible recessive disorder and calculate carrier risk for each partner.

▪ Test for carrier status if feasible.

▪ Offer prenatal diagnosis if both partners are carriers, or if carrier status cannot be determined.

▪ If there is no likely significant family history, the risk of a major problem in the offspring of first cousins is increased only to 5 per cent (3 per cent risk additional to a background risk of 2 per cent). Risks are closer to background for more distant consanguinity.

Prenatal diagnosis and fetal carrier status

Prenatal testing by DNA analysis in recessive conditions will usually gratuitously identify whether a non-affected fetus is a carrier (like its parents) of one of the recessive genes. There are no easy ethical guidelines as to whether or not this information should be reported: perhaps the decision should rest with the parents individually in each case.

2 X-linked recessive

Duchenne/Becker muscular dystrophies

1/3000 males are born with a mutation in the dystrophin gene at Xp21, resulting in either Duchenne (DMD) or Becker (BMD) muscular dystrophy. 1/2000 women are carriers.

Boys with DMD often first present with delayed onset of walking (after 18 months) and subsequent frequent falling. Weakness of proximal muscles progresses to requirement for a wheelchair by 12 years. Death from cardio-respiratory failure usually occurs by 25 years. BMD has a milder course with hip weakness in young adult men progressing to wheelchair requirement often by 40 years.

A few female carriers may exhibit much milder muscle weakness, or exceptionally a full presentation (e.g. with Turner's syndrome (45,XO), with X-autosome translocation, or as a monozygous twin).

Direct DNA testing is possible in the 70 per cent of families where the dystrophin gene mutation is readily detected as a deletion of one or more whole exons. Mutation analysis in the remaining 30 per cent of cases is time consuming and costly, and indirect DNA marker analysis is employed.

Fresh mutation accounts for 1/3 boys affected by DMD; in 2/3 cases the mother is a carrier. A higher proportion of BMD mothers are carriers.

Male partner affected with BMD (or DMD)
- Study DNA sample from affected man for deletion in dystrophin gene.
- Prenatal test is unhelpful as no son will be affected, all daughters will be carriers.

Previous affected son
- Study a DNA sample from the affected boy for dystrophin deletion. If a deletion is detected offer CVS, knowing the accuracy is 100 per cent from DNA testing.
- Check serum creatine kinase (CK) in the mother on two occasions. A level 'in the normal range' may help reduce her risk, but never excludes carrier status.
- Any DMD boy's mother shown to be at very low risk of carrier status remains with a 15 per cent risk of germinal mosaicism for a dystrophin mutation, and should be offered CVS.
- If no deletion (or other mutation) is identified in the affected boy, take DNA also from any normal brothers and the mother. Prenatal diagnosis will usually be possible using indirect polymorphic DNA markers. A relatively high error risk due to a 12 per cent recombination risk across the dystrophin gene is minimised by using markers from each end and from the middle of the gene, but thereby slowing the analysis.
- From CVS, parents are reassured if the fetus is female, but investigation and reporting of carrier status of a female fetus is a subject of current ethical debate.

• A full family study is always indicated to identify other carriers prospectively, or to offer reassurance.

Family history of DMD or BMD

• Refer to clinical geneticist for full family DNA and CK study to determine carrier risk for sisters or other female relatives.

• Pre-pregnancy referral is required for full investigation.

• If the affected male has a known dystrophin gene deletion, accurate prenatal diagnosis can be offered from CVS if carrier risk cannot be excluded.

3

Fragile-X syndrome

Fragile-X is the commonest cause of genetic mental retardation in males after Down syndrome. The incidence is 1/2500 males. Although all males expressing the fragile-X chromosome (at Xq28) in low rolate lymphocyte cultures have retardation, a proprotion of men proven to be obligate carriers of the fragile-X gene mutation have normal intelligence.

Around 1/3 of carrier women have mental retardation, though usually to a lesser degree than in men. These tend to be the women showing larger expansions.

The fragile-X gene mutation is an expansion of a tandemly repeated CGG triplet base sequence in the fragile-X gene at Xq28. The severity of retardation correlates with the number of copies of the triplet repeat.

Specific diagnostic testing from DNA analysis is now possible and can be offered prenatally. The size of a triplet expansion in a placental sample correlates with that in the fetus, but may not be identical. The expansion size tends to increase with each generation, particularly during meiosis in the female.

Family history of fragile-X

• Confirm that diagnosis in the affected male (or female) is supported by demonstrating an expanded CGA triplet base sequence.

• Test the at-risk female consultand by DNA analysis for evidence of CGG expansion.

• If no expansion is found, reassure her that she is not a carrier. If she has an expansion she can be offered a specific prenatal test from CVS.

• If CVS shows a male with CGG expansion, the likelihood is for significant retardation, as even if expansion in the placenta were small it may be greater in some fetal tissues (e.g. fetal brain).

- If CVS shows a female with CGG expansion, she will be a carrier, but 1/3 can have retardation. Counselling is difficult. One option may be to offer fetal blood sampling to study size of expansion detected there, and also to determine the proportion of cultured lymphocyte exhibiting the fragile-X site, since this also correlates with retardation in female carriers.

- Referral to a clinical geneticist is essential for optimal interpretation and for pursuing a full family study to identify other carrier women or reassure those who are not.

Other X-linked recessive conditions

Generally the approach to carrier assessment and prenatal diagnosis in other X-linked recessive conditions is the same as in Duchenne muscular dystrophy, i.e. a combination of pedigree assessment with biochemical, haematological or clinical tests as applicable, to give an initial guide to likelihood of carrier status, but with the more definitive carrier testing coming from DNA studies. In most cases this is by indirect linked polymorphic marker analysis and therefore requires a full family study for interpretation, but increasingly individual genes are being characterised and direct mutation analysis from comparison with the affected male in the family is becoming possible. A full family study through a clinical genetics service also allows the opportunity for prospective identification of other carriers in the family, or for reassuring women who are not.

Prenatal diagnosis should in general be considered only after evaluation of carrier risks and assessment of likely informativeness of the test. Examples include haemophilia and X-linked retinitis pigmentosa.

Haemophilia

Activity/antigen ratio can be used to alter the relative likelihood of carrier status but is not an absolute test. Several polymorphic DNA markers (from Xq28), and now specific factor VIII gene mutations are used for more definitive carrier and prenatal tests.

X-linked retinitis pigmentosa

Clinical assessment including electroretinogram is combined with polymorphic indirect DNA marker study for carrier testing, but this is complicated by genetic locus heterogeneity. Prenatal diagnosis from DNA markers would therefore require a thorough and complete family study prior to its consideration.

3 Autosomal dominant conditions

Counselling for the 50 per cent risk to offspring of someone with an autosomal dominant condition is complicated by the variability of expression and even incomplete penetrance which is observed in many such disorders. Also, apparently isolated cases may arise from new mutation, but not necessarily.

Alternatives which could lead to recurrence are:

- Non-penetrance in one parent
- Germinal mosaicism in one parent
- Autosomal recessive phenocopy
- Also the assumed paternity could be incorrect.

Neurofibromatosis Type I

For 75 per cent of people with type I neurofibromatosis (NF) it remains as a cosmetic, but sometimes disfiguring, skin problem. A large head is often associated and some degree of learning difficulty is experienced by 30 per cent. The genetic concern is whether an affected offspring may be one of the remaining 25 per cent with complications which include plexiform neuroma, tibial pseudarthrosis, limb overgrowth, optic glioma or other tumour.

Affected prospective parent

The NF gene located on chromosome 17q has now been characterised, but as yet mutations have only been discovered in a small proportion of cases (around 5 per cent). Direct mutation testing cannot yet be used routinely for prenatal diagnosis. Prenatal diagnosis can be offered only where there is a clear family history and where DNA samples can be obtained from other family members in order to establish the linkage phase of close DNA polymorphic markers. The severity of affected status, or any increased risk of complications cannot be determined, except by detecting a specific complication on subsequent fetal ultrasound scan.

Previous affected child

Around 30 per cent of cases of NF arise from new mutation.

- Examine both parents of an affected child, including for Lisch nodules on the iris.
- NF is fully penetrant but the possibility of germinal mosaicism leaves a small residual recurrent risk (around 2 per cent) when the parents are unaffected. At present, while the genetic fault in an individual case is unlikely to be identifiable, prenatal diagnosis is not a practical option in this situation.
- If one parent has NF a prenatal diagnosis by DNA polymorphic marker analysis could be offered from CVS, but samples from both parents and the previously affected child would be required first to establish which DNA probes would be informative.

Family history of NF

Since NF is considered to show full penetrance, full examination of a prospective parent will establish whether or not their children would be at 50 per cent risk. A family DNA study could help in the few cases of doubt.

Myotonic dystrophy

Myotonic dystrophy (DM) is important for its relatively high prevalence (approximately 1/5000), its extreme variability of presentation with anticipation (increased severity in each subsequent generation), for the increased anaesthetic risk, and in obstetrics and gynaecology for an increased incidence of sub-fertility, whereby some undiagnosed couples are enrolled for fertility treatment. Classically the condition presents with weakness of facial, neck and distal muscles, associated with myotonia of grip, and often with an overall apathy or lack of energy. Cardiac conduction defects, cataracts and frontal balding are all frequent by middle age.

Congenital onset, which is seen in the affected children of some symptomatic mothers, can present *in utero* with paucity of fetal movement, polyhydramnios and premature delivery of a baby who may have joint contractures (talipes or arthrogryposis) and severe congenital hypotonia with respiratory and feeding difficulties. Prolonged ventilation of a full-term neonate may be required. The congenital-onset is invariably associated subsequently with some degree of mental retardation.

The DM gene is located on chromosome 19q, and as with fragile-X syndrome it is now known that the gene defect causing DM is an expansion of a tandemly repeated CTG triplet base sequence. The degree of expansion correlates with the severity of presentation, being largest in babies with congenital onset. The CTG repeat sequence invariably increases in length when inherited from a female, sometimes to a considerable degree. At male meiosis a lesser expansion usually occurs, but occasional reduction in size may also be seen. The CTG expansion provides a direct and specific diagnostic DNA test for myotonic dystrophy which can be employed in assessing presymptomatic status of those with a family history of DM, and in providing specific and accurate prenatal testing from CVS at 11 weeks' gestation.

For an affected person

- Take a DNA sample from the affected prospective parent and from their spouse. The sex of the affected person and the size of CTG expansion give a guide as to the likely degree of further expansion, and hence severity, in their offspring. Onset almost invariably occurs at a younger age in an affected son or daughter than in the parent.
- Specific prenatal diagnosis can be offered from CVS. The CTG expansion size in chorionic villi may give some guide to expected severity in the offspring if the pregnancy were to continue. Perhaps paradoxically it seems that many of the more severely affected parents decide against having a prenatal test or to terminate an affected fetus if a test is done.

For an affected mother with a previous congenitally-affected baby

- Take DNA sample from the baby (if possible) and both parents.
- Further offspring (male or female) have a 50 per cent risk of DM, and almost without exception would also present with the congenital-onset form.
- Prenatal diagnosis from CVS is now always possible.

Family history

- Take the full family history.
- Obtain a DNA sample, if possible from a known affected member, to confirm CTG expansion.
- Take the full past history and examine consultand for signs of DM, especially grip and percussion myotonia; EMG and slit lamp examination are probably now no longer necessary.
- Discuss pre-symptomatic testing from DNA with them; i.e. future implications, life insurance aspects, etc.
- Take a DNA sample if they wish to proceed.

- If the sample is found to show no CTG expansion total reassurance can be given regarding their offspring, and prenatal testing can be avoided.
- If the sample does show a CTG expansion further counselling will be needed in its own right; a specific prenatal test is also possible.

Huntington's chorea

Huntington's chorea (HC) is arguably one of the most devastating of hereditary conditions. Symptomatic onset can be from 12 to 70 years, but usually commences between 30 and 60 years. The triad of symptoms of involuntary movement (chorea), mood changes (usually depression) and dementia may not each occur in every case, but any one of these may lead to family breakdown. Currently there is no treatment. As with myotonic dystrophy, anticipation may be the rule for age at onset in a subsequent generation when it is the father who is passing on the dominant gene.

The genetic fault in HC is also now known to be the expansion of a tandemly repeated CAG triplet sequence in the Huntington gene on chromosome 4p. While this can now provide a specific and accurate differential diagnostic test in symptomatic cases, its potential use in prenatal testing is overshadowed by the inevitability of a prenatal test also being a predictive test for the unwitting parent. Pre-symptomatic predictive testing should only be offered following careful counselling guidance from a Clinical Genetic Service, and would rarely be sanctioned within the time-pressures of someone presenting already in a pregnancy.

A form of prenatal testing (exclusion testing) based on indirect linked polymorphic DNA markers can often still be offered if the relevant unaffected (or affected) grandparent is available for a DNA sample. Then if the couple would wish to terminate a pregnancy where the risk to the fetus is shown to be increased from 25 per cent to 50 per cent this can be made possible by demonstrating whether the fetus has inherited one copy of the HC gene region from their affected or unaffected grandparent on that side of the family. The family DNA study should ideally be made prior to the onset of a pregnancy in order to determine DNA probe informativeness.

Family history of HC or affected HC patient

- Genetic or pregnancy advice should **always** be with the involvement of a Clinical Genetic Service.

- A full family history should be taken.
- A reported family history should be verified where possible from medical records, etc.
- DNA should be obtained (or located) from one affected family member to confirm typical CAG expansion.
- Following referral for genetic counselling it will be ascertained whether the patient is thinking about a pre-symptomatic test for themselves or not.
- Neurological examination is made only if the patient wishes for this degree of clinical predictive guidance.
- Pre-symptomatic testing is performed following a minimum of three counselling sessions, and only when the geneticist and the patient both feel that there has been sufficient thought and preparation for it.
- If the patient and their partner elect for fetal exclusion testing rather than pre-symptomatic prediction, DNA samples are collected from both of the couple and from the patient's parent(s). If both parents are deceased fetal exclusion testing cannot be offered.
- For someone who is already known to carry a faulty HC gene (i.e. is pre-symptomatic) definitive prenatal diagnosis from CVS can be offered. The couple must, however, be very sure that they would wish to request termination if the fetus proves to be affected, as otherwise a child could be growing up knowing, or with their parents knowing, that they would inevitably develop HC.

Other autosomal dominant conditions

Prenatal diagnosis can now be offered in many other dominant conditions, mostly by DNA analysis from CVS. Although rapidly increasing in number, as yet specific diagnosis from direct mutation detection can be made for only a few conditions. These include peroneal muscular atrophy with slowed nerve condution (CMT type Ia), some families with dominant retinitis pigmentosa, familial polyposis coli, and new mutation cases of facioscapulohumeral muscular dystrophy. In most dominant conditions prenatal diagnosis would be performed using indirect linked polymorphic DNA markers and therefore require a family study before knowing whether the prenatal test would be informative. Examples include adult polycystic kidney disease, familial retinoblastoma and Marfan's syndrome.

In any dominant condition, apart from cases arising from new mutation, one parent will by definition always be affected. Perhaps because of this, it is invariably a minority of such families who request prenatal diagnosis, and the clinician has no authority to try to influence this situation.

CHROMOSOMAL INHERITANCE

Previous baby with chromosome disorder

It is essential to recheck the karyotype report on the previous affected baby. Aneuploidy (single extra or missing whole chromosomes) or triploidy have a reassuringly low recurrence risk; for structural chromosome anomalies (translocations, inversions, ring chromosomes, extra marker chromosomes) the recurrence risk may be much higher.

Trisomy: (t21, t18, t13)

Parents' chromosomes

Parents' chromosomes do not have any increased risk of abnormality and there is no indication for routine karyotyping of parents. The recurrence risk, which is predominantly for t21 is 1 per cent, or twice the age-dependant risk, whichever is the greater, i.e. the risk is 1/100 for a mother aged 38 years or younger, 1/50 at 40 years and 1/25 by 44 years.

Triploidy and trisomies (other than those above) identified from early pregnancy loss

There is no evidence to suggest that the risk for producing a chromosomally abnormal liveborn infant is significantly increased above age-dependant risk.

Mosaic trisomy (i.e. for chromosomes 8, 9, 13, 18, 21, 22)

The recurrence risk in most cases is very much lower than the 1 per cent figure, as the non-disjunction occurs during post-zygotic mitotic cell division.

Translocation trisomy

The karyotypes of both parents must be checked. If normal, recurrent risk is possibly around 2 per cent (from the possibility of parental germinal mosaicism for a balanced translocation), and is probably independent of maternal age. A full family study should be commenced if one parent has a balanced translocation.

Sex chromosome anomaly

If simple aneuploidy (e.g. XO, XXY, XYY, XXX) parental karyotype is not indicated. The recurrence risk is 1 per cent or lower, and shows much less correlation with parental age than for autosomal trisomy. Structural sex chromosome anomalies (e.g. ring X or Xq duplication as an isochromosome) require parental karyotyping.

Structural chromosome anomaly

Parental karyotyping is essential if not already done to identify cases with balanced chromosome rearrangements in one parent. If parents have normal karyotypes the recurrence risk of previous *de novo* anomaly is that for parental germinal mosaicism (around 2 per cent). For children with microdeletion syndromes, study of parental karyotype requires the appropriate laboratory technique.

Parent with balanced chromosome rearrangement

The risk of liveborn offspring with chromosomal anomaly will depend on the nature of the individual rearrangement, and genetic advice should be sought in each case. Generally the risk of chromosomal abnormality in conceptus will be of the order of 50 per cent, and the smaller the sections of chromosome material which are involved the greater is the likelihood of a fetus with chromosomal imbalance surviving to term. A 13/14 Robertsonian (centromere to centromere) chromosome translocation may be an exception in having a relatively low risk of resulting in fetal trisomy or monosomy.

Prenatal testing is usually strongly advisable, usually by 11-week CVS, but for rearrangements likely to result in early miscarriage rather than fetal survival a second trimester amniocentesis may be more appropriate. Referral to clinical genetics for study of the extended family is also indicated.

Some chromosomal variants (e.g. small pericentric inversion on chromosome 9) are normal population variants and do not have any associated risk of fetal chromosome abnormality.

Other family history of chromosome disorder

The nature of the disorder should be ascertained. If it is a simple trisomy or sex chromosome aneuploidy the risk to the presenting prospective parent is not increased above the age-appropriate population level. If it is a structural rearrangement, the risk depends on the karyotype analysis in intervening relatives in the family. Only if the parent remains in line should chromosome testing be offered, and then the parent's chromosomes should be checked before considering a prenatal test.

Chromosome translocation accounts for only 5 per cent of cases of Down's syndrome babies born to mothers under 30 years, and <5 per cent to older women: in only 1/3 of these cases is there a familial risk. Therefore give reassurance of likely low risk if the karyotype of the index case cannot be confirmed as simple t21, but offer to karyotype the consultand if anxiety remains.

Previous recurrent miscarriage

For any couple with three or more first trimester pregnancy losses both parents should be karyotyped, especially if the result might influence whether or not they would wish for prenatal chromosome testing. If both partners have normal karyotype there is no increased indication for a prenatal test, indeed perhaps the reverse. If one partner has a balanced rearrangement from which the unbalanced offspring would inevitably miscarry, invasive prenatal testing may also be inappropriate.

Prospective parent with a clinical chromosome disorder themselves

XXX, XYY

Both have normal fertility. It is rare for the extra sex chromosome to be passed on to the fetus, and the overall risk of XXX or XXY from an XXX mother, or of XXY or XYY from an XYY father is around 4 per cent at most. Prenatal diagnosis should be discussed but offered at the parents' discretion.

Trisomy 21

Pregnancy can occur in women with Down's syndrome. The fetus has a 50 per cent risk of similar t21. Discovery of pregnancy would often lead to request for termination irrespective of the feasibility of prenatal diagnosis.

ALTERNATIVE REPRODUCTIVE OPTIONS

Termination of pregnancy (TOP) is an option for only some couples. For many
- no prenatal test is available, **or**
- TOP is unacceptable, **or**
- TOP is unacceptable if the fetus has a significant chance of being normal.

Some may consider
- **Postponing pregnancy** in anticipation of genetic research enabling future prenatal testing. Consider storage meantime of DNA samples from key family members.
- **Artificial insemination by donor sperm (DI)** for autosomal recessive or dominant inheritance where the father is a faulty gene carrier. For CF, sickle cell or thalassaemia the proposed donor sperm should be tested for carrier status.
- **Egg donation** for X-linked recessive, dominant or mitochondrial inheritance where the mother is a faulty gene carrier, or remains at-risk: also where inheritance pattern in an affected child is uncertain. Consider appropriateness if mother is affected or pre-symptomatic (e.g. in myotonic dystrophy or Huntington chorea).
- **Adoption** although parental age and illness-risk may be adverse factors.
- **IVF and pre-implantation embryo selection**: prenatal diagnosis either fully or partially informative using PCR techniques, but the couple is opposed to termination or already requiring IVF (e.g. sexing alone in X-linked recessive disorder).

Future population screening

Population screening for carrier or pre-symptomatic status is inevitably going to become possible in many genetic conditions. Informed debate is required for consideration of the ethical, scientific and social aspects of any proposed policy, in addition to the financial considerations. Anticipated candidate conditions for eventual introduction to the pre-pregnancy or antenatal population are.
- Autosomal recessive carriers:
  cystic fibrosis
  spinal muscular atrophy (gene yet to be identified)

sickle-cell, ß-thalassaemia ⎱
Tay–Sachs disease   ⎰ in certain racial groups.

- X-linked recessive carriers:
  Duchenne/Becker MD
  fragile-X.
- Dominant pre-symptomatic status:
  myotonic dystrophy.

4 Medical Disorders of Pregnancy

4

4

4.1 Cardiovascular disorders of pregnancy
Cardiovascular physiology in pregnancy

Blood pressure (BP) is proportional to cardiac output and systemic vascular resistance.

Since the fall in the latter is greater in early pregnancy than the rise in the former, the systolic blood pressure (SBP) falls slightly in early pregnancy but rises again in late pregnancy. The diastolic blood pressure (DBP) is well below non-pregnant levels from early in pregnancy. It returns to those levels after 30 to 32 weeks' gestation.

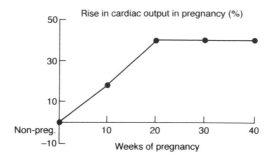

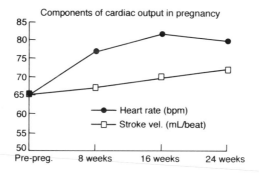

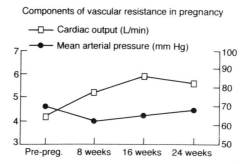

Fig. 4.1.1 Cardiac output in pregnancy.

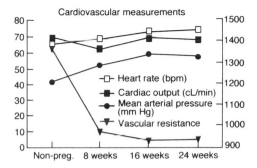

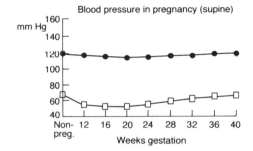

Fig. 4.1.1 *Continued*

Among the factors reducing vascular resistance and controlling BP are the balance between vasodilatory prostacyclin (PGI$_2$) and vasoconstrictive thromboxane A$_2$ (TXA$_2$), and oestrogen induced increase in nitric oxide synthesis in blood vessels.

The normally pregnant woman is relatively refractory to vasopressor agents, i.e. her BP does not rise in response to a small dose of a vasopressor.

MEASUREMENT OF BLOOD PRESSURE

The criteria to be fulfilled are:
- The women should be relaxed and in a semi recumbent position with slight lateral tilt (to avoid supine hypotension).

- The blood pressure cuff should be at level of the heart.
- A standard (12×23 cm) cuff is suitable only for arm circumference less than 35 cm. (Too small a cuff in an obese individual leads to falsely high reading.)
- DPB is measured at the muffling of sounds (Korotkoff Phase 4) rather than their disappearance (Korotkoff Phase 5). However, this is not the convention in the USA where Korotkoff Phase 5 defines DPB.

Note: Automated recordings of blood pressure record levels at Korotkoff Phase 5 and may give a slightly low reading for diastolic blood pressure.

The blood pressure normally falls during sleep, both in the pregnant and non-pregnant woman. In women developing pre-eclampsia, the evening fall is at first lost and later the circadian pattern is reversed with the appearance of nocturnal hypertension. This is important when diagnosing and treating hypertension in pregnancy, e.g. it may be necessary to give increased dosages of anti-hypertensives at night.

HYPERTENSION IN PREGNANCY

Hypertensive disorders of pregnancy are a major cause of maternal death in the UK, responsible for 27 deaths, 14 of which were associated with eclampsia in the 1988–1990 triennium. Seven of the 27 deaths occurred before 33 weeks' gestation. Twelve were due to cerebral haemorrhage, and ten due to pulmonary complications and adult respiratory distress syndrome occuring between 4 and 21 days after delivery. **A blood pressure of 170/110 mm Hg is an obstetric emergency and requires treatment**. (See Table 4.1.1 for the classification of severity of hypertension.)

Table 4.1.1 Severity of the hypertension.

	Systolic BP (mm Hg)	Diastolic BP (mm Hg)
Mild/moderate	140–165	90–105
Severe	⩾170	⩾110

DEFINITIONS

Definition of hypertension

- Two consecutive BP readings of 140/90 mm Hg and over four or more hours apart or an increase of SBP >30 mm Hg and of DBP >15 mm Hg over the earliest recorded reading in pregnancy. The combination of a diastolic blood pressure of >90 mm Hg, combined with a systolic minus diastolic differential of 25 mm Hg over the booking blood pressure are more discriminatory for pre-eclampsia. Perinatal mortality and morbidity begin to rise associated with those levels. The level of DBP is of greater prognostic significance than SBP for the fetus.
- In the first trimester of pregnancy two per cent of women have a blood pressure at or above 140/90 mm Hg. In the second half of pregnancy up to 20 per cent of pregnant women may have an occasional blood pressure reading of 140/90 mm Hg or higher. In only one per cent of women does the blood pressure exceed 170/110 mm Hg.
- A diastolic blood pressure of more than 90 mm Hg measured after 20 weeks of pregnancy is suggestive of pregnancy induced (or gestational) hypertension. A diastolic blood pressure of 90 mm Hg is 3 standard deviations above the mean for mid pregnancy, 2 standard deviations above the mean for 34 weeks but only 1.5 standard deviations above the mean at term.

Definition of proteinuria

- A 24 hour urine collection containing 0.3 g or more of protein.
- Two random mid-stream urine (MSU) or catheter specimens containing '2 plus' (equivalent to 1 g albumin/L; see Table 4.1.2) or more on a reagent strip.
- A urinary tract infection must be excluded if a dipstick test shows 1+ or more of protein.

CLASSIFICATION OF HYPERTENSION IN PREGNANCY

The main purpose is for medical audit. All systems are arbitrary and unsatisfactory to some extent. The International Society for the Study of Hypertension of Pregnancy (ISSHP) suggest the following:

Table 4.1.2 The measured correlation in g/L of protein as observed on dipstick testing of urine.

Protein (+)	g/L
Trace	0.1
1+	0.3
2+	0.3–1.0
3+	3.0
4+	10.0

Gestational hypertension and/or proteinuria

Hypertension and/or proteinuria developing during pregnancy, labour or the puerperium in a previously normotensive non-proteinuric woman subdivided into:

- Gestational hypertension (without proteinuria)
- Gestational proteinuria (without hypertension)
- Gestational proteinuric hypertension (pre-eclampsia).

Each of these can develop during pregnancy, in labour, or in the puerperium.

Chronic hypertension and chronic renal disease

Hypertension and/or proteinuria in a women with either chronic hypertension or chronic renal disease present before, diagnosed during, or persisting after pregnancy subdivided into:

- Chronic hypertension (without proteinuria)
- Chronic renal disease – proteinuria with/without hypertension
- Chronic hypertension with superimposed pre-eclampsia (proteinuria developing for the first time in pregnancy in a woman with known chronic hypertension).

Women with hypertension and/or proteinuria when first seen before 20 weeks' gestation (who do not have a hydatidiform mole) are classified under this heading.

Unclassified hypertension and/or proteinuria

Hypertension and/or proteinuria found either:

- at first booking examination at or after 20 weeks of pregnancy in a woman without known chronic hypertension or chronic renal disease; **or**
- during labour, pregnancy or the puerperium but where insufficient information is available to permit classification.

The classification in pregnancy is provisional and should be reviewed at the end of the puerperium.

PRE-ECLAMPSIA

Pre-eclampsia is a multi-system disorder peculiar to human pregnancy, usually characterised by hypertension, renal impairment and fluid retention. Proteinuria and some degree of intravascular coagulation are not uncommon. The primary pathology is endothelial damage. It may be due to a failure of maternal adaptation to the presence of trophoblast. As a result:

- Plasma volume does not expand normally; the net effect is a reduced maternal plasma volume.
- Prostanoid production is abnormal, e.g. there is a relative reduction of endothelial production of prostacyclin (PGI_2) compared to thromboxane. This affects systemic vascular resistance as evidenced by:

continued responsiveness to vasopressors;

the development of hypertension.

There is a resulting cascade effect on virtually every system in the body. Among these effects are:

1 **Vascular endothelium**. Vasospasm damages the endothelium resulting in platelet adherence and fibrin deposition.

2 **Kidney**. Glomular damage (including swelling of the endothelial cells) is the cause of proteinuria. A rise in plasma urate is an early feature of pre-eclampsia. In severe cases creatinine clearance and urinary output fall.

3 **Coagulation**.

- Platelet turnover is increased which can result in larger platelets on a blood film and a fall in platelet count which can be severe in some cases (see below).
- Disseminated intravascular coagulation (DIC) is a rare but serious end point in some cases.
- Haemolysis can also occur.

4 **The liver**. Fibrin deposits in the sinusoids can cause hepato-cellular damage. The epigastric pain and vomiting associated with fulminat-

ing pre-eclampsia are due to effects on the liver. In some cases jaundice and severe liver damage can follow, often out of proportion to other signs and symptoms. (DIC is also present.)

5 **Cardio-pulmonary effects**. Severe pre-eclampsia is a high cardiac output state with inappropriately high systemic vascular resistance and hyperdynamic left ventricular function. Cardiac failure and pulmonary oedema can complicate the most severe cases.

6 **Central nervous system**. Among the signs of CNS involvement are atypical headache, hyper-reflexia, visual disturbances and ankle clonus. Vasoconstriction of cerebral vessels occurs, probably as a protective mechanism against severe hypertension. At a mean arterial pressure of about 130 to 150 mm Hg this mechanism begins to fail, and small vessel walls are damaged and disrupted. This leads to cerebral oedema, haemorrhages and infarcts – all associated with eclampsia, a major cause of maternal death.

7 **Feto/placental effects**. These occur as a result of:

▪ Relative lack of trophoblast infiltration of the walls of maternal spiral arterioles during development of the placenta.

▪ Failure of normal development of the uteroplacental circulation.

▪ Aggregation of platelets, fibrin and lipid-laden macrophages ('acute atherosis') within unadapted spiral arterioles.

Pre-eclampsia is, therefore, the commonest cause of intra-uterine growth retardation (IUGR) in non-malformed infants and of elective pre-term deliveries.

MANAGEMENT OF HYPERTENSIVE DISORDERS OF PREGNANCY

Points to remember

▪ Pre-eclampsia is a disease with a wide spectrum of severity.

▪ It rarely develops before 20 weeks and may progress rapidly and become fulminating.

▪ Beware of the symptomatic manifestation of pre-eclampsia (see below); symptoms indicate the need for delivery.

▪ Once persistent proteinuria occurs, symptoms (and the need to deliver) tend to arise within two weeks.

The degree of risk to mother and fetus with raised blood pressure and/or proteinuria are related to:

▪ the underlying cause;

- the stage of pregnancy at onset;
- the severity of the hypertension and associated maternal signs and symptoms;
- the presence or absence of IUGR.

Principles of management

1 Routine antenatal care (see Table 4.1.3 for risk factors)
- Measure BP and test for proteinuria at each visit.
- Women at increased risk of pre-eclampsia should be weighed.
- Hypertension requires further assessment.

Table 4.1.3 Risk factors for severity of pre-eclampsia.

Maternal	Fetal
Small risk	Multiple pregnancy
First pregnancy or new partner	Hydatidiform mole
Previous pre-eclampsia	Large placenta
Maternal age less than 20 or over 35	Triploidy
Family history of pre-eclampsia or eclampsia (daughters of eclamptic women are 8 times more likely to have pre-eclampsia and complications)	Trisomy 13, 18
Underweight and short	
Migraine	
Moderate risk	
Chronic hypertension	
Severe risk	
Collagen vascular disease	
Diabetes	
Chronic renal disease	

2 Treatment of hypertension
- Severe hypertension (e.g. $\geqslant 170/110$ mm Hg) results in loss of auto-regulatory control within the cerebral vasculature. The resulting hyperperfusion can result in serious damage.
- Therefore, blood pressure at or over 170/110 mm Hg must be treated to reduce the risk of maternal cerebral haemorrhage (see below). The

main justification for treating gestational hypertension at levels between 150/110 and 170/110 mm Hg is to at least delay progression towards the higher levels.

- Treating moderately increased blood pressure (140/90 to 160/100 mm Hg) neither prevents super-imposed pre-eclampsia nor directly benefits the fetus.
- Pre-existing hypertension will continue to require treatment.
- Having excluded any other complicating factor, isolated mild hypertension can be managed as an outpatient from routine clinics.

3 Pre-eclampsia

Severity of pre-eclampsia

Table 4.1.4 shows the three stages of pre-eclampsia.

- The objective is to make the diagnosis in stage 1, admit in stage 2 and proceed to delivery before the onset of stage 3.
- Stage 1 disease can be managed in a day assessment unit as long as platelet levels are not falling or liver function is not abnormal.
- Stage 2 disease requires admission and assessment on the day of detection.
- **Stage 3 disease is an obstetric emergency**.
- Pregnant women complaining of headache, epigastric pain and tenderness and vomiting should be considered to have symptomatic (fulminating) pre-eclampsia until proved otherwise (Table 4.1.5).

Table 4.1.4 The severity of pre-eclampsia and recommended management depending on presence or absence of symptoms and signs. (Reproduced with permission from Redman, C.W.G. (1989) Hypertension in pregnancy. In *Obstetrics* (Ed. by A. Turnbull & G. Chamberlain), p. 523, Churchill Livingstone, London.)

	Stage 1	Stage 2	Stage 3
Hypertension	Yes	Yes	Yes
Proteinuria	No	Yes	Yes
Symptoms	No	No	Yes
Eclampsia	No	No	Possible
Typical duration	2 weeks–3 months	2–3 weeks	2 hours–3 weeks
Timing of admission	Elective	Same day	Emergency
Likely timing of delivery	Not before 38 weeks	34–36 weeks?	Soon after stabilisation

Table 4.1.5 Symptoms and signs of pre-eclampsia (stage 3, i.e. severe disease).

Muzziness in the head
Lethargy and slow verbal responses
Nausea and vomiting
Headache
Epigastric pain and tenderness
Sudden oliguria
Visual disturbances
Ankle clonus

Biochemical and haematological features of pre-eclampsia

1 Renal function

Proteinuria   This is a sign of generalised endothelial damage in the kidney. It is associated with increased perinatal mortality rate and intrauterine growth retardation. Although dipstick testing is used, (see Table 4.1.3) in the clinical situation, proteinuria should be quantified with a 24 hour collection.

False positive results can be due to contamination of the urine by vaginal discharge or by chlorhexidine, highly alkaline or very concentrated urine (specific gravity >1.030). False negatives may occur if the urine is very dilute (specific gravity <1.010).

Prolonged proteinuria may cause hypoalbuminuria (<28 g/L) and can result in nephrotic syndrome.

The absence of proteinuria does not absolutely preclude severe disease.

Elevated plasma urate levels (>0.35 mmol/L)   See Table 4.1.6 for specific plasma urate levels for gestation. These help to distinguish women with pre-eclampsia from gestational hypertension and chronic hypertension alone. There is a higher perinatal mortality rate

Table 4.1.6 Abnormal levels of uric acid for gestation.

Gestation (weeks)	Uric acid levels (mmol/L)
28	0.3
32	0.35
36	0.40
40	0.45

in women with elevated plasma urate levels and hypertension than in those with hypertension alone.

Plasma creatinine   Levels above 80 micromol/L are abnormal and above 100 micromol/L are grossly abnormal in the absence of pre-existing renal disease.

Plasma urea   Levels are more variable, but values above 6 mmol/L correspond to possible renal impairment and above 7 mmol/L probable renal impairment.

2 Haematology

Platelets   Counts of $<150 \times 10^9$/L are low for pregnancy and falling levels are indicative of some degree of DIC. **Counts $<100 \times 10^9$/L are clinically worrisome**. An increase in platelet size (>9/femtolitre) suggests a rapid turnover which occurs in severe pre-eclampsia.

Packed cell volume   A haematocrit of greater than 0.35 is a sign of haemoconcentration, associated with vasoconstriction and failure of expansion of plasma volume which are at the heart of pre-eclampsia.

3 Liver

Pre-eclampsia can cause hepatic sinusoidal fibrin deposition with focal parenchymal necrosis and periportal polymorph nuclear infiltration. Obstructive jaundice may occur from the hepatocellular oedema.

Liver function tests should be measured at least weekly in stage 2 disease and at least daily in stage 3 disease. An elevated aspartate transaminase (AST >40 IU/L) suggests liver damage in pregnancy. Although alkaline phosphatase (ALP) is normally elevated in pregnancy, it and gamma glutamyl transaminas (GGT) rise a few days after the maximum severity of disease and after the AST has returned to normal. The initial rise in AST can be due to damage to other cells and tissues such as red blood cells, heart, skeletal muscle, kidney and pancreas.

Other complications of pre-eclampsia

1 Cerebral involvement

One of the most dangerous features of pre-eclampsia, cerebral haemorrhage, is the most important cause of maternal death from hypertensive disease. Cerebral disturbance is the cause of eclamptic seizures. The average blood pressure of the woman with eclampsia is usually high (170–190/110–120 mm Hg) but not necessarily so.

2 *The fetus*

Fetal investigations are described in Chapter 6.

3 *HELLP syndrome*

This is an acronym for **H**aemolysis, **E**levated **L**iver Function Tests, and **L**ow **P**latelets. Its features are shown in Table 4.1.7. It is a severe form of pre-eclampsia.

- It affects up to 12 per cent of women with severe pre-eclampsia and the incidence may be increasing. Maternal and fetal morbidity and mortality are high if it is not recognised and treated promptly.

4

Table 4.1.7 Features of pre-eclampsia and HELLP syndrome.

Signs
Pregnancy induced hypertension (may not be very high in HELLP syndrome)
Excessive weight gain (>1 kg/week)
Generalised oedema
Pulmonary oedema
Laryngeal oedema
Ascites

Abnormalities of organ systems
Acute renal cortical and tubular necrosis
Periportal hepatic necrosis, haematoma underneath liver capsule that may rupture
Disseminated intravascular coagulation
Placental abruption

Biochemical abnormalities
Hyperuricaemia
Proteinuria
Hypocalcaemia
Haemolysis – decreasing haematocrit
Thrombocytopaenia ($<100 \times 10^9$/L)
Increased liver enzymes AST $\geqslant 48$ IU/L
                         Alanine aminotransferase $\geqslant 24$ IU/L
                         LDH $\geqslant 164$ IU/L
Increased fibrin degradation products
Decreased serum antithrombin III

Fetal abnormalities
Intrauterine growth retardation
Intrauterine hypoxaemia
In utero fetal asphyxia and death

- It may be insidious in onset and is often not clinically recognised at presentation.
- The presenting symptom is often epigastric pain and tenderness.
- Hypertension and proteinuria may not be present initially.
- Liver function tests (LFTS) and platelet counts must be carried out if the condition is suspected.
- AST rises first and lactate dehydrogenase (LDH) 24–48 hours post-delivery. LDH >600 IU/L indicates very severe disease.
- Most women with liver involvement in pre-eclampsia have worsening thrombocytopaenia until many hours after delivery. The platelet count gradually returns to normal after delivery. LDH and AST may continue to increase for a few days after delivery.
- Management of these women needs to be a team effort in which obstetrician, midwives, haematologists, internists and anaesthetists work together.

The priorities of management are:
- early detection;
- delivery as soon as is safe for the mother;
- correction of haematological defect;
- high dependency/intensive care.

ANTIHYPERTENSIVE THERAPY

Blood pressure requires treatment at levels at or above 170 mm Hg systolic and/or 110 mm Hg diastolic to prevent cerebral haemorrhage.

This level of blood pressure is an obstetric emergency.
The aim of therapy is to gain control in the short term and maintain it long enough after delivery until the risk of extreme hypertension and eclampsia has receded.

For long term control the choice of antihypertensive is **methyldopa**, **nifedipine** or **beta adrenergic blocking agents** (beta-blockers). The aim is to use the drug which is safe in pregnancy, has a quick onset of action and allows some titration of dose–response and can safely be combined with a second drug if needed.

Hypertension will often improve within 24 hours after delivery but may increase again at around 48–72 hours post-partum. Antihypertensives should be continued for at least three days after delivery.

Hypertension may persist and require treatment for some weeks after delivery.

Antihypertensive treatment may be reduced or stopped 2–3 weeks after discharge. This decision can be made by the general practitioner.

Methyldopa

Methyldopa is an agonist of alpha$_2$ adrenoreceptors in the brainstem, and thus reduces sympathetic outflow.

Its use in women with mild to moderate hypertension (140–170/90–110 mm Hg) is associated with a reduction in the occurrence of severe hypertension and its potential complications during pregnancy and the immediate puerperium.

Dose of methyldopa

- Loading dose of 500–1000 mg.
- 250–750 mg four times per day.
- Maximal dose 3 g per day.
- *Side effects:* Sedation for first 24 hours and tiredness thereafter.
- Methyldopa is established as a safe drug to use in pregnancy, by long term follow up of the children of treated mothers.

Calcium channel blockers

This class of drugs reduces blood pressure by antagonising calcium channels in smooth muscle and causing vasodilation.

Nifedipine

Although not licensed for use in pregnancy, it is valuable in the treatment and control of hypertension in pregnancy.

- It is potent with rapid onset when given orally. It interferes with excitation–contraction coupling by blocking calcium influx into smooth muscle cells.
- The major and sometimes debilitating side effects are flushing, headache and oedema.
- It can be given in three forms for both the acute and long term control of blood pressure in pregnancy.

Commence nifedipine by giving the capsule:

- **Capsules (10 mg)** act within 10–15 minutes. Treatment should commence with this preparation. Dose: 10 mg twice daily increasing up to 20 mg three times per day (at the higher dose, slow release tablets are preferable). Maximal dose: 60 mg/day.

- **Slow release tablets (20 mg)**. The onset of action is slower (about 60 minutes) but they have a sustained release, producing a prolonged effect. Dose: 20 mg 8 hourly (maximum dose).
- **True long acting preparation (20–30 mg tablets)**. Some women do not absorb this form of the drug. Therefore the change from one preparation to this long acting form of the drug requires careful observation.

Note: The combination of beta-blockers and nifedipine is very potent. Nifedipine lowers systemic vascular resistance. Normally with such a loss of resistance, the fall in blood pressure is prevented by the reflex increase in heart rate. If a beta-blocker is present, heart rate does not increase, so the fall in blood pressure is greater.

4

Beta-blockers

Beta-blockers are competitive antagonists to the effects of endogenous catecholamines on beta-adrenoreceptors. They may have partial agonist effects.

No single beta-blocker can be considered superior to others for use in pregnancy, despite the theoretical claims for cardioselectivity and alpha-agonist activity.

Labetalol and oxprenolol have been studied to the greatest extent in pregnancy. The use of atenolol has been associated with IUGR.

Oxprenolol

- An effective single oral agent for the management of hypertension in pregnancy.
- It is particularly useful in inhibiting the reflex tachycardia which can occur in 30 per cent of women taking nifedipine which then blunts the hypotensive response (but see note above).
- Dose: 40 mg to 320 mg twice daily. Tablets come in 40 mg and 160 mg dosages.

Labetalol

- A combined alpha- and beta-blocking agent (beta>alpha) which can be effective as a single agent.
- Dose: 100 to 200 mg 8 hourly orally.
- Some women do not respond and it can cause postural hypotension.

THE ACUTE CONTROL OF SEVERE HYPERTENSION

It is important to stabilise all patients with blood pressure above 170/110 mm Hg before delivery or transfer.

If caesarean section under general anaesthetic is planned, intubation can cause a further acute rise in blood pressure leading to cerebrovascular accident and cardiac failure.

Nifedipine

Nifedipine may be used in the first instance together with loading doses of methyldopa (500–1000 mg) if blood pressure reaches 170/110 mm Hg.

- Give nifedipine 10 mg every 30 minutes until the blood pressure is under 160/100 mm Hg. Give methyldopa if there is no improvement after three doses.

Hydralazine

Hydralazine a vasodilator directly inhibiting the contractile activity of smooth muscle. Although no longer the first drug of choice because of its short action and side effects it is an alternative to nifedipine and methyldopa in the acute control of blood pressure.

- Dose: 10 mg intramuscularly (which may be combined with an oral loading dose of methyldopa 500–1000 mg). Its effects only last for 1–2 hours. The hydralazine can be repeated every 2–3 hours or infused continuously intravenously, until the action of methyldopa begins 6–8 hours later. Do not use more hydralazine than 300 mg in 24 hours.
- Hydralazine is best used as intermittent intramuscular or intravenous injections of 10–20 mg for transient rises in blood pressure where oral nifedipine cannot be given.
- If used as an infusion make up 50 mg hydralazine in dextrose 5 per cent to a volume of 100 mL. This gives 0.5 mg/mL. Start at 10 drops per minute (5 mg/hour). Increase by doubling the dose every 30 minutes until the blood pressure is controlled. Maximum dose is 40 mg/hour or 80 drops per minute. Aim to keep the blood pressure under 170/110 mm Hg.
- If necessary the effectiveness of hydralazine can be enhanced by methyldopa, causing sympathetic inhibition which blocks the reflex tachycardia that develops as the blood pressure falls.

▪ *Side effects:* Hydralazine causes a prolonged activation of nora-drenaline release which may result in headaches, anxiety, rest-lessness, shakiness, vomiting and hyper-reflexia (and therefore mimics impending eclampsia). These effects are more likely to be troublesome with continuous intravenous infusion. It can also cause an increase in intracranial pressure because of dilating the capacitance vessels in the cerebral circulation. This is not desirable with the possibility of impending eclampsia, where intracranial pressure may already be increased. Cardiac output increases because of increased venous return. A marked tachycardia always occurs.

Labetalol

▪ Give an immediate bolus loading dose of 50–100 mg intravenously and 50 mg every 30 minutes until the blood pressure is less than 160/100 mm Hg.

▪ For an infusion make up 200 mg labetalol in dextrose 5 per cent to a volume of 100 mL (i.e. 2 mg/mL). Commence at 10 drops per minute (20 mg/hour). Increase by doubling the dose every 30 minutes until the blood pressure is controlled. Maximum dose is 160 mg/hour or 80 drops per minute.

Alternatives for control of refractory blood pressure (only to be used in conjunction with specialist advice)

Diazoxide

▪ Its role is in the management of acute hypertension when small intravenous boluses (50 mg) or infusions enable the controlled reduction of blood pressure.

▪ It acts directly upon smooth muscle to decrease peripheral resistance.

▪ Generally, 300 mg in a 20 mL solution is required.

▪ The maximum dose is 4 ampoules of 300 mg in 24 hours.

Sodium nitroprusside

▪ A potent and direct dilator of both arterial and venous circulation. It improves maternal haemodynamics when cardiac failure and hyper-tension coexist.

▪ Dose: 0.3–1.0 microgram/kg body weight per minute. As soon as a response is obtained, the dose should be titrated to individual requirements at between 0.5 and 1.0 microgram/kg/minute (average 3 microgram/kg/min). Usually 200 microgram/minute (range 20–400 microgram/minute) is sufficient to maintain the blood pressure at a level 20–30 per cent lower than the pre-treatment diastolic blood pressure.

Glyceryl trinitrate (GTN)

- An alternative to sodium nitroprusside.
- Use a syringe pump with 50 mg diluted in 5 per cent dextrose to give 1 mL/hour set on the pump, equivalent to 0.25 microgram/kg/min. This solution can be made up with the help of a normogram (Fig. 4.1.2). This relates the concentration to be prepared in the syringe to the patient's body weight.

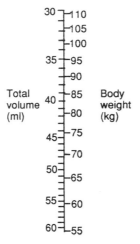

Fig. 4.1.2 A normogram for the correct solution and dosage of glyceryl trinitrate. (By G.W. Burton (1986). Reproduced from Thomas, T.A. (1989) Resuscitation of the obstetric patient. In *Cardiopulmonary Resuscitation*, (Ed. by P.J.F. Baskett), p. 293. Elsevier Science Publishers BV, Amsterdam.

Angiotension converting enzyme inhibitors (e.g. Captopril)

- These drugs are potent anti-hypertensive agents which inhibit the conversion of angiotensin I to angiotensin II, thereby reducing the concentration of this vasoconstricting peptide.
- Their use has been associated with a high incidence of intrauterine

death in pregnant animals and oligohydramnios, fetal anuria, and stillbirth when used in humans late in pregnancy.

▪ Therefore they should not be used in young women wishing to become pregnant, and if they are being taken when the woman becomes pregnant an appropriate alternative should be given.

MANAGEMENT OF ECLAMPSIA

It is of no proven benefit to use an anticonvulsant prophylactically, i.e. in the patient who has not had an eclamptic seizure. Clinical signs of hyper-reflexia and clonus are unreliable and therefore anticonvulsants are not indicated to treat these signs.

If a convulsion has occurred magnesium sulphate rather than diazepam or phenytoin is the treatment of choice for control of eclampsia. In the eclampsia trial group collaborative study it has been shown that women allocated magnesium sulphate had a 52 per cent lower risk of recurrent convulsions than those allocated diazepam and a 67 per cent lower risk than those allocated phenytoin. In addition women given magnesium sulphate are less likely to need ventilation, to develop pneumonia or to need intensive care support.

Magnesium sulphate

Mechanism of action

Magnesium sulphate reverses the excessive cerebral vasoconstriction that occurs in pre-eclampsia and for many is the drug of choice for eclampsia. It can be given intramuscularly or intravenously.

Regimen

▪ Give 4 g (8 mL of 50 per cent magnesium sulphate solution diluted with 12 mL sterile water) intravenously to stop the convulsions.

This should produce a peak maternal plasma concentration of 5–9 mg/dL. Levels will fall to about 3–4 mg/dL within 60 minutes. Within 90 minutes about 50 per cent of the infused magnesium moves into bone and other cells. By four hours 50 per cent of the infused dose is excreted into the urine.

▪ Follow this by 10 g of magnesium sulphate intramuscularly (10 mL of 50 per cent magnesium sulphate solution into each buttock) to prevent recurrence of convulsions.

▪ If convulsions recur give a further 2 g of magnesium sulphate intravenously over 3 min.

▪ A further 5 g of magnesium sulphate should be given intramuscularly every 4 hours for the first 24 hours after delivery provided that on assessment by the medical staff the respiratory rate is >16/minute, the urine output is >25 mL/hour and knee jerks are present.

Alternative regimen
▪ A continuous intravenous maintenance dose of 2 g/hour results in therapeutic plasma magnesium levels of 4–8 mg/dL.

The therapeutic to toxicity ratio is low (Table 4.1.8). Magnesium sulphate has been associated with cardiorespiratory arrest and, if given intravenously, with neonatal hypermagnesaemia.

Antidote: calcium gluconate – 1 g intravenously.

Phenytoin

▪ Phenytoin has been used for the control of seizures in the pregnant woman with variable results.
▪ **Give as a loading dose of 18 mg per kg pregnant weight** intravenously. Phenytoin should be given slowly because of the risk of cardiovascular collapse or central nervous system depression. Give half the dose over 20 minutes and the remainder over 40 minutes. **Electrocardiogram monitoring is necessary**.
▪ Oral phenytoin 200 mg is given after 12 hours and continued until 48 hours after delivery.
▪ The intravenous preparation is very alkaline and irritant to the veins, but should not be diluted to avoid precipitation.
▪ Check phenytoin levels two hours after commencing the infusion. The therapeutic level is 40–80 micromol/L. Give an additional intravenous bolus dose as indicated below:

Serum phenytoin level	Additional i.v. dose
20–30 micromol/L	300 mg
30–40 micromol/L	200 mg

▪ A trough level should be taken 24 hours after commencing phenytoin. Then commence oral phenytoin and measure trough levels daily as follows:

Serum phenytoin level	Maintenance dose
<40 micromol/L	250 mg 8 hourly
40–70 micromol/L	200 mg 8 hourly
>70 micromol/L	200 mg 12 hourly

Chlormethiazole
This is now the least popular anticonvulsant for eclampsia. It is given

Table 4.1.8 Magnesium toxicity.

Signs	Plastma level of magnesium (mg/dL)
Loss of patella reflexes, nausea, feeling of warmth, flushing, somnolence, double vision, slurred speech and weakness	9–12
Muscular paralysis and respiratory arrest	15–17
Cardiac arrest	30–35

as an 0.8 per cent solution with a loading dose of 40–100 mL to stop convulsions and then 60 mL per hour to keep the patient drowsy but rousable. Neonatal depression is likely if the total dose exceeds 12 g.

OBSTETRIC MANAGEMENT

When should a woman with pre-eclampsia be delivered?

- Symptomatic pre-eclampsia, regardless of gestation, requires delivery as soon as the mother's condition is stable.
- Women with proteinuric pre-eclampsia should not be undelivered beyond 36 weeks.
- It may also be indicated to deliver women with non-proteinuric pre-eclampsia at 38–40 weeks, but avoid inducing all women with hypertension indiscriminately before term.
- Difficult management decisions occur with stage 2 pre-eclampsia between 26 and 34 weeks.

Absolute indications for delivery

- Pre-eclampsia becomes symptomatic (stage 3).
- The fetus is compromised (e.g. diminished growth, abnormal biophysical profile and absent end-diastolic flow on Doppler ultrasound, short term fetal heart rate variability <3 ms).
- The maternal blood pressure cannot be controlled with the mother on maximal antihypertensive therapy.
- The platelet count is less than 50×10^9/L.
- Plasma creatinine has risen from normal levels to more than 120 micromols/L.
- There is evidence of liver damage.

Intrapartum care

During delivery avoid giving oxytocin with large doses of 5 per cent dextrose and water because of the risk of hyponatraemia and convulsions. In the third stage of labour, avoid giving ergometrine because it may precipitate a hypertensive crisis. Use syntocinon 5 units intravenously instead.

Postpartum care – intravenous fluid replacement

- **Fluid replacement should be no more than 1 mL/kg per hour**
- **Urine output should be at least 0.5 mL/kg/hour**.
- Pre-eclamptic patients are at considerable risk of adult respiratory distress, because pre-eclampsia is a 'leaking capillary syndrome'. It is essential in these patients to **avoid iatrogenic fluid overload**, which can happen easily because they have a decreased intravascular volume.
- If oliguria occurs assess the aetiology. A reduction in urine output is to be expected post-operatively and after the arterial pressure has been effectively reduced by antihypertensive drugs. Exclude pre-renal failure associated with blood loss at delivery and renal failure associated with DIC.
- Assess whether there is pre-renal failure by giving a safe fluid challenge of up to five 100 mL aliquots of Hartmann's solution over 2 hours. It should only be repeated after careful assessment of the patient's overall fluid status (i.e. addition of input, losses and output over a time period). Acute renal failure is diagnosed if the urine output is less than 30 mL/hour (0.5 mL/kg/hour) which persists for 8 hours or more.
- Insert a CVP line if oliguria is uncorrected by a fluid challenge or if there has been extensive blood loss at delivery. **Maintain at 4 cm H_2O**. It should not be greater than **10 cm H_2O**. If an oliguric woman does not respond to volume replacement acute tubular necrosis may have already occurred.
- Women with severe pre-eclampsia are best cared for post-delivery in a high dependency unit and sometimes an intensive care unit.
- A woman who has had severe pre-eclampsia should be assessed at hospital 6 weeks post-delivery. Blood pressure and renal status should be examined. A renal ultrasound/intravenous urogram should be done where there is persisting renal impairment with or without protei-

nuria. Occasionally a renal biopsy is required on advice from a nephrologist.

PREVENTION OF PRE-ECLAMPSIA

What is the role of low dose aspirin?

The results of the CLASP (collaborative low dose aspirin) randomised trial suggest that low dose aspirin 60–80 mg per day does not alter the severity of pre-eclampsia or the incidence of growth retardation.

DIFFERENTIAL DIAGNOSIS OF HYPERTENSION

- Essential hypertension – a diagnosis of exclusion.
- Underlying renal disease.
- Renal artery stenosis.
- Coarctation of the aorta.
- Cushing's syndrome.
- Conn's syndrome – primary aldosteronism diagnosed by hypokalaemic alkalosis and hypertension.

PHAEOCHROMOCYTOMA

Phaeochromocytoma is rare, but is associated with fetal and maternal mortality in up to 20 per cent of cases. It is often difficult to diagnose because the symptoms and signs may be attributed to other causes (see Table 4.1.9).

Pregnant women with severe, intermittent or atypical hypertensive problems should be investigated. Women at high risk are those with neurofibromatosis and multiple endocrine neoplasia (MEN type 2).

Table 4.1.9 Symptoms and signs of a phaechromocytoma.

Paroxysmal headaches, palpitations, and increased perspiration
Arrhythmias, postural hypotension
Severe or intermittent hypertension, hypertension associated with paroxysmal symptoms, hypertension in the first half of pregnancy, hypertension and abnormal glucose tolerance or diabetes mellitus
Chest or abdominal pain
Cardiovascular collapse
Hyperglycaemia

Investigations and diagnosis

- A 24 hour urine specimen is collected into an acid bottle for analysis of catecholamines.
- Levels of free catecholamines should be:
  Noradrenaline   <556 nanomol/24 hours
  Adrenaline   <136 nanomol/24 hours.
- The creatinine level should be checked on the 24 hour specimen to check for completeness and should be about 10 mmol/L.
- If the first test is negative but clinical suspicion persists, three 24 hour specimens are required before the diagnosis can be excluded with certainty.
- There are no dietary restrictions required on the basis of assay interference. **Notify the laboratory if the woman is on any drugs that may interfere with the assay, e.g. methyldopa**.
- A definitive diagnosis is made by CT scan.

Management of unstable hypertension

- **Phenoxybenzamine**, an irreversible alpha-adrenoreceptor antagonist, protects against the effects of the sudden release into the circulation of large amounts of catecholamine from the tumour.
- Dose: 10 mg twice daily increasing by 10–20 mg up to 20 mg four times daily until hypertension is controlled.
- New specific alpha$_1$ (but not alpha$_2$) antagonists (derived from prasozin) such as Doxazosin, Terazosin and Trimazosin, can be used. They are long-lasting but do not produce irreversible block.
  Once a day dosage with Doxazosin 2 mg nocte produces sufficient alpha blockade.
- Labetalol may also be used, particularly for an adrenaline secreting tumour.
- **Beta-blockade should not be used without prior alpha blockade as unopposed alpha-adrenergic activity may lead to generalised vasoconstriction and a steep rise in blood pressure**.

Surgical excision

- This is ideally done before 23 weeks gestation.
- After 24 weeks gestation uterine size makes abdominal exploration and access to the tumour difficult unless the woman is delivered.

Optimal results are obtained if surgery is delayed until the fetus is mature. Elective caesarean section is required and should be performed under adrenergic blockade, followed by surgical exploration and removal of the tumour.

• Because of the possibility of incomplete removal of tumour, recurrences and metastases (which may not develop for many years), follow up with measurements of urinary catecholamines is essential. Malignancy occurs in 10 per cent and is more common when the tumour site is extra-adrenal.

CARDIAC DISEASE IN PREGNANCY

Cardiac disease may be present before or diagnosed *de novo* in the pregnancy on the basis of signs and symptoms (see Table 4.1.10). It is the third leading cause of maternal mortality in the UK with 21 deaths between 1988 and 1990 (DHSS, 1994).

The incidence of heart disease in pregnancy is about 1 per cent.

The maternal heart in pregnancy

• Between about eight and thirty weeks' gestation changes occur in the maternal blood volume and circulation that increase the cardiac workload (output) by about 30–50 per cent. This persists throughout the rest of the pregnancy.

• Cardiac output increases from 3.5 to 6 L/min in early pregnancy. Heart rate increases by 10 per cent in pregnancy.

• Among the physiological changes observed are warm extremities, a large pulse volume, tachycardia and slightly elevated jugular venous pressure.

• The cardiac apex is slightly displaced due to slight cardiomegaly and elevation of the diaphragm by the enlarging uterus. Normal flow murmurs may be produced, i.e. a pulmonary systolic murmur and third heart sound.

Important points about cardiac disease in pregnancy

• A cardiac physician should be consulted early in the pregnancy.

• Women with cardiac disease are at greatest risk of decompensation in the mid-trimester, during labour and in the immediate postpartum period.

Table 4.1.10 The history, signs and symptoms of heart disease in pregnancy.

History

Breathlessness on slight effort or at rest (orthopnoea)

Syncope – due to severe aortic stenosis or sub-aortic stenosis
  Hypertrophic cardiac myopathy
  Fallot's tetralogy or Eisenmenger syndrome
  Dysrhythmias

Chest pain – the commonest cause in pregnancy is gastro-oesophageal reflux; myocardial ischaemia is rare in pregnancy; chest pain may occur with severe aortic stenosis or HOCM

The hyperdynamic circulation of pregnancy causes alterations in the cardiovascular system which may mimic heart disease

Types of murmur and heart disease

Mid diastolic – mitral stenosis

Pan systolic – ventricular septal defect, mitral regurgitation or tricuspid regurgitation

Late systolic – mitral regurgitation, mitral valve prolapse or hypertrophic cardiomyopathy

Ejection systolic murmur
  Louder than grade 3 out of 6 – aortic stenosis
  Varies with respiration – pulmonary stenosis
  Associated with other abnormalities, e.g. ejection clicks – valvular, pulmonary and aortic stenosis

Signs of heart failure

Pulmonary oedema

Cyanosis

(Finger clubbing if chronic)

Pulse deficit

Signs of endocarditis – splinter haemorrhages

- Women with valvular stenosis are less likely to tolerate the cardiovascular changes of pregnancy than women with incompetent valves.

- Women with prosthetic heart valves require full anticoagulation throughout pregnancy.

- Iron should be given to prevent anaemia developing during the pregnancy.

Rheumatic disease

Mitral stenosis

Mitral stenosis is the most important rheumatic disease. It is detected by the characteristic mid-diastolic murmur. The severity of the symptoms are related to the degree of stenosis.

Symptoms of mitral stenosis are: dyspnoea on effort and orthopnoea in severe cases, chest pain (like that of angina), palpitations or atrial fibrillation and fatigue. Electrocardiogram (ECG) changes with mitral stenosis are: P mitrale, right ventricular hypertrophy and right axis deviation.

Congenital heart disease

The majority of symptomatic congenital cardiac lesions have been corrected surgically by the time pregnancy occurs. Those with persistent pulmonary hypertension are the most dangerous, but small septal defects or a persistent ductus arteriosus are well tolerated. Hypertrophic obstruction cardiomyopathy (HOCM) may also give cause for concern in pregnancy.

Risks to the mother from heart disease in pregnancy

- Maternal mortality is more likely where pulmonary blood flow cannot be increased due to obstruction within the pulmonary blood vessels or at the mitral valve.
- This occurs in Eisenmenger syndrome (maternal mortality 30–50 per cent) and primary pulmonary hypertension (maternal mortality 40–50 per cent).
- Well managed pregnancy is not detrimental to the long term health of the woman with heart disease (if she survives pregnancy itself).
- The incidence of congenital heart disease in the babies of mothers with congenital heart disease is between 3 and 14 per cent.

Investigations for heart disease

Chest X-ray

Women with normal hearts in pregnancy show slight cardiomegaly, increased pulmonary vascular markings and distension of the pulmonary veins.

Electrocardiography

In pregnancy T wave inversion of lead 3, ST segment changes and Q waves which would be considered pathological normally occur frequently. The ECG diagnoses dysrhythmias.

Echocardiography

This has no radiation hazard.

Indications for cardiac surgery in pregnancy

Failure of medical treatment with a surgically correctable lesion in the presence of intractable heart failure or debilitating symptoms.

4

Antenatal care

The priorities are to prevent anaemia, infections (particularly respiratory) and heart failure. Care is ideally provided jointly by cardiologist and obstetrician.

Antibiotic prophylaxis for heart disease in labour is given in Table 4.1.11.

Table 4.1.11 Antibiotic prophylaxis to avoid endocarditis in labour.

Prior to anaesthesia give:
  Amoxycillin 1 g
  and Gentamicin 120 mg

6 hours after delivery give:
  Amoxycillin 500 mg 6 hourly
  and Gentamicin 80 mg 12 hourly

For those who are penicillin sensitive give:
  Vancomycin 1 gm one i.v. injection or
  Vancomycin 500 mg × 2 injections 12 hourly given over 60 minutes each because
    of the risk of idiosyncratic hypotensive reactions

Treatment of heart failure (see Table 4.1.12)

This is a medical emergency and its resolution takes priority. The main elements are:

- Oxygen by face mask.
- Digoxin controls the heart rate in atrial fibrillation, supraventricular tachycardias and acutely in heart failure. Digoxin and

Digitoxin cross the placenta, producing similar drug levels in the fetus within five minutes of intravenous administration.

- The loading oral dose is 7.5 mg to 10 mg.
- Most patients will be maintained on 0.125–0.75 mg digoxin daily. In those with increased sensitivity to the adverse effects of digoxin, a dose of 0.625 mg daily or less may be enough.
- Monitor digoxin levels by taking blood 6 hours after the last dose.
- Therapeutic levels in serum are 0.8 nanogram/mL (1.0 nanomol/L) to 2.0 nanogram/mL (2.56 nanomol/L). Levels above 3.0 nanogram/mL (3.74 nanomol/L) are toxic.
- Digoxin is secreted in breast milk but therapeutic maternal blood levels are unlikely to cause harm to the neonate. Hypokalaemia is a possible consequence so monitor neonatal potassium levels.

Table 4.1.12 Risk factors for heart failure.

Anaemia
Arrhythmias
Hypertension
Hyperthyroidism
Infections, particularly urinary tract infection.
Multiple pregnancy

Diuretics

Frusemide

Frusemide is a loop diuretic used to treat pulmonary oedema. The dose is 20 to 50 mg given by slow intravenous injection (the rate should not exceed 4 mg/minute).

Thiazide

An oral thiazide may also be used in mild to moderate heart failure. It can cause hypokalaemia.

Other measures

Treat pulmonary oedema with opiates such as morphine to reduce anxiety and to decrease venous return by causing venodilatation. Also use aminophylline if there is associated bronchospasm.

Life threatening pulmonary oedema which does not respond to drug therapy may be helped by mechanical ventilation and in other nonresponsive cases cardiac surgery should be considered if the lesion is operable.

Dysrhythmias

The mainstays of treatment are digoxin, quinidine and beta-adrenergic blocking agents (e.g. propanolol or oxprenolol) used only after consultation with a cardiologist. Newer drugs such as verapamil, diltiazem or amiodarone can be used if necessary. Fetal supraventricular tachycardia can be treated *in utero* with amiodarone or verapamil.

Pregnancy in women with artificial heart valves

The major problem is anticoagulation. There are two possible regimens, neither of which is ideal.
▪ Regimen 1 Give oral Warfarin to 37 weeks, then admit and transfer to continuous intravenous heparin to produce heparin levels of 0.4 to 0.6 units/mL.
▪ Regimen 2 Use a high dose continuous subcutaneous infusion of heparin to achieve heparin levels as above.

If pre-term labour supervenes while the woman is taking Warfarin she should be given fresh frozen plasma (FFP) 10 to 15 mL/kg (usually 3 packs) intravenously. The risk of viral transmission is extremely low in the UK. Prothombin complex is an expensive alternative which is virus free. FFP works quickly compared to Vitamin K which takes several hours. Heparin therapy should also be commenced.

Warfarin can be used after delivery. It is not excreted in significant quantities in breast milk.

Myocardial ischaemia

This is a rare complication of pregnancy.
▪ Severe central retrosternal pain may indicate cardiac ischaemia, especially if associated with exercise. It may radiate to the arms or neck and cause nausea.
▪ A strong family history of myocardial infarction at a young age or a known hyperlipidaemia would give strong grounds for suspicion of an ischaemic cause for such pain.
▪ An ECG must be carried out and may show ST segment depression and symmetrical T wave inversion.

Management of women with heart disease during labour

The principles are:

- Monitor fluid balance strictly and do not overload with intravenous (particularly crystalloid) fluids.
- Nurse propped up to avoid supine hypotension due to venocaval compression from the gravid uterus.
- All emergency drugs must be available for immediate treatment of heart failure, including oxygen, digoxin, frusemide and aminophylline.
- Epidural analgesia must be used with extreme care but is definitely contraindicated if:

  there is a major obstruction to the outflow tract;
  the woman is on anticoagulants;
  Eisenmenger syndrome or HOCM are present.

- Assisted delivery (preferably by vacuum extractor) may be necessary if the woman has impaired exercise tolerance.
- Avoid ergometrine for the management of the third stage to prevent a sudden increase in venous return to an already strained heart. Therefore give syntocinon only to prevent post-partum haemorrhage (PPH).

Puerperial cardiomyopathy

This is a congestive cardiomyopathy of unknown aetiology which may develop late in pregnancy or typically in the puerperium.

The symptoms are fatigue, dyspnoea and oedema with signs such as peripheral cyanosis, small pulse volume, low blood pressure with small pulse pressure, raised jugular venous pressure, gallop rhythm, functional mitral and/or tricuspid regurgitation and pleural effusions.

ECG changes include a sinus tachycardia and non-specific T wave changes.

One third of women recover permanently; for the remainder, there may be progression and recurrence in subsequent pregnancies.

BIBLIOGRAPHY

Belfort, M.A. & Moise, K.J.J. (1992) Effect of magnesium sulfate on maternal brain blood flow in preeclampsia: a randomized, placebo-controlled study. *American Journal of Obstetrics & Gynecology*, **99**, 554–556.

De Swiet, M. (1989) Heart Disease in Pregnancy. In *Medical Disorders in Obstetric Practice* 2nd ed., (Ed by M. De Swiet) pp 198–248. Blackwell Science Ltd, Oxford.

Department of Health and Social Security (1994) Hibbard, B.M., Anderson, M.A., Drife, J.O., Tighe, J.R., Sykes, K., Gordon, G., Pinkerton, J.H.M., Miner, D., Botting, B. *Report on Confidential Enquiry into Maternal Death in the UK 1988–1990*. HMSO, London.

Dommisse, J. (1989) Phenytoin sodium and magnesium sulphate in the management of eclampsia. *British Journal of Obstetrics & Gynaecology*, **97**, 104–109.

Chua, S. & Redman, C.W.G. (1991) Are prophylactic anticonvulsants required in severe pre-eclampsia? *The Lancet*, **337**, 250–251.

Cockburn, J., Moar, V.A., Ounsted, M. & Redman, C.W.G. (1982) Final report of the study on hypertension during pregnancy: the effects of specific treatment on the growth and development of the children. *The Lancet*, **i**, 647–649.

Hampton, J. (1986) *The ECG Made Easy*. Churchill Livingstone, Edinburgh.

Hutton, J.D. James, D.K. Stirrat, G.M., Douglas, K.A. & Redman, C.W.G. (1992) Management of severe pre-eclampsia and eclampsia by U.K. consultants. *British Journal of Obstetrics & Gynaecology*, **99**, 554–556.

Kumar, P.J. & Clark, M.L. (1990) *Clinical Medicine*. Balliere Tindall, London.

Macdonald, R. (1991) Editorial: Aspirin and extradural blocks. *British Journal of Anaesthesia*, **66**, 1–3.

Martin, J.N. (1991) The natural history of HELLP syndrome: patterns of disease progression and regression. *American Journal of Obstetrics & Gynecology*, **164**, 1500–1513.

Redman, C.W.G. (1976) Fetal outcome in trial of antihypertensive treatment in pregnancy. *The Lancet*, **2**, 753–756.

Redman, C.W.G. (1989) Hypertension in pregnancy. In *Obstetrics* (Ed. by A.C. Turnbull & G. Chamberlain), pp 515–541. Churchill Livingstone, London.

Redman, C.W.G., Beilin, L.J. & Bonnar, J. (1977) Treatment of hypertension in pregnancy with methyldopa: blood pressure control and side effects. *British Journal of Obstetrics & Gynaecology*, **84**, 419–426.

Rosevear, S.K. & Liggins, G. (1986) Platelet dimensions in pregnancy-induced hypertension. *New Zealand Medical Journal*, **99**, 356–357.

Ryan, G., Lange, I.R. & Naugler, M.A. (1989) Clinical experience with phenytoin prophylaxis in severe preeclampsia. *American Journal of Obstetrics & Gynecology*, **161**, 297–304.

Swanton, R.H. (1984) *Cardiology*. Blackwell Scientific Publications, Oxford.

Thomas, T.A. (1989) Resuscitation of the obstetric patient, In *Cardio-pulmonary Resuscitation* (Ed. by J.F. Baskett) pp 275–294. Elsevier Science Publishers BV, Amsterdam.

Weinstein, L. (1982) Syndrome of haemolysis, elevated liver enzymes and low platelet count: a severe consequence of hypertension in pregnancy. *American Journal of Obstetrics & Gynecology*, **142**, 159–167.

4

4.2   Systemic lupus erythematosus

Systemic lupus erythematosus (SLE) is a multisystem autoimmune disease. Table 4.2.1 gives the clinical features of the syndrome as devised in 1982 by the American Rheumatism Association. SLE is diagnosed if an individual has four out of the eleven criteria present either serially or simultaneously during an interval of observation. In addition, the presence of antiphospholipid antibodies – anticardiolipin and lupus anticoagulant – without the full clinical syndrome of SLE identify a group of women at high risk of adverse pregnancy outcome.

Table 4.2.1 Clinical features of SLE to aid diagnosis of the syndrome. (Source Tann *et al.* (1982).)

Facial butterfly rash
Discoid rash
Photosensitivity
Oral or nasopharyngeal ulceration
Nonerosive arthritis involving two or more peripheral joints
Pleurisy or pericarditis
Psychosis or seizures

Proteinuria >0.5 g/day (or 3+) or cellular casts
One of the following haematological disorders:
   Haemolytic anaemia, with reticulocytosis
   Leukopenia WBC <4000/mm^3 on two or more occasions
   Lymphopenia <1500/mm^3 on two or more occasions
   Thrombocytopenia <100 000/mm^3

Immunological disorder
   (1) Positive LE cells
   (2) Antibody to native DNA in abnormal titre
   (3) Antibody to smooth muscle nuclear antigen
   (4) Chronic false positive syphilis serology for 6 months
Antinuclear antibody in abnormal titre

CLINICAL IMPLICATIONS OF SLE

SLE is an important condition in pregnancy because of the association with a whole series of complications, of which the most significant are:

- Pre-eclampsia
- Recurrent miscarriage
- Fetal loss
- Thrombosis
- Thrombocytopenia
- Fetal growth retardation
- Placental abruption
- Congenital heart block.

It may also cause a Coombs' positive haemolytic anaemia, livido reticularis, pulmonary hypertension, transverse myelitis and valvular heart disease.

Venous thrombosis is the most commonly reported complication. Clotting occurs in medium or larger vessels resulting in, for example, pulmonary emboli, hepatic infarction, hepatic or portal vein thrombosis, mesenteric infarction, or acute adrenal insufficiency.

Cerebral thrombosis may be venous (venous sinus, retinal vein), arterial (cerebral infarction), or embolic (secondary to endocarditis).

SLE is a cause of heart block in the fetus associated with anti-Ro antibodies.

Lupus anticoagulant or inhibitor

Lupus anticoagulant (LA) is an immunoglobulin which prolongs one or more of the *in vitro* phospholipid-dependent tests of coagulation. It is an inhibitor of the coagulation pathway which paradoxically results in an increased risk of arterial and venous thromboembolism.

The presence of LA is associated with several manifestations of SLE but many patients with LA do not have SLE and it can therefore complicate pregnancy in the absence of overt disease.

Tests for lupus anticoagulant
- Activated partial thromboplastin time (APPT)
- Kaolin clotting time (KCT)
- Dilute Russell viper venom time (dRVVT)
- Tissue thromboplastin time (TTT)

The APTT test is the most generally available, but its sensitivity for lupus anticoagulant depends on the phospholipid content of the reagent which varies widely. The physiological increase in factor VIII levels during pregnancy tend to shorten the APTT and may mask a positive LA test.

The KCT is a sensitive and specific test for lupus anticoagulant and may be used to monitor the response to corticosteriods. Residual platelet contamination may produce false-negative results in all tests for lupus anticoagulant. To avoid this, plasma samples should be separated immediately and centrifuged.

The dRVVT is a sensitive test and is not altered by pregnancy-induced changes in coagulation factors.

Confirmatory tests demonstrate prolonged coagulation times that are not due to a coagulation factor deficiency and that the inhibitor is directed to lipid antigens. Factor deficiencies are usually excluded by the addition of fresh frozen plasma (FFP) to the abnormal plasma samples. If the prolonged clotting time is corrected completely a circulating anticoagulant has not been demonstrated.

Anticardiolipin assay

- Anticardiolipin is an antiphospholipid antibody closely related to lupus anticoagulant
- Results are measured in immunoglobulin G (IgG) or immunoglobulin M (IgM) antiphospholipid antibody units (GPL or MPL units). An abnormal IgM anticardiolipin is >5 MPL units and an abnormal IgG anticardiolipin is >5 GPL units.

>80 GPL/MPL is a high positive, 20–80 GPL/MPL medium positive and 5–19 GPL/MPL low positive.

- The higher the titre of anticardiolipin antibody, the greater the risk of thrombosis, thrombocytopenia and fetal loss.

Antiphospholipids with or without clinically apparent SLE

The prevalence of these antibodies in a low risk obstetric population is given in Table 4.2.2.

Table 4.2.2 Prevalence of antiphospholipid antibodies in a low risk population of pregnant women. (Source Pattison *et al.*, (1993).)

	Incidence (per cent)
Antiphospholipid antibodies	2–4
Anticardiolipin antibodies	1
Lupus anticoagulant	1.2
Antinuclear antibodies	3.2

Antiphospholipid (APL) antibody and lupus anticoagulant are present in almost 50 and 30 per cent, respectively, of patients with SLE.

The antibodies do not have the same clinical significance, though both are associated with recurrent fetal loss and/or thrombotic episodes.

Pregnancy outcome associated with abnormal serology

Up to 90 per cent of women with lupus anticoagulant have one or more fetal losses.

The presence of APL antibodies is associated with adverse pregnancy outcome (perinatal morbidity and mortality up to eight times normal, increased incidence of pre-eclampsia, growth retardation and fetal distress) in 50 percent of women.

High titre anticardiolipin antibodies are associated with poor pregnancy outcome (e.g. up to five times the mean are associated with fetal loss).

The poor prognosis is compounded if there is renal involvement. A creatinine clearance of less than 65 mL/minute/m^3 or proteinuria >2.4 g in 24 hours is ominous. A serum creatinine of >132 micromol/L is associated with a 50 per cent fetal loss rate.

Treatment of women with SLE or positive serum antiphospholipid antibodies

Optimal treatment is empirical and disputed. Laboratory tests do not completely predict pregnancy outcome. Among the treatment options are corticosteroids (usually high doses), azathiaprine, plasma exchange or infusions of immunoglobulin.

▪ Aim to keep the KCT under 250 s. Lupus antibodies often become negative but suppression of anticardiolipin antibodies is more difficult.

REGIMEN FOR TREATMENT OF ANTIPHOSPHOLIPID SYNDROME

This is shown in Fig. 4.2.1.

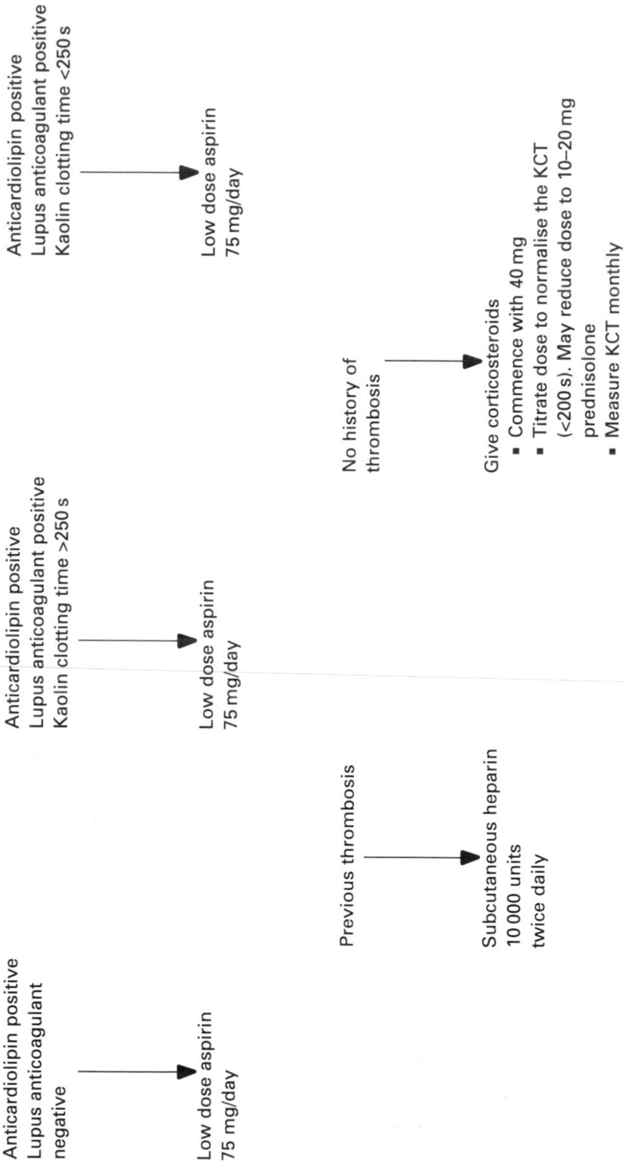

Anticardiolipin positive
Lupus anticoagulant negative
Low dose aspirin 75 mg/day
Anticardiolipin positive
Lupus anticoagulant positive
Kaolin clotting time >250 s
Low dose aspirin 75 mg/day
Previous thrombosis
Subcutaneous heparin 10 000 units twice daily
No history of thrombosis
Give corticosteroids
Commence with 40 mg
Titrate dose to normalise the KCT (<200 s). May reduce dose to 10–20 mg prednisolone
Measure KCT monthly
Anticardiolipin positive
Lupus anticoagulant positive
Kaolin clotting time <250 s
Low dose aspirin 75 mg/day

Fig. 4.2.1 Treatment for women with antiphospholipid antibodies with a history of pregnancy loss.

Indications for steroid treatment

Use steroids only if there is a clinical history of an adverse obstetric outcome. Definitive knowledge of mechanism and success rate for aspirin + prednisolone treatment is lacking.

Risks of corticosteroid treatment

- Iatrogenic Cushing's syndrome
- Severe acne
- Increased gestational diabetes mellitus
- Vertebral osteopenia
- Isolated reports of posterior capsular cataract, and increased risk of listeriosis, pneumonia, miliary tuberculosis.

Lupus anticoagulant may be suppressed by intravenous immunoglobulin (IVIg). It has only been used where steroid and aspirin therapy has been unsuccessful and has not been subject to randomised controlled trials. IVIg probably does not inhibit APL antibody production, but may block Fc or alter antibody receptor binding. It is also very expensive.

It may be given as Sandoglobulin by i.v. infusion every 3–6 weeks from 12 weeks of pregnancy in patients with a bad obstetric history and where there is persistent lupus anticoagulant activity despite low-dose aspirin and maximal steroid therapy.

A history of arterial or venous thromboembolism indicates the need for subcutaneous heparin throughout pregnancy for prophylaxis (see Section 4.9) in addition to aspirin and corticosteroid treatment, if indicated.

Overall treatment in women with a history of adverse outcome should result in a livebirth rate for all forms of treatment of at least 66 per cent.

FETAL CONGENITAL HEART BLOCK

Anti Ro antibodies

An IgG autoantibody to soluble ribonucleoprotein is found in about 24 per cent of SLE patients. Sixty per cent of women who deliver a baby with congenital heart block have anti-R_o antibodies.

The IgG is deposited in the fetal heart, initiating immune inflammatory responses leading to fibrosis and calcification of the atrioventricular node and bundle of His, endocardial fibroelastosis, cardiomyopathy and multiple structural abnormalities. The critical damage occurs during cardiac organogenesis at 6 weeks of pregnancy.

Monitoring the fetus and timing of delivery

Congenital heart block can be diagnosed before delivery from routine auscultation of the fetal heart and subsequent cardiotocography when bradycardia is observed. Detailed ultrasound examination of the fetal heart reveals atrioventricular dissociation confirming complete heart block and any structural heart disease, present in 15–20 per cent of cases.

4

THROMBOCYTOPENIA IN PREGNANCY

The causes of low platelets in pregnancy are:

1 Pregnancy associated thrombocytopenia (platelet count 100–150×10^9/L)

2 Autoimmune (idiopathic) thrombocytopenia (ITP)

3 Alloimmune thrombocytopenia (ATP) causing neonatal autoimmune thrombocytopenia (NAIT)

Platelet physiology

- Platelets have a life span of 7–10 days and are anuclear cells derived from megakaryocytes.
- Clinical effects do not appear until the platelet count falls below 50×10^9/L.
- Increased platelet turnover may be recognised by examining the numbers of large platelets (greater than 9 femtolitre).

Pregnancy associated thrombocytopenia

This is thought to be due to increased sequestration of platelets in pregnancy. Pregnancy-associated thrombocytopaenia occurs in about 8 per cent of the population with no significant maternal/fetal morbidity. The maternal platelet count is less than the usual lower limit of normal (150×10^9/L). An isolated finding of levels down to 100×10^9/L is acceptable and does not require intervention.

Any other cause of low platelets such as SLE, pre-eclampsia or drug reactions due to, e.g. ampicillin, aspirin, carbamazapine, heparin, methyldopa, nitrofurantoin, phenytoin or sodium valproate, should be excluded.

Essential differences between ITP and ATP

ITP can be a serious maternal disorder but very little threat to the fetus other than depressed platelet counts at birth. The risk to the mother is serious obstetric **haemorrhage**, especially with very low platelet counts.

ATP causes **neonatal autoimmune thrombocytopenia (NAIT)** which is a very serious fetal disease with no maternal consequences. These cases should be managed by a team skilled in intrauterine transfusion procedures.

4

AUTOIMMUNE THROMBOCYTOPENIA (ITP) (IDIOPATHIC THROMBOCYTOPENIA)

The incidence is 1/1000 pregnancies. Low maternal platelet count, generally diagnosed in the first half of pregnancy, is likely to be due to immune thrombocytopenia (ITP). IgG antibodies cross the placenta and cause transient fetal thrombocytopenia usually lasting for up to a week (though it occasionally persists for up to four months). A diagnosis of autoimmune thrombocytopenia is confirmed by the presence of antiplatelet antibodies.

Major postpartum risks include **haemorrhage** (incidence 5–26 per cent) which is correlated with the degree of thrombocytopenia. Intradural haematoma is a risk with epidural cannula. It should not occur if the platelet count is greater than $50 \times 10^9/L$ and clotting characteristics are normal. Maternal platelet count is a poor predictor of neonatal thrombocytopenia.

10–15 per cent of babies of affected mothers will have a platelet count of less than $50 \times 10^9/L$ at delivery. This has no associated significant morbidity. However, the perinatal mortality for a baby with ITP is 5 per cent. Intracranial haemorrhage occurs in less than 1 per cent of all cases, the risk being confined to the 3 per cent of severely affected babies with platelet counts of less than $50 \times 10^9/L$. Caesarean section is not necessarily protective.

Antenatal management of ITP

- If the platelet count is greater than 100×10^9/L at booking repeat at 26–28 weeks, at monthly intervals and just before anticipated delivery.
- If the platelet count falls below 100×10^9/L, then measure it weekly.
- If the platelet count is less than 50×10^9/L or if there is bleeding, check tests of coagulation: prothrombin time, activated partial thromboplastin time to exclude any additional coagulation defect. Serum platelet autoantibodies are measured either indirectly as those free in the serum (the more sensitive technique) or directly as the amount of antibody that is platelet bound (platelet associated IgG (PAIgG).

4

Treatment

For a maternal platelet count below 20×10^9/L or 50×10^9/L approaching delivery, give prednisolone 1 mg/kg/day (60–80 mg/day). This will increase the platelet count to over 50×10^9/L within three weeks in most cases. After a response occurs taper the dose to the lowest that will maintain the platelet count $>70 \times 10^9$/L.

Alternatively immunoglobulin therapy – 400 mg/kg/day intravenously – gives a rapid increase in maternal platelet count, which lasts for at least two weeks. The object of this treatment is to raise maternal platelet count, by decreasing platelet autoantibody synthesis.

Delivery

Because there is no correlation between fetal and maternal platelet counts or fetal platelet counts and maternal antibody levels, there is no evidence that caesarean section confers benefit on the fetus, to avoid the risk of intracranial haemorrhage.

Cordocentesis is not indicated for ITP.

If the maternal platelet count is less than 30×10^9/L, then cover labour and delivery with a platelet transfusion. Each unit raises the platelet count by approximately 10×10^9/L.

ALLOIMMUNE THROMBOCYTOPENIA (ATP) CAUSING NEONATAL ALLOIMMUNE THROMBOCYTOPENIA (NAIT)

This condition is like rhesus haemolytic disease, except that the fetal platelets are the target of the allo antibodies with an incidence of 1/1000 to 1/5000 pregnancies. The most important specific antigen is the PlA1 system. The diagnosis is confirmed by identifying a normal maternal platelet count in a PlA1 antigen negative mother and PlA1 positive partner. Maternal plasma also contains an antibody to paternal and fetal platelets.

One in fifty caucasian women is PlA1 negative (2 per cent). Of their partners 98 per cent will be PlA1 positive and of these only 5 per cent will be heterozygous. Despite this, most PlA1 negative women do not become sensitized. High risk factors for becoming sensitized are the HLA types of the mother – HLA-DR3, HLA-B8 and DRW52.

The major risk is of fetal intracranial haemorrhage which occurs in 15–20 per cent of affected pregnancies. Screening of all pregnancies is not available and first affected pregnancies are seldom detected unless, for example, ultrasound happens to be carried out and identifies brain damage as a result of intracranial haemorrhage. Haemorrhage causes porencephaly (hypoechogenic areas) due to fluid replacing brain tissue. This has a bad prognosis with neurological deficit in up to 25 per cent of cases and a mortality rate of about 15 per cent.

Women who have had one affected pregnancy and who are found to have anti-platelet antibodies should be referred to a specialist centre for consideration of cordocentesis. This test is associated with significant risk and must only be carried out in recognised fetal medicine centres.

Antenatal management of NAIT

- Platelet and HLA typing and testing for platelet alloantibodies should be carried out in the following situations:
  a previously affected baby;
  female relatives of women who have delivered an affected baby;
  neonatal thrombocytopenia;
  unexplained porencephaly;
  hydranencephaly.

- After a first affected pregnancy 75–90 per cent of subsequent pregnancies are as, or more severely, affected than the first.
- Not only is the risk of haemorrhage greater in these babies, but it is less likely to be related to the absolute platelet count.

Management of alloimmune thrombocytopenia

- Cordocentesis (at 22 weeks) identifies the PlA1 antigen of the fetus, determines fetal platelet level and can be a means of treatment.
- Cordocentesis may be done up to monthly if necessary.
- Immunoglobulin 1 g/kg/week may be given intravenously to the mother for the severely thrombocytopenic baby (platelet count $<50 \times 10^9$/L. This may increase the platelet count by a mean of 70×10^9/L.
- Steroid treatment is of no benefit to the fetus with alloimmune thrombocytopenia.
- Direct platelet transfusion can be given to the baby during cordocentesis to cover labour and delivery.
- Regular antenatal ultrasound examinations should be done to identify fetal intracranial haemorrhage.

Risk of late cordocentesis

- Fetal loss rate 1 per cent.
- Early morbidity (cord haematoma, fetal bradycardia necessitating delivery) 5 per cent.

Risk to the fetus

- The risk of intracranial haemorrhage is small if the platelet count is above 50×10^9/L in the fetus.
- Intracranial haemorrhage may occur antenatally from the second trimester onwards in 4 per cent or during labour in 10 per cent of cases.
- Intracranial haemorrhage may be recurrent.
- Labour is hazardous to the fetus with alloimmune thrombocytopenia (in contrast to autoimmune ITP) because of the risk of intracranial haemorrhage.
- Much of the high perinatal mortality and morbidity is associated with intracranial haemorrhage after vaginal delivery of a baby with unsuspected alloimmune thrombocytopenia.
- Delivery can either be achieved by elective caesarean section or induction of labour at term after intravascular platelet transfusion to the baby by cordocentesis.

MYASTHENIA GRAVIS

Myasthenia gravis is due to auto antibodies against acetylcholine receptors, with complement-dependent destruction of the post synaptic portion of the neuromuscular junction. Incidence in the general population is 1/20 000. The effect of pregnancy on the disease has been reported as no change in status in approximately one third of cases, with exacerbations in a further third and remission in one third. Myasthenia gravis may adversely affect the pregnancy, with an incidence of elective pre-term delivery of up to 40 per cent. The signs and symptoms are difficulty in speaking, swallowing, clearing secretions, diplopia and ptosis.

- Between ten and twenty per cent of babies of mothers with myasthenia gravis will develop transient neonatal myasthenia gravis due to the transplacental passage of anti-acetyl-cholinesterase antibodies. In utero myasthenia gravis may produce hydramnios, decreased movement and contractures.

Uterine smooth muscle is not involved and therefore labour is not affected by the condition. However, since the voluntary muscles involved in expulsion may be weakened assisted delivery may be required.

Treatment in pregnancy

- Pyridostigmine 240–1500 mg/day in divided doses given every 3–8 hours. If an increased dose is required as the pregnancy progresses decrease the medication interval before increasing the individual dosage.
- Side effects of anti-cholinesterase drugs include nausea, vomiting, diarrhoea and increased oral and bronchial secretions.
- Corticosteroids may also be of benefit.
- In labour use a parenteral route (intravenous or intramuscular) to avoid erratic absorption of the acetylcholine receptor (AChR) drug.
- Drugs to be avoided because they exacerbate or cause muscle weakness in patients with myasthenia gravis include both beta sympathomimetic and beta-blocking agents, gentamicin, tetracycline, halothane and ether, and trichloroethylene. The antibodies are transferred in breast milk.

BIBLIOGRAPHY

Birdsall, M.A. & Pattison, N.S. (1993) Antiphospholipid antibodies in pregnancy: clinical associations. *British Journal of Hospital Medicine*, **50**, 251–260.

Browning, J. & James, D. (1990) Immune thrombocytopenia in pregnancy. *Fetal Medicine Review*, **2**, 143–157.

De Sweit, M. (1989) Systemic lupus erythematosus and other connective tissue diseases. In: *Medical Disorders in Obstetric Practice*, 2nd ed., (Ed. by M. De Swiet) pp 408–425. Blackwell Scientific, Oxford.

Lockshin, M.D., Druzin, M.L. & Qamar, M.A. (1989) Prednisone does not prevent recurrent fetal death in women with antiphospholipid antibody. *American Journal of Obstetrics & Gynecology*, **160**, 439–443.

Lockwood, C.J. Romero, R., Feinberg, R.F., Clyne, L.P., Coster, B. & Hobbins, J.C. (1989) The prevalence and biological significance of lupus anticoagulant and anticardiolipin antibodies in a general obstetric population. *American Journal of Obstetrics & Gynecology*, **161**, 369–373.

Lubbe, W.F., Palmer, S.J. Butler, W.S. & Liggins, G.C. (1983) Fetal survival after prednisone suppression of maternal lupus anticoagulant. *The Lancet*, **1**, 1361–1363.

Lubbe, W.F.& Liggins, G.C. (1984) Lupus anticoagulant in pregnancy. *British Journal of Obstetrics & Gynaecology*, **91**, 357–363.

Pattison, N.S., Chamley, L.W., McKay, E.J., Liggins, G.C. & Butler, W.S. (1993) Antiphospholipid antibodies in pregnancy: prevalence and clinical association. *British Journal of Obstetrics & Gynaecology*, **100**, 909–913.

Scott, J.R., Rote, N.S. & Branch, D.W. (1987) Immunologic aspects of recurrent abortion and fetal death. *Obstetrics & Gynecology*, **70**, 645–656.

Tann, E.M., Cohen, A.S., Aries, J.F., Masi, A.T., McShane, D.J., Rothfield, N.F., Schaller, J.G., Talal, N. & Winchester, R.J. (1982) The 1982 revised criteria for the classification of systemic lupus erythematosus. *Arthritis & Rheumatism*, **25**, 1271–1277.

Triplett, D.A. (1989) Antiphospholipid antibodies and recurrent pregnancy loss. *American Journal of Reproduction & Immunology*, **20**, 52–67.

4.3   Diabetes in pregnancy

Diabetes is either insulin or non-insulin dependent. It can be present before pregnancy (established, insulin dependent diabetes) or be induced by pregnancy (gestational diabetes), which disappears after the pregnancy.

The main objectives of management of diabetes in pregnancy (either pre-existing or gestational) are to keep the blood glucose level below 7.5 mmol/L 1–2 hours after a meal and less than 5.0 mmol/L before a meal.

The aim of normoglycaemia is to prevent maternal and fetal complications. Although the definition of what are 'normal' and 'abnormal' blood glucose levels in pregnancy is not universally agreed and the evidence that perinatal morbidity and mortality are improved by treatment of gestational diabetes is not clear, the principle of treatment of raised glucose levels seems reasonable to prevent complications in babies of diabetic mothers, particularly macrosomia.

4

DIAGNOSIS OF GESTATIONAL DIABETES

The diagnosis of gestational diabetes is based on measurement of blood glucose levels (not fructosamine or glycosylated haemoglobin (HbA1$_c$), which are monitoring measurements.

The blood glucose values used here are based on venous plasma samples. Whole blood values are 10–15 per cent lower, while capillary values are 7–8 per cent higher. Check with your local laboratory what samples are used for analysis.

Screening for gestational diabetes?

Two main strategies have been proposed:
1 Opportunistic screening based on 'risk markers'.
2 Routine screening.

1 Screening based on 'risk markers'

Impaired glucose tolerance should be screened for in the following situations:
- significant glycosuria on two occasions antenatally;
- mother, father or siblings with diabetes;
- previous infant >90th centile for gestational age and sex;
- previous unexpected perinatal death;
- maternal obesity (>20 per cent over ideal weight or over 90 kg);
- polyhydramnios.

2 Routine screening

A random blood glucose greater than 6.1 mmol/L within 2 hours of eating or >5.6 mmol/L at more than 2 hours should be investigated with an oral glucose tolerance test.

These levels represent the 99th centile for the normal population, i.e. it identifies 1 per cent of normal women as being abnormal.

Glucose tolerance test

- The best time for testing is 28 weeks' gestation.
- After 12 hours of fasting a blood sample is taken.
- 75 g of glucose in 200–250 mL of water (or equivalent volume of e.g. 'Lucozade') is drunk over 5 minutes.
- A further blood sample is taken after 2 hours.
- The 95th centile for blood glucose in the third trimester of pregnancy is **5.2 mmol/L fasting and 9.0 mmol/L 2 hours after a 75 g load** (see Table 4.3.1).
- Women with levels greater than these require further assessment of **impaired glucose tolerance** using 'glucose profiles'.

Table 4.3.1 Reference values for a 75 g oral glucose tolerance test in pregnancy.

	Blood glucose level after 2 hours (mmol/L)[a]		
	Normal	IGT[b]	Diabetes mellitus
2nd Trimester	<7.8	7.8–11.0	>11.0
3rd Trimester	<9.0	9.0–11.0	>11.0

[a] Blood glucose levels two hours after a 75 g oral glucose tolerance test.
[b] Impaired glucose tolerance. IGT is treated as vigorously as clearcut diabetes.

GLUCOSE PROFILES

- Blood glucose is measured before (pre-prandial) and 2 hours after (post-prandial) each meal and before going to bed. This amounts to seven tests per day.
- If glucose levels are greater than 7.5 mmol/L, initial advice should be given about a high fibre diet with correct calorific intake and carbohydrate content (see below).
- Repeat the profile two weeks later.
- If levels remain elevated, commence a once daily injection of

insulin, e.g. Protophane 10 units (an Isophane insulin). (It may be given at night if the blood sugar in the morning is high.)

- Increase the dose to achieve the desired fasting glucose levels before next injection dose.
- Approximately 10 per cent of women with gestational diabetes require treatment with insulin.
- Continue management as shown below.

Insulin therapy for pre-existing diabetes

- Insulin is normally given as injections of short acting insulin 30–45 minutes before each of the three main meals and intermediate acting before bed. Also commonly used is a twice daily short and intermediate combination e.g. Actrapid and Protophane/Monotard (see Table 4.3.2).

Table 4.3.2 Insulin dosage adjustment for fluctuations of glucose.

If elevated before:	Then increase:
Breakfast	Evening intermediate acting (exclude Somogyi effect)
Lunch	Morning short acting
Dinner	Morning intermediate acting
Bedtime snack	Evening short acting

Note: Too short an interval between short acting insulin and any meal time runs the risk of post-prandial *hypoglycaemia*. Therefore, make sure that insulin is given 45 minutes (ideally) before a meal, but 30 minutes as a compromise.

- In general a twice daily injection regimen is divided as follows:

Split the total daily dose to give a 2:1 ratio of morning to evening dose.

Then split the morning and evening dose 2:1 ratio of intermediate to short acting (see Table 4.3.3).

- However, with human insulins, a 50/50 ratio between long acting and short acting insulins is common and night time dose may exceed morning requirements.
- Long acting insulins (e.g. Ultratard) are difficult to use in pregnancy and patients are generally switched to intermediate types.
- **Aim for a blood glucose level of <5.0 mmol/L pre-prandial and <7.5 mmol/L post-prandial (i.e. 1–2 hours after a meal).** Table 4.3.4

shows how the insulin dose should be adjusted for fluctuations in blood glucose levels.

- Review the blood glucose profiles twice weekly.

Typical testing schemes

- A 7 point profile weekly (before and 1–2 hours after each meal and pre-bed) **or** a twice weekly 4 point profile (before each meal and bed).

Table 4.3.3 An example of a twice daily insulin regimen of intermediate and short acting insulin in divided doses.

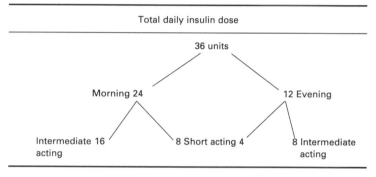

Total daily insulin dose

36 units

Morning 24   12 Evening

Intermediate 16   8 Short acting 4   8 Intermediate
acting   acting

Table 4.3.4 Types of insulin, their peak activity (hours from time of injection) and useful duration of action.

Type of insulin	Peak activity (hours)	Useful duration (hours)
Short acting 　Velosulin 　Actrapid 　Humilin S	1–2	4–8
Intermediate acting 　Insulatard 　Protophane 　Monotard 　Humilin I	2–4	12–24
Long acting (avoid in pregnancy) 　Ultratard 　Ultralente	8	20–48

Note: Within-patient variation of insulin absorption and sensitivity can be as great as 50 per cent.

- Additional profiles should be done if the mother is unwell or if hypo- or hyperglyaemia are suspected.
- Test urine for protein and ketones if mother is unwell or blood glucose >17 mmol/L.

Morning hyperglycaemia

This may be due to nocturnal **hypo**glycaemia: check blood glucose at 03.00 hours. If it is less than 3 mmol/L reduce appropriate insulin, e.g. bedtime and intermediate acting. If the 03.00 hours value is high, increase the evening dose of insulin progressively. *Note:* The pre-bed snack may well need to be increased concurrently.

Diabetic control

- Education, input and support from a diabetes specialist nurse and advice from a dietitian are essential.
- Measure blood glucose pre-prandially. Some post-prandial measurements need to be done to avoid excessive glucose peaks.
- Aim to achieve normoglycaemia (see above).
- Check glycosylated haemoglobin in each trimester and fructosamine monthly or at each visit.
- **Glycosylated haemoglobin (HbA1$_c$)** is the amount of glucose associated with the haemoglobin molecule. The normal value of HbA1$_c$ is less than 7.5 per cent.
- Fructosamine should be less than 2.4 mmol/L (but check local assay levels).
- Home capillary samples can be checked by collecting small samples into micro-collecting tubes or using specially treated filter strips (available from the laboratory).

DIET

The recommended diet for diabetic women is:
- 30 kilocalories (126 kilojoules) per kilogram actual body weight (2300–2400 kilocalories, 9660–10080 kilojoules) to be consumed as 50–55 per cent carbohydrate, 10–15 per cent protein and 30–35 per cent fat (ideally 1/3 saturated, 1/3 mono-unsaturated and 1/3 poly-unsaturated). Unrefined carbohydrate may need to be increased dur-

ing pregnancy, particularly the bed-time snack, to prevent hypoglycaemia.

▪ Calorie intake should be balanced throughout the day: e.g. 25 per
cent breakfast, 30 per cent lunch, 30 per cent dinner and 15 per cent
bed-time snack.

▪ A high fibre diet is recommended.

DIABETIC MANAGEMENT DURING LABOUR AND DELIVERY

Consider induction of labour from 38 weeks' gestation or earlier if the
diabetes is uncontrolled or insulin requirements have reduced, suggesting altered fetal requirements. Give careful consideration to the
mode of delivery. Consider elective caesarean section in women with
a history of infertility or miscarriage, poor diabetic control, vascular
complications, or a baby estimated to be larger than 4.2 kg.

'Uncomplicated' diabetic pregnancies

Management of diabetes in labour

When the mother is admitted in established labour or with an artificial rupture of the membranes (ARM) and syntocinon infusion,
implement the following:

▪ Nil by mouth.

▪ Establish intravenous infusions with 500 mL 5 per cent dextrose
with 10 mmol KCl at 100 mL/hour and short-acting insulin in normal
saline (50 units actrapid in 50 mL saline) at approximately 2 units per
hour. Adjust this rate to keep capillary blood glucose at 4–7 mmol/L.

▪ Monitor with hourly capillary glucose or more frequently if glucose
levels are abnormal and the dose of insulin needs to be changed (see
Table 4.3.5).

▪ Reduce insulin infusion to 1 unit per hour following delivery.

▪ Check blood glucose, urea and electrolytes on admission, before
caesarean section and 4 hourly in labour.

Induction with prostaglandin (or latent phase of spontaneous labour)

Normal diet and usual twice daily insulin on antenatal ward until in
established/active labour when proceed as for vaginal delivery.

Table 4.3.5 Sliding scale for insulin infusion rate according to capillary blood glucose levels.

Glucose level (mmol/L)	Action
<3	Stop insulin
3–4	Reduce insulin rate by $\frac{1}{2}$–1 U/hour
4–7	Continue insulin at same rate, usually 1–3 U/hour)
7–10	Increase insulin by 1 U/hour
>10	Increase insulin by 2 U/hour[a]

[a] May need larger increases particularly if obese, dehydrated or on steroids.

Elective caesarean section

- Normal diet and insulin the evening before.
- Urea and electrolytes on admission.
- Nil by mouth from midnight.
- Capillary glucose at 08.00 hours.
- Intravenous infusion at 500 mL 5 per cent dextrose with added 10 mmol KCl at rate 100 mL/hour from 08.00 hours.
- Intravenous infusion of quick acting insulin from 08.00 hours at 1–3 units per hour initially.

Post delivery

After delivery insulin requirements drop rapidly

- Give i.v. 5 per cent dextrose, KCl and insulin as above until able to eat and drink normally.
- Then stop insulin infusion, give normal diet and daily subcutaneous insulin at a reduced dosage (usually one third of pre-delivery dose) but at the same frequency.
- Monitor diabetic control with blood glucose measurements and adjust insulin doses as necessary.
- Encourage breast feeding.
- Routine postnatal management.
- Six week follow-up appointment. Ensure appointments for routine diabetic care are re-established. Carry out an oral glucose tolerance test for gestational diabetics to document return to normality.

MATERNAL COMPLICATIONS FROM DIABETES

Perinatal mortality need not be increased in gestational diabetics or those with frank diabetes providing glucose control is tight and the pregnancy is adequately monitored. Good glycaemic control before conception is essential to decrease the increased spontaneous abortion rate in diabetic women.

- **Congenital malformations** occur in 4–11 per cent of diabetics compared to 1–2 per cent of the normal population. For example, the incidence of heart defects is about 25 per 1000, compared with 8 per 1000 in babies of non-diabetic mothers. The critical period for malformations is 3–6 weeks after conception (5–8 weeks after last period). The incidence of major malformations is correlated with elevations of first trimester glycosylated haemoglobin, and is also linked to pre-existing diabetic microvascular disease.

- **Preterm labour and delivery** occurs in up to 50 per cent of diabetic pregnancies – 75 per cent are planned and 28 per cent spontaneous.

- **Pre-eclampsia** (12 per cent) – especially those with microvascular disease.

- **Traumatic delivery** and increased risk of caesarean section associated with macrosomia.

- **Hyperglycaemia** (>10 mmol/L) and **ketoacidosis** (>1+), or **hyperosmolar non-ketotic coma** – these need to be controlled as a matter of urgency.

- Peripheral, visceral or autonomic **neuropathy**.

- **Retinopathy** includes background retinopathy of microaneuryms, hard exudates and haemorrhages. Pre-proliferative include intraretinal microvascular abnormalities and areas of hypoperfusion and cotton wool spots. Vitreous haemorrhage may occur. Examine the fundi in each trimester. Laser therapy is indicated for proliferative retinopathy. Pregnancy accelerates progression of retinopathy, although it usually regresses after delivery. There is a risk of retinal detachment. Pre-retinal or vitreous haemorrhage – clinically presents as sudden unilateral change (cobwebs, clouding or loss of vision).

Expulsive efforts during the second stage of labour should be avoided in women with proliferative retinal change. Also avoid labour if there is a risk of pre-retinal haemorrhage (unless it has been treated by laser).

- **Nephropathy** is associated with hypertension, prematurity, lower birth weights and an increase in perinatal mortality. A serum creatinine >250–300 micromol/L is incompatible with a successful pregnancy.

COMPLICATIONS FOR THE BABY OF THE DIABETIC MOTHER

- Congenital malformations (especially cardiac and musculoskeletal).
- Macrosomia – up to 30 per cent of babies weigh above 90th centile.
- Intrauterine growth retardation may occur, particularly in the presence of maternal microvascular disease.
- The perinatal mortality rate is 4–5 times greater than normal. In many cases the cause of fetal death is unknown but is likely to be 'metabolic' rather than asphyxial.
- Birth trauma.
- Cardiomyopathy and congestive cardiac failure.
- Respiratory distress.
- Hypoglycaemia (less than 2 mmol/L) occurs in 50 per cent within 12 hours if not closely observed.
- Hypocalcaemia less than 1.7 mmol/L (in 25–50 per cent).
- Hypomagnesaemia.
- Jaundice serum.
- Polycythaemia.
- The risk of diabetes in later life is five to twenty times background rate.

IMMEDIATE CARE OF THE NEWBORN INFANT

- Feed at 60 mL/kg gradually increasing to 90 mL/kg.
- Monitor blood glucose level with a meter (e.g. Glucometer™) or strip (e.g. Dextrostix™) hourly for 6 hours, 2 hours before feeds for the next 8 hours and then 4 hourly before feeds until 48 hours has passed.
- If blood glucose <1.0 mmol/l infuse 10 per cent dextrose. If 1–2 mmol/L give glucagon 300 microgram/kg (approximately 1.0–1.5 IU) This usually gives a response in 30 minutes which lasts 6–8 hours. If haematocrit >0.70 – exchange transfusion.

PRE-PREGNANCY MEDICAL MANAGEMENT OF DIABETES MELLITUS

Pre pregnancy medical monitoring of the insulin dependent diabetic is essential.

- Optimise glycaemic control for three cycles prior to conception as this reduces the congenital malformation rate.

- Ideally, the HBA1$_c$ and fructosamine should be normal over three cycles, but advice needs to be tailored to the individual.
- The non-insulin dependent diabetic woman on oral hypoglycaemics should be started on insulin before pregnancy.
- Treat retinopathy.
- Check renal function: urea and electrolytes, creatinine, uric acid.
- Check rubella status.
- Offer vitamin supplements containing folate.

BIBLIOGRAPHY

Brudenell, M. & Doddridge, M.C. (1989) *Diabetic Pregnancy*, Churchill Livingstone, Edinburgh.

Hatem, M., Anthony, F., Hogston, P., Rowe, D.J.F. & Dennis, K.J. (1988) Reference values for 75 g oral glucose tolerance test in pregnancy. *British Medical Journal*, **296**, 676–678.

Kucera, J. (1971) Rate and type of congenital anomalies among offspring of diabetic women. *Journal of Reproductive Medicine*, 7, 61–70.

Mitchell, S.C., Sellmann, A.H., Westphal, M.G. & Park, J. (1971) Etiologic correlates in a study of congenital heart disease in 56,109 births. *American Journal of Cardiology*, **28**, 653–657.

Glucose tolerance in pregnancy – the WHO and How of testing. *The Lancet* (editorial), 19 November, 1988, pp. 1173–1174.

4.4   Infections in pregnancy

DIAGNOSIS OF INFECTION IN THE FETUS

- The fetus elaborates IgM in response to antigen exposure *in utero*, and detection of specific IgM antibody in cord blood is the best diagnostic test for congenital infections.
- Specific IgM is only detected after 20 weeks' gestation.
- Non-specific IgM level at or over 18 mg per 100 mL also suggests intrauterine infection.
- For the diagnosis of fetal infections 1–4 mL of fetal blood is obtained

by cordocentesis (see p. 205). A blood film and karyotyping should also be done.

MATERNAL AND FETAL VIRAL INFECTIONS

Rubella

Rubella is a togavirus and the only member of the genus *Rubivirus*.
- Naturally acquired infection confers life-long immunity.
- Re-infection may occasionally occur in those with vaccine-induced immunity.
- Rubella status should be checked in all women when they attend for antenatal booking.
- Lack of immunity is suggested by a rubella antibody level of less than 15 IU.
- Non-immune women should be vaccinated **after** the pregnancy is complete. There is a high rate of seroconversion so routine post-immunisation testing is not indicated.
- About 2 per cent of pregnant women under 35 years of age are susceptible to rubella because they have not been offered or have refused vaccine, or due to failed seroconversion after vaccination.

Risk of vaccination in pregnancy

Although there is no evidence of fetal damage following vaccination of susceptible women in early pregnancy, vaccination should not knowingly be carried out during pregnancy.

Clinical presentation

- The incubation period is 14–18 days.
- Ten per cent of infections in caucasian women are subclinical.
- Mild infection is characterised by generalised rash which may be preceded by cartarrh and enlargement of the posterior cervical, post-auricular and suboccipital lymph nodes and prodromal symptoms such as malaise and fever for 1–2 days before the rash develops.
- The rash is discreet at first – pinpoint macular lesions, that first appear on the face, trunk and limbs.
- The woman is infectious during the last week of the incubation period and for about a week after the onset of the rash.
- The virus produces an anti-mitotic effect upon infected cells which leads to retardation in cell division. The result is major malformation

if it occurs during the critical stage of organogenesis (e.g. deafness and retinopathy occur in babies following maternal infection between 13 and 16 weeks' gestation).

Diagnosis and investigation

- Test the mother for rubella specific IgM.

Rubella specific IgM is usually detectable by four days after onset of illness and remains detectable for at least one month.

Re-infection (usually asymptomatic) may be detected serologically, by demonstrating a significant rise in antibody titre, following close exposure to rubella. A specific IgM response may also be detected, but this is often transient and at a low level.

Management of the pregnant woman in contact with rubella whose immune status is unknown

If antibody is detected in the serum within 10 days of contact, the woman is immune and there is no fetal risk.

- Obtain serum from the acute phase of illness for the detection of antibodies and test for IgM.
- Obtain a serum sample 7–10 days later and measure any rise in antibodies.

Serological tests performed on women well after the incubation period (more than 5–7 days after the onset of illness) will show no rise in antibody titre, although the presence of high titres may indicate recent rubella infection. IgM testing will help to sort this out.

If an earlier blood sample is available (e.g. booking blood) and antibodies are present in both samples, at the same concentration, then the woman is immune. Seronegative women should be tested weekly for four weeks after their last contact.

There should be no diagnostic problem if the woman has presented within six weeks of onset of the illness or contact.

Pregnant women presenting with a rash should have full serological investigation.

Pregnant women with a record of vaccination and who present with a rash should be investigated because of the possibility of vaccine failure. On subsequent exposure to rubella virus there is a typical primary antibody response with IgG seroconversion and a high concentration of specific IgM which persists for at least six to eight weeks. Loss of natural rubella immunity occurs rarely. In such cases, re-infection with wild rubella virus or revaccination produces a booster rather than a primary response, characterised by a rise in IgG antibody with a negative or low level of IgM.

If re-infection is diagnosed (almost invariably following vaccine induced immunity), cordocentesis should be performed for specific IgM antibody testing. However, IgM may not appear in fetal blood until 23 weeks, despite intrauterine infection early in pregnancy. Culturing rubella virus from amniotic fluid may take up to six weeks and is relatively insensitive. The technique of chorionic villus sampling together with nucleic acid hybridisation has been used successfully to diagnose congenital rubella infection in the first trimester. The risk of fetal infection from maternal re-infection is about 5–10 per cent.

Prognosis and neonatal considerations

Primary rubella infection in the first trimester of pregnancy leads to fetal infection and congenital abnormalities in 80–90 per cent of cases. If the infection occurs in the fourth month the risk to the fetus is 50–60 per cent and of congenital abnormalities is 20–25 per cent. After the fourth month, fetal infection is common but damage is rare, and limited to deafness.

The commonest defects associated with congenitally-acquired rubella are cataracts, heart defects and sensorineural deafness. Cardiac and eye defects are especially common if infection occurs at the time of critical organogenesis   eight weeks. The earlier the infection in pregnancy, the greater the risk of multiple defects.

Congenitally infected children may themselves act as reservoirs of infection. At six months of age 20–30 per cent of them may still be excreting the virus from the nasopharynx.

Cytomegalovirus

Cytomegalovirus (CMV) is a DNA virus, the largest of the herpes viruses. CMV is transmitted in adults by sexual or salivary contact, occasionally from urine and blood transfusion. It remains latent throughout life, being shed intermittently and may reactivate. Up to 12 per cent of health women excrete the virus during pregnancy and of those 1–2 per cent have a primary infection (see Table 4.4.1).

The risk of congenital defects is very low following secondary maternal infection. Less than 0.5 per cent of babies in the United Kingdom will excrete the virus at birth.

Table 4.4.1 The incidence of fetal infection after maternal CMV infection.

1–2 per cent of pregnancies have a primary infection.
30–40 per cent of cases of infection cross the placenta.
Therefore 100 infected fetuses for every 300 infected mothers.
3 per cent of fetuses are damaged at birth with severe handicap such as microcephaly, etc.
7 per cent of fetuses have less impairment which is not detected until later.
90 per cent of fetuses will not show any damage, although they are infected.

The clinical syndrome associated with CMV infection may include intrauterine growth retardation, jaundice, hepatosplenomegaly, microcephaly, chorioretinitis, purpuric skin lesions, and thrombocytopenia or haemolytic anaemia.

Clinical presentation
Maternal primary infection in pregnancy is usually asymptomatic. Asymptomatic recurrent infection may also occur.

Diagnosis and investigation
CMV is diagnosed from culture of the virus from the urine or throat swabs in transport medium. Detection of CMV-specific IgM and IgG antibodies in a single blood sample suggests a recent or current infection. Seroconversion in the period between two blood samples also indicates current infection. A combination of culture and fluorescein or enzyme-labelled monoclonal antibodies to early antigens will detect viral nuclear antigens within 24–48 hours. IgM persists for up to 16 weeks following primary infection.

Fetal infection (10 per cent of cases only) can be diagnosed by fetal blood sampling after 20 weeks' gestation and finding specific IgM-positive blood cultures and elevated gamma-glutamyl transferase.

Prognosis
If a mother has a primary infection of CMV in pregnancy there is a three per cent chance of the baby having CMV related damage, of which half will be limited to unilateral or bilateral hearing loss. If fetal infection is confirmed, the risk of damage rises to 10 per cent, but failure to isolate the virus does not guarantee that the baby is not affected.

Management

There is no safe anti-viral agent which can be used to alter the outcome. Termination of pregnancy is not routinely indicated.

Herpes simplex virus (HSV)

- Infection can occur with herpes type 1 and 2.
- Seventy per cent of genital infections are caused by herpes type 2. The incidence of neonatal herpes is about 1 case per 40 000 live births.
- Reactivation is more common than primary infection in pregnancy.

Clinical presentation

Local symptoms such as pain, rash, dysuria, and discharge and systemic symptoms such as fever, headaches, and generalised aches. The rash starts as erythema, followed by painful vesicles, which burst to leave shallow ulcers that heal in 7–10 days. Vesicles continue to occur for up to two weeks and the entire illness may last up to four weeks.

Seventy per cent of babies with neonatal herpes simplex virus are born to mothers with no history of genital lesions. Most neonatal cases result from primary maternal HSV infection around the time of delivery.

Diagnosis and investigation

Aspirate fluid from the lesions and place on a glass slide and send for microscopic identification.

Prognosis and the neonate

Neonatal herpes simplex virus infection may be localised to the skin, eye or mouth or it may be generalised involving the brain, liver, adrenals, lungs and other organs. Without anti-viral treatment about 70 per cent of babies with localised herpes simplex virus infection will develop disseminated infection.

Maternal treatment

- **Primary infection: oral acyclovir (200 mg five times daily for 10 days)** started within 6 days of onset of rash, reduces the time to healing, the duration of viral shedding and pain.
- Treat painful lesions with solacaine cream three times daily. Advise salt baths – one handful of salt in the bath or 1 teaspoon per 600 mL of water. This acts as a disinfectant and promotes healing. Oral analgesia may be required.

- **Secondary infection** may not need treatment although the woman often requests it. Use acyclovir 200 mg q.d.s.
- If recurrent attacks are frequent specialist advice is required.

Prevention of neonatal HSV infection

Transmission rate to babies are greatest among mothers with active, primary genital herpes at delivery. Their risk is 50 per cent if they are delivered vaginally so caesarean section is advocated in this group.

The risk to the baby of an asymptomatic woman with a history of recurrent genital herpes is low and the baby should be delivered vaginally.

When a mother with recurrent genital herpes has active genital lesions at term vaginal delivery can still be justified but the possible small increased risk of infection (particularly in the presence of florid lesions) can be used to justify delivery by caesarean section.

Prognosis

It is too late to treat symptomatic babies with acyclovir. Any baby delivered vaginally in a mother with primary herpes should be started on acyclovir immediately. Babies delivered vaginally in mothers with recurrent herpes should also be treated with acyclovir.

Varicella zoster

It occurs rarely in pregnancy but may cause miscarriage in the first trimester and damage neuronal cells causing denervation of developing organs and extremities. This can cause microcephaly, hydrocephaly, optic atrophy, chorioretinitis, microphthalmia and damage to the cervical and lumbosacral plexi causing hypoplasia of the extremities and dysfunction of the urethral and anal sphincters.

Pregnant women with varicella are at risk of severe viral pneumonia.

Treatment

- Treat viral pneumonia with **acyclovir** intravenously, 15 mg/kg 8 hourly for seven days. The therapeutic level of acyclovir in the serum is thought to be between 10 and 20 mg/mL.
- Anti-varicella-zoster-immunoglobulin (VZIg), 250 mg i.m. should be given to newborn babies after delivery if they have been born to

women who develop chickenpox within seven days before until seven days after delivery.

■ If a non-immune mother is exposed to chickenpox, 1 g of VZIg can be given i.m., in order to attenuate the illness in the mother.

Prognosis and neonatal considerations

Sixty per cent of babies will acquire chickenpox if their mothers have chickenpox between seven days before until seven days after delivery.

There is a 30 per cent mortality of babies if chickenpox occurs in the mother within four days of delivery.

Parvovirus B19

It is a species specific small non-enveloped DNA virus, 20–25 namometres in size which infects erythroblasts, inhibiting mitosis, but not the stem cells necessary for recovery. It causes erythema infectiosum (Fifth disease, slapped cheek syndrome).

The virus is transmitted by nasal droplet. A viraemia develops on day 5–7 and lasts until day 10–15. It causes a mild febrile illness common in schoolchildren between the ages of 5 and 15. Approximately 35–50 per cent of the general population is susceptible to parvovirus B19. Infection should be suspected if there has been a local outbreak or the mother has polyarthralgia or a lacy rash.

B19 infections occur in <1 per cent of pregnancies. The risk of transmission to a susceptible adult in the household of an infected child is 50 per cent. To a teacher during an outbreak in a school, it is 20 per cent. The risk of presumed parvovirus related fetal deaths in women infected during the first 20 weeks of pregnancy is 3–9 per cent.

Clinical presentation in the mother

A non-specific febrile illness may occur. The rash occurs 7–18 days after inoculation and after disappearance of viraemia the rash may be non-specific. In typical cases it has a 'slapped cheek' appearance with an erythematous lacy rash on the trunk and extremities. By then the subject is no longer infectious.

Clinical presentation in the fetus

Most women with B19 infection in pregnancy have normal infants, but it is associated with inhibition of fetal erythropoiesis. The result is severe fetal anaemia, ascites and hydrops.

Fetal infection is diagnosed by demonstrating viral DNA in fetal blood. Specific IgM is often negative. The prognosis of the infected fetus is poor. Untreated hydrops caused by parvovirus causes fetal or neonatal death. It may be treated successfully by intravascular fetal blood transfusion.

Diagnosis

- Suspect infection from clinical history.
- Look for B19 antigen or DNA in the serum within three days of the onset of clinical symptoms.
- IgM antibodies are present in 90 per cent of women 4–7 days after the onset of symptoms; they peak at 30 days and persist for up to four months.
- IgG antibodies appear approximately 7–10 days after symptoms and persist for several years. Antibodies may not prevent infection but lessen the degree of viraemia and protect the fetus.
- After three days (and especially after the rash has developed) these tests will be negative. If this is the case look for anti-parvovirus B19 IgM antibody, which indicates recent infection.
- Once the mother presents with fetal hydrops, the serum may no longer contain the B19 IgM. The presence of B19 IgG is not helpful, since it persists for months to years after infection. Pair sera for evidence of IgG seroconversion.
- Infection can be associated with an otherwise unexplained increase in maternal alphafetoprotein (AFP).

Fetal complications

Hydrops fetalis   The fetal red blood cell life span is only 45–70 days in the second trimester and haemolysis caused by virus can be severe. Anaemia results in high output cardiac failure and tissue hypoxia leading to hydrops. Myocarditis may occur. Infiltration of the liver with erythropoietic tissue may lead to portal hypertension and hypoproteinaemia, due to impaired protein synthesis. This may explain the persistence of acites despite normal haemoglobin levels after intrauterine transfusion.

Pulmonary hypoplasia   This may occur secondary to pleural effusions or compression by the enlarged liver.

Clinical management

- If a woman is exposed to parvovirus, establish her immune status.

- Look for evidence of recent infection.
- If tests show the pregnant woman has been infected, monitor by fetal ultrasound and maternal alphafetoprotein to try to assess the effects on the fetus.
- Correct the fetal anaemia with intrauterine transfusion.

Hepatitis B virus (HBV)

Marker	Definition
HB_sAg	Hepatitis B surface antigen
HB_sAb	Antibody to HB_sAg
HB_cAg	Core antigen
HB_cAb	Antibody against core antigen
HB_eAg	Hepatitis B_e antigen
HB_eAb	Antibody against HB_eAg

Most adults with acute HBV infection recover fully and become immune. Ten per cent become carriers of the virus. HBV infection can be transmitted to the baby at birth from mothers who have recently had acute HBV infection (whether symptomatic or asymptomatic) or from those who are $HB_sAg +$ carriers and who are eAg + /eAb –, eAg – / eAb –.

The risk of transmission from an eAg + mother is 90 per cent, an eAg –/eAb – mother 40 per cent and from an eAb + mother 10 per cent.

Diagnosis

The reverse passive haemagglutination assay is used.

If a pregnant woman is $HB_sAg +$ do further investigations to distinguish acute cases from carriers and highly infectious individuals from those of low infectivity. The infectivity is assessed by enzyme-linked immunosorbent assay (ELISA) or radioimmunoassay (RIA) for e antigen/antibody status. Acute cases have high titres of anti-HBV core (HB_cAb) IgM.

Prevention

At least 90 per cent of perinatal infections can be prevented if the baby is given active/passive immunisation at birth.

Give hepatitis B immunoglobulin (HBIg) 200 IU at birth to the baby of any woman who is $HB_sAb +$ and eAg + or has no e antibody. In addition, give the first dose of vaccine within 12 hours on the contralateral side to the HBIg and subsequently at 0, 1 and 6 months of age. Check the antibody status of the baby at one year. If antibodies are undetectable give a booster dose of vaccine.

Human papilloma (warts virus) infection

This is the most commonly acquired sexually transmitted disease. The incubation period is usually 1–3 months but may be up to two years.

Warts grow in pregnancy and should be effectively treated in the third trimester.

Treatment

- Podophyllin and podophyllotoxin have been associated with an adverse pregnancy outcome, so are contraindicated in pregnancy.
- Treat once or twice weekly with trichloracetic acid. It is important to paint the area of the wart and the underlying skin base. Warn the patient that this may hurt.
- The treatment is usually effective with 1–2 applications.
- Check the patient 2–3 weeks later to ensure regression of all warts. Subsequent therapy may be required because of the growth of microwarts that have not been visible on first presentation.
- If regression has not occurred by 20 weeks' gestation, leave them to grow. They will be easier to treat after delivery.
- Patients with a history of treatment for vulval, vaginal or cervical warts, should have cervical cytology performed at yearly intervals.

Human immunodeficiency virus (HIV)

Definition

HIV-1 is a retrovirus. It is composed of core (p 18, p 24, and p 27) and surface (gp 120 and gp 41) proteins, genomic RNA and the reverse transcriptase enzyme, surrounded by a lipid bilayer envelope. HIV gains access to host cells via the binding of its surface protein gp 120 to CD4 receptors on helper T lymphocytes, B lymphocytes, macrophages, lymph nodes, Langerhans cells of the skin and some brain cells. The virion then fuses directly with the host cell membrane, an action apparently mediated by the gp 41 surface protein. Once inside its reverse transcriptase converts its RNA genome to DNA which is incorporated into the host genome. The host cell is killed during HIV replication which results in depletion of helper T lymphocytes and subsequent immunodeficiency associated with clinical disease.

Aetiology

HIV infections are most commonly acquired through intravenous drug use. In the United Kingdom, heterosexually acquired AIDS is not common except where the partner is in a high risk group. Vertical transmission to the fetus occurs in between 15 and 40 per cent. Babies will carry passively acquired HIV IgG antibody for up to 15 months, so determination of infective status is difficult. High levels of maternal antibody to HIV envelope glycoprotein gp 120 reduce the risk of the baby being infected. The risk of vertical transmission is increased in the presence of depressed helper T cell counts, elevated suppressor T cell count, anaemia, lymphocytopenia, p 24 antigenaemia with elevated levels of β 2 microglobulin and low absolute maternal CD4 cell count.

Impact of pregnancy on progression and maternal HIV infection

Pregnancy **may** increase the risk of progression to symptomatic HIV disease by accelerating the depletion of CD4 cells. CD4 count of less than $300/mm^3$ are associated with an increased risk of serious opportunist infections in pregnancy.

In 40 per cent of HIV positive pregnant women the virus can be detected in cervical secretions.

Approximately half of the women identified as HIV infected during pregnancy will progress to AIDS in 2–6 years.

Strategies to reduce vertical transmission

Transmission of HIV from the mother to the baby can occur in utero, during labour or delivery and by breast feeding. Up to 70 per cent of transmission probably occurs in late pregnancy or labour.

Caesarean section may reduce the transmission risk by up to 50 per cent but post-operative morbidity is more common and severe in HIV infected women.

Zidovudine is an inhibitor of the reverse transcriptase enzyme of HIV thus preventing viral DNA incorporation into the host genome. It reduces opportunistic infections and prolongs survival in AIDS patients. It has been shown to reduce the risk of vertical transmission by approximately two thirds in pregnant women with mildly symptomatic HIV disease and no previous antiviral treatment if given to the mother antenatally and intrapartum to the newborn (Connor *et al.*, 1994). This substantial potential benefit is to be balanced against the unknown long-term risk. There is as yet no evidence of an increased incidence of serious adverse effects on the baby.

The current suggested policy is as follows but it will need to be reviewed in the light of further experience.

1 Deliver all HIV positive pregnant women by caesarean section.

2 Treat HIV positive women who are symptomatic (but with no previous retroviral therapy and with a CD4 cell count $>200/\text{mm}^3$) using zidovudine as follows:

- 100 mg orally five times daily antenatally from 14 weeks' gestation.
- During labour 2 mg/kg i.v. over 1 hour then 1 mg/kg/hour until delivery.
- The woman who presents late for or has had no antenatal care should be commenced on treatment as soon as possible.

3 Treat the babies of the above with zidovudine 2 mg/kg orally six hourly for six weeks.

4 Avoid breast feeding in all HIV positive women.

5 Seek specialist help especially in those women who have symptoms associated with HIV infection or a CD4 count $\leqslant 500/\text{mm}^3$.

RISK OF HIV AND HEPATITIS INFECTION TO MEDICAL PERSONNEL

HIV

HIV is less transmissible than hepatitis B virus, requiring hollow needles and larger volumes of blood. The risk of HIV seroconversion after a single needlestick or sharps injury involving known HIV infected blood less than 0.5 per cent. Injury from a suture needle or other solid needle has not been reported.

Intact skin and mucous membranes are important defences against HIV. The estimated risk of transfer of HIV from an infected surgeon to a patient range from 1:48 000 to 1:1 000 000. If the patient proves to be HIV positive or refuses tests, and a surgeon has a needle stick injury, the surgeon should be tested for HIV antibody at three and six months. Safe sex techniques should be used until the HIV test has been known to be negative at three months. If any influenza-like illness that might represent seroconversion occurs after the incident the surgeon must stop invasive procedures and have an antibody test.

Zidovudine is the only drug considered to offer the possibility of modifying the risk of infection with HIV after an inoculation incident.

Hepatitis B

Surgeons are at greatest risk of acquiring hepatitis B from patients who are HB$_e$Ag positive. Without prophylaxis the risk may be greater than 30 per cent after a single exposure by needle stick or sharps injury to eAG + infected blood. Hepatitis B may be acquired from exposure of broken skin to blood from an e antigen positive carrier. The risk after full immunisation is virtually zero.

All surgeons should be immunised against hepatitis B and be known to have hepatitis B virus antibodies >100 IU.

4

Universal precautions to be taken for all patients

- Have vaccination against hepatitis B.
- Cover all cuts and abrasions with waterproof dressings.
- Do not pass sharps from hand to hand.
- Do not use hand needles.
- Do not guide needles with fingers.
- Do not resheath needles.
- Dispose of all sharps safely into approved containers.
- Put disposables and waste in yellow clinical waste bags for incineration.

Additional precautions when caring for known HIV and hepatitis B virus positive and high risk patients

- Consider non-operative management.
- Remove unnecessary equipment from theatre.
- Observe highest level of theatre discipline.
- Have only experienced surgeons and health care works in theatre.
- Use double gloves, high efficiency masks, eye protection, boots, impervious gowns and closed wound drainage.
- Use disposable anaesthetic circuitry or appropriate method of decontamination.
- Disinfect theatre floor with hypochlorite.

OTHER MATERNAL AND FETAL INFECTIONS

Listeriosis

Definition

Listeria monocytogenes is a Gram-positive, coryneform bacterium that can produce human, animal and fetal infections. Incidence in the UK is 1 in 20 000 births.

In 1990 there were only 24 confirmed cases associated with pregnancy in over 700 000 births in England and Wales. In some cases, although the fetus is severely affected, the mother may exhibit no symptoms at all.

Listeria monocytogenes is one of the few pathogens which can form colonies at 4°C, the average temperature of a domestic fridge. It survives in the soil, vegetation and establishes itself in carrier or diseased animals. **Pregnant women should not eat foods at high risk of containing listeria**. These include soft ripened cheeses (such as brie, camembert and blue vein), and pate. Cook-chilled meals and ready-to-eat poultry need to be heated to at least 70°C for two minutes to kill the bacillus.

Clinical presentation

Maternal infection may be silent or present as a 'flu like illness associated with fever, rigors, generalised pain, pharyngitis, myalgia, back pain, diarrhoea and urinary tract symptoms (but with sterile urine). The incubation period may be from two days to six weeks. Rates of intrautine or neonatal death may be as high as 50 per cent. A characteristic feature is the presence of meconium staining of the liquor despite prematurity.

A live born infant may develop meningitis, encephalitis, pneumonia, conjunctivitis and petechial or other skin rashes.

Diagnosis and investigation

Listeria monocytogenes may be cultured in blood and from genital tract and urine. It is important to state the clinical suspicion of listeria, since the microbiologist may have to use special techniques, without which listeria may not be isolated and identified. Stool specimens are not useful. Up to 5 per cent of healthy individuals may carry listeria in the gut without ill effects. Samples of meconium-stained liquor may be examined for listeria.

If listeriosis is suspected, samples should be taken from the neonate, stillborn fetus, or other products of conception. These include blood, CSF, tracheal or gastric aspirate and meconium and swabs from eye, ear and nose. Samples of placenta should be taken for culture before the tissue is fixed and the remainder sent for histology. Serological tests for listeria antibodies in maternal or cord blood are neither specific nor sensitive enough to make the diagnosis.

Treatment

Ampicillin in high dose 6–8 g/day. Success depends on the degree of infection at the time of presentation.

Group B streptococcal (GBS) infection

The incidence is 1–4/1000 births. 15–20 per cent of women carry the organism in the vagina at the time of delivery; 40–70 per cent of the babies of these mothers become colonised and of these only about 1 per cent develop evidence of infection. Risk factors for infection include prematurity, low birthweight, prolonged rupture of membranes and intrapartum fever.

The mortality rate from perinatal infection of the babies can be as high as 80 per cent despite early recognition of symptoms and prompt treatment. Of those babies who survive GBS meningitis, half will have severe neurological sequelae.

Treatment of the baby is penicillin – 200 000 units/kg/day for 10 days.

Prevention

Culture of vaginal swabs from all pregnant women and treatment of carriers is neither effective nor advisable. Recolonisation usually occurs after treatment of carriers of GBS.

Toxoplasmosis

Toxoplasma gondii is an obligatory intracellular protozoan which is elongated or sickle shaped at approximately $3 \times 4 \times 6$–7 micrometre^3. It is common and widespread in man. In the United Kingdom, 25 per cent of women infected are 'immune'. In France, more than 70 per cent of women are immune. The principal route of transmission is eating undercooked meat, especially lamb. It can also be transmitted from household pets. Thus pregnant women should not eat raw meat and should wear gloves if it is necessary to handle the cat litter.

Clinical presentation

It is usually either asymptomatic or associated with minor symptoms and signs, e.g. lymphadenopathy with 'glandular fever' like cells in the blood.

Diagnosis and investigation

Blood samples should be sent for Sabin–Feldman dye test, indirect haemagglutination test, and specific tests for IgG and IgM. A repeat sample will be required.

Fetal infection can be diagnosed by fetal blood sampling (but only after 20 weeks' gestation) and demonstration of specific IgM and IgG, abnormal levels of liver enzymes, thrombocytopenia, and isolation of the parasite.

Effects on the fetus/neonate

Transmission rates to the fetus vary from 25 per cent in the first trimester to 65 per cent in the third. The incidence of severe fetal infection falls from 75 per cent early to negligible in late pregnancy.

Infection in the first trimester is more likely to lead to severe consequences for the baby. Sixty per cent of infections occur in the third trimester but most infected newborns have no overt clinical infection. Some of these develop complications later. Among the consequences of fetal infections are: fetal death, growth retardation, chorioretinitis, blindness, hydrocephalus, microcephalus, mental retardation, epilepsy, intracerebral calcification, hepatosplenomegaly and deafness. There is a significant reduction in fetal complications if toxoplasmosis infection is diagnosed and treated.

Treatment

- Treat the mother with spiromycin – 3 g daily for three weeks.
- If fetal infection is confirmed give **sulphadiazine 3 g/day and pyrimethamine 50 mg/day** (plus vitamin supplements in the form of yeast tablets 8 g/day, or folinic acid 5 mg twice weekly) for three weeks. For the rest of pregnancy continue the above alternately for three weeks each.
- If there is no fetal infection treatment with spiramycin is sufficient.

Candidiasis

Candida is a fungus. The incidence of candidiasis rises in pregnancy due to increasing oestrogen levels and the concomitant increase in acidity of the vaginal pH (normal 4.5).

Diagnosis and investigation

- Take high vaginal swabs. Candida has a typical 'cottage cheese' appearance occurring as white plaques. It may be severely itchy or asymptomatic.
- Recurrent candida infection may be associated with occult diabetes. Therefore measure the serum glucose level in such cases.

Treatment

- Give clotrimazole pessaries (100 mg or 200 mg) and cream (1%) for three days. If there is a history of persistent/recurrent candida infections, give a six day course. For prophylaxis, give one 500 mg pessary (e.g. with concomitant antibiotic treatment).
- Clotrimazole is a broad spectrum antifungal agent. It also has activity against trichomonas, staphylococci, streptococci and bacteroides. It has no effect on the endogenous lactobacilli whose numbers can influence vaginal infections.
- The cream should be adequate to treat the often severe pruritus which may be profound. Advise also the therapeutic (healing and antiseptic effects) of a salt bath – one handful of salt in the bath. Alternatively, for douching the area – 1 teaspoon of salt in 600 ml (1 pint) of water.
- Treat the male partner twice daily with clotrimazole cream.

Gonorrhoea

Aetiology

Gonorrhoea is caused by aerobic Gram-negative intracellular diplococci (commonly occurring in pairs). Organisms are spread from mucosal areas. In women the cervical and urethral mucosae are commonly infected.

Clinical presentation

- Up to 50 per cent are asymptomatic
- Gonorrhoea causes acute pelvic inflammation.

Diagnosis and investigation

A Gram-stained smear will often show characteristic kidney or bean shaped Gram-negative intracellular diplococci.

Rapid transport of the specimen to the laboratory in Stuart's or Amie's media is necessary. The specimen is inoculated onto highly nutrient agar plates. (Thayer–Martin also contains vancomycin, colistin and nystatin or lincomycin.) The gonococci typically form semi-translucent grey colonies of oxidase-positive Gram-negative diplococci in 24–48 hours.

Treatment

Where there is a low risk of resistant strains in the community and non-penicillinase resistant gonococcus use:

- **amoxycillin** 3.0 g orally with 1 g probenecid orally, **or**
- aqueous **procaine penicillin** 2.4 megaunit intramuscularly with 1 g probenecid orally.
- If the woman is hypersensitive to penicillin use **spectinomycin** 2 g i.m.

If resistant strains are more common (e.g. occurring in more than 5 per cent of the population) give:

- ofloxacin 400 mg twice daily for ten days;
- cefotaxime 1 g i.m.; **or**
- erythromycin 500 mg twice daily orally for 14 days.

For disseminated and adnexal infections the following can be used:

- amoxil 500 mg three times daily for 14 days after a loading dose of 3 g with probenicid 1 g;
- cefotaxime 1 g i.v. 8 hourly for seven days;
- ceftriaxone 1 g i.m. or i.v. every 24 hours for seven days;
  or, if penicillin sensitive,
- spectinomycin 2 g i.m. every 12 hours for seven days.

Treatment of infants born to infected mothers

- Benzyl penicillin 50 000 units i.m. single dose or ceftriaxone 50 mg/kg i.v. or i.m. as a single dose.
- Penicillin eye drops q.d.s. and i.m. penicillin as above.

Frank neonatal infection is treated using one of the following:

- ampicillin 62.5 mg/kg/day i.m. in four divided doses (100 mg for babies more than 10 days old);
- **benzyl penicillin 100 000** units/kg/day in two to four divided doses

(150 000 units/kg/day) for meningitis or for babies more than 10 days old;

- cefuroxime 30 mg/kg/day i.m. in two doses;
- cefriaxone 25–50 mg/kg/day i.v. or i.m. as a single daily dose.

Treatment should be for a minimum of 7 days or 14 days of meningitis is diagnosed.

Ophthalmia neonatorum should be treated using antibacterial ointment or drops. The mother and father of all affected babies should be treated and any further contact traced.

Trichomoniasis

Trichomonas vaginalis is an ovoid flagellate protozoan parasite recognised by its characteristic jerking movement in wet preparation. It is sexually transmitted and is often associated with simultaneous yeast or gonococcal infection.

Clinical presentation

Trichomonas causes an irritating, persistent vaginitis, which worsens during menses and pregnancy when the vagina is more alkaline. The main symptom is an itchy or irritating greenish yellow, frothy, malodourous discharge. Clinical examination reveals reddened vaginal and cervical mucosa with petechial haemorrhages and extensive cervical erosion.

Diagnosis and investigation

The characteristic motile protozoa can be seen on wet mount preparations of specimens taken from the genital tract.

Treatment

Metranidazole 400 mg twice daily (but not during the first trimester of pregnancy because of potential teratogenicity).

Treponemal infections

Syphilis, yaws and pinta are all caused by treponemes which are indistinguishable morphologically and serologically.

Clinical apparent syphilis is rare in pregnancy in developed countries but failure to diagnose it can have severe long term effects in the mother and the baby. Routine antenatal screening is therefore still indicated.

Screening for syphilis

Blood is taken at the booking antenatal visit for VDRL (Venereal Disease Reference Laboratory) and TPHA (*Treponema pallidum* haemagglutination) tests.

More specific tests are needed if:

- screening tests are positive,
- there is a history of contact,
- there is clinical evidence of syphilis.

FTA (abs) (fluorescent treponemal antibody – absorbed) is the most sensitive test for syphilis.

Biological false positive reactions (BFPR) are much commoner than true infections and can occur as a result of pregnancy itself, after blood transfusion or associated with other conditions (e.g. systemic lupus erythematosus). FTA (abs) is negative in BFPR detected by other tests.

Treatment of syphilis

Early syphilis

- Aqueous procaine penicillin 900 000 units daily for 14 days, for primary and secondary syphilis and for three weeks in late syphilis;
or
- benzathine penicillin G 2.4 g in a single dose, if the patient is unable to come every day. Give a further stat dose. Use it also as a booster when treating primary and secondary and late syphilis, as a booster dose at weekends or if the patient is not able to attend on the odd occasion.

Latent syphilis

- Aqueous procaine penicillin as above; **or**
- benzathine penicillin – dose as above for three weeks.
  If the mother is allergic to penicillin use
- erythromycin 500 mg 6 hourly for three weeks.

Follow up

Repeat serology monthly for the remainder of the pregnancy. Re-treat any women who shows evidence of re-infection or serological relapse.

Following the pregnancy check VDRL, TPHA and FTA titres monthly for six months, three monthly for another six months and twice a year for two years.

Congenital syphilis

This condition can have serious effects on every organ and system of the developing fetus. Transplacental transmission occurs in 80–90 per cent in the first year of untreated infection. If untreated 25–30 per cent of fetuses will die *in utero* and a similar number post-natally. Forty per cent of the survivors will develop late symptomatic syphilis. After the second year of infection transmission to the fetus is rare. Infection is commoner in the first and second trimester. There were less than 20 cases of fetal infection in the UK from 1971 to 1987.

Adequate treatment of the mother is highly effective in preventing or reducing transmission. FTA (IgM) is used to detect neonatal infection. Treatment is by crystalline penicillin G 50 000 units/kg i.e. 50 mg/kg intramuscularly in a single daily dose.

BIBLIOGRAPHY

Best, J.M., Banatvala, J.E., Morgan-Capner, P. & Miller, E. (1989) Fetal infection after maternal reinfection with rubella: criteria for defining reinfection. *British Medical Journal*, **299**, 773–775.

Best, J.M. & Banatvala, J.E. (1990) Rubella. In: *Principles and Practice of Clinical Virology*, (Ed. by A.J. Zuckerman, J.E. Banatvala & J.R. Pattison) 2nd edn. pp 337–374. Chichester: John Wiley.

Brown, Z.A., Vontver, L.A., Benedetti, J., Critchlor, C.W., Sells, C.J., Berry, S. & Corey, L. (1987) Effects on infants from the first episode of genital herpes during pregnancy. *New England Journal of Medicine*, **317**, 1246–1251.

Connor, E.M., Sperling, R.S., Gelber, R., Kiselev, P., Scott, G., O'Sullivan, M.J., Van Dyke, R., Bey, M., Shearer, W., Jacobson, R.L., Jimenez, F., O'Neil, E., Bazin, B., Delfraissy, J.-F., Culnane, M., Coombs, R., Elkins, M., Moye, J., Stratton, P. & Balsley, J. (1994) Reduction of maternal–infant transmission of HIV-1 with Zidovudine treatment. *New England Journal of Medicine*, **331**, 1173–1180.

Joint Working Party for the Hospital Infection Society and the Surgical Infection Study Group (1992) Risks to surgcons and patients from HIV and hepatitis: guidelines on precautions and management of exposure to blood or body fluids. *British Medical Journal*, **205**, 1357–1343.

Peckham, C.S., Chin, K.S., Colman, J.C., Henderson, K., Hurley, R. & Preece, P. (1983) Cytomegalovirus infection in pregnancy: preliminary findings from a prospective study. *Lancet*, **i**, 1352–1355.

Public Health Laboratory Service Working Party on Fifth Disease (1990) Effective study of human parvovirus (B19) infection in pregnancy. *British Medical Journal*, **300**, 1166–1170.

Van Elsacker-Niele, A.M.W., Salimanas, M.M.M., Weiland, H.T., Vermey-Keers, C., Anderson, M.J. & Versteeg, J. (1989) Fetal pathology in human parvovirus B19 infection. *British Journal of Obstetrics & Gynaecology*, **96**, 768–775.

4.5   Neurological disorders of pregnancy

4

EPILEPSY

The effect of pregnancy on epilepsy is unpredictable for any woman. The best indication is the degree of control beforehand. The longer the period without seizure before pregnancy the smaller the likelihood of fits during it.

Greater seizure frequency may be due to altered drug handling or metabolism, e.g.

- plasma clearance is more rapid due to increased blood flow through liver and kidney, etc.,
- the plasma volume increases causing a relative reduction in drug levels,
- decreased gastrointestinal absorption,
- change in material pH (mild respiratory alkalosis) causes increased renal excretion.

Isolated seizures do not usually cause harm to the fetus, but status epilepticus may result in a high fetal and even maternal mortality.

Among the fetal effects can be dysmorphic facies (see below) and distal digital hypoplasia associated with phenytoin or carbamazepine exposure. There is also an increased incidence of neural tube defects of 1–2 per cent of fetuses exposed to valproic acid in the first trimester.

Pharmacological treatment of epilepsy

The main objectives are to use the smallest number of drugs (one only if possible), at the lowest dosage required to prevent convulsions.

The most commonly prescribed drugs are **carbamazepine** and **phenytoin**. Sodium valproate is best avoided because of the risk of neural tube defects. If, however, valproate is the only possible choice (e.g. for a specific type of epilepsy) exclude a neural tube defect in the fetus.

Check blood levels monthly.

Supplementation with folic acid 5 mg before and during pregnancy may decrease the incidence of birth defects. With women who are epileptic and in the childbearing age group, start a multivitamin tablet with folic acid 0.5–1 mg when contraception is stopped.

Anticonvulsant medication

Phenytoin sodium (dilantin)

Average dose is 400 mg/day in a single or divided dose. Up to 1200 mg/day may be required to maintain a therapeutic blood plasma level of **10–20 microgram/ml**. If seizures continue despite therapeutic medication levels with only one drug a second drug may be needed.

Phenobarbital

Average daily dose is 100 mg twice daily or three times daily. Therapeutic level is 10–20 microgram/mL. Measure the phenobarbital level after it has been taken for two weeks.

Clinical implications

Phenytoin can be associated with the **fetal hydantoin syndrome** which consists of craniofacial and limb abnormalities. Carbamazepine (tegretol) may cause craniofacial defects and fingernail hypoplasia, and valproic acid may result in fetal neural tube defects. All medications appear to increase the risk of mental retardation. Anticonvulsant drugs taken during the first trimester double the baby's risk of a major congenital malformation such as cleft lip, cleft palate, congenital heart disease. **However, seizures are a greater risk to the mother and fetus**.

Management of generalised tonic clonic status epilepticus in pregnancy

- Commence oxygen by face mask at a flow rate of 8 L/minute.
- Perform an ECG. Watch for the ECG changes of atrial and ventricular conduction depression or ventricular fibrillation.

- Insert an intravenous line and start an i.v. fusion of normal saline with vitamin B complex. Give a bolus of 50 mL 50 per cent glucose and 100 mg of thiamine i.m. Infuse diazepam i.v. 5 mg/minute to a total dose of 40 mg or until the seizure stops. Diazepam is only effective for 15–20 minutes. Commence i.v. phenytoin, infuse a total dose of 18 mg/kg body weight for 24 hours. If seizures persist, commence i.v. phenobarbital, 20 mg/kg at a rate no greater than 100 mg/minute until seizures stop or a loading dose of 20 mg/kg is given.
- Insert an endotracheal tube and monitor vital signs.

Management in labour

Anticonvulsant therapy can be given parenterally, e.g. phenytoin 100 mg every 6–8 hours i.v. (in normal saline) or phenobarbital 60 mg i.m. or i.v. every 6–8 hours. Because factors II, VII, IX and X are decreased in babies of mothers on anticonvulsant therapy, consider giving vitamin K 10 mg i.m. to reduce the risk of neonatal haemorrhage.

BELL'S PALSY

A facial paralysis sometimes occurs in the third trimester or the first two weeks post-partum. The closer the onset to birth, the better the prognosis for complete spontaneous recovery. The cause is presumed to be viral. A brief course of hydrocorticosteroid therapy may help those patients with complete weakness.

PITUITARY ADENOMAS

Usually pituitary tumours cause primary or secondary amenorrhoea, but ovulation induction with fertility drugs will enable women with a prolactinoma to become pregnant.

Five per cent of microadenomas less than 10 mm in diameter become symptomatic during pregnancy; 15–35 per cent of macroadenomas and extrasellar adenomas enlarge. Headache tends to precede visual field defects by one month. Visual acuity and visual field should be examined clinically. CT or MRI scanning is indicated if visual field defects develop. Measuring prolactin levels is not useful in pregnancy. If vision is impaired give bromocriptine. If despite treatment, the visual acuity is less than 20/50 or if bitemporal hemianopia encroaches upon nasal sectors, surgery may be indicated. Among the differential diagnosis of a pituitary mass found in the postpartum period is a lymphocytic hypophysitis.

BIBLIOGRAPHY

Delicio, D.J. (1985) Seizure disorders in pregnancy. *New England Journal of Medicine*, **312**, 559.

Kochenour, N.K., Morris, G.E. & Sawchuk, R J. (1980) Phenytoin metabolism of pregnancy. *Obstetrics & Gynecology*, **56**, 577–582.

MacGregor, J.A., Guberman, A. & Amer, J. (1987) Idiopathic facial nerve paralysis (Bell's palsy) in late pregnancy and the puerperium. *Obstetrics & Gynecology*, **69**, 435–438.

Molich, M.D. (1985) Pregnancy in the hypoprolactinaemic woman. *New England Journal of Medicine*, **312**, 1364.

Saunders, M. (1989) Epilepsy in women of childbearing age. *British Medical Journal*, **299**, 581.

4.6   Renal disease in pregnancy

RENAL PHYSIOLOGY

In pregnancy there is an increase in glomerular filtration rate (GFR) because of volume expansion. GFR and effective renal plasma flow (ERPF) increase by 50–80 per cent compared to the non-pregnant state.

Creatinine clearance is increased to 150–170 mL/min/1.73m^2 (1.35–2.20 mL/s/1.73m^2) (m is the standardisation for body size incorporating weight and height) by the end of the second timester of pregnancy. Values for creatinine considered normal in the non-pregnant woman, may be abnormal in pregnancy. Plasma levels of **creatinine** greater than **75 micromol/L** and **urea** greater than **4.5 mmol/L** require further investigation in renal function. The normal ranges for urea and creatinine in pregnancy are given in Table 4.6.1.

Abnormal proteinuria is >500 mg/24 hours. Some loss of protein is

Table 4.6.1 Creatinine and urea: mean levels pre-pregnancy and in pregnancy, and levels in renal disease.

	Pre-pregnancy	Pregnancy	Renal disease
Creatinine			
(micromol/L)	62	44	80
(mg/dL)	0.7	0.5	0.9
Urea			
(mmol/L)	4.5	3.2	5.0
(mg/dL)	13	9	14

due to the increase in GFR and ERPF. Women with underlying renal lesions may have marked increments in protein excretion during pregnancy, which should not be misconstrued as exacerbation of disease.

Abnormal plasma urate levels are >300 micromol/L (5.0 mg/dL).

The normal glucose excretion is 20–100 mmol/day – up to ten times the non-pregnant. Two thirds of healthy pregnant women will have glycosuria on dipstick testing to a degree conventionally considered clinically significant. Increases in GFR and ERPF may also explain the increased excretion of solutes, glucose, amino acids, water soluble vitamins and protein.

Acid–base regulation

A mild alkalaemia is present in pregnancy. Arterial blood pH increases to 7.42–7.44. P_{CO2} decreases from 36 mm Hg to 31 mm Hg. Plasma bicarbonate decreases by approximately 4 mmol/L. Values of 18–22 mmol/L are normal.

Plasma osmolality decreases early in pregnancy and at week 10 reaches a nadir of 8–10 mmol/kg below the non-pregnant value which is maintained through to term.

Dilatation of the renal tract in pregnancy

Kidney size increases by 1 cm. Urine volumes may vary because of large quantities of urine remaining in dilated collecting system. Urinary obstruction or stasis may explain why pregnant women with asymptomatic bacteriuria are more prone to develop pyelonephritis.

Vesico-ureteral reflux further disposes pregnant women to symptomatic infection.

URINARY TRACT INFECTION (UTI)

True bacteriuria is defined as > 100 000 bacteria of the same species per millilitre of urine. The commonest infecting organism is *Escherichia coli* (90 per cent).

Other organisms frequently responsible include species of *Klebsiella, Proteus*, coagulase-negative *Staphylococcus* and *Pseudomonas*.

Asymptomatic bacteriuria

Defined as true bacteriuria without subjective evidence of a urinary tract infection. It occurs in 5–7 per cent of pregnant women, 40 per cent of whom will develop symptomatic ascending infection and acute pyelonephritis. Prompt treatment early in pregnancy can prevent most cases of acute pyelonephritis.

Ampicillin or a cephalosporin are the antibiotics of choice (a single dose of amoxycillin 3 g orally is usually effective).

Treat coagulase-negative infection (*Staphylococcus albus*) with flucloxacillin 250 mg t.d.s.

Avoid

- **Sulphonamides**, because they competitively inhibit the binding of bilirubin to albumin and can increase the risk of neonatal hyperbilirubinaemia.
- **Nitrofurantoin** should be avoided in late pregnancy because of the risk of haemolysis due to deficiency of erythrocyte phosphate dehydrogenase in the newborn.
- **Tetracyclines** are contraindicated during pregnancy because they predispose to dental staining and rarely may cause acute fatty liver.

While **trimethoprim** is a folic acid antagonist it remains an extremely effective antibiotic for urinary tract infections and may be used in pregnancy with folic acid supplements. It can be used as a low dose prophylaxis (100 mg dose *nocte* combined with folic acid 5 mg) in women with a long term history of urinary tract infection.

Acute pyelonephritis

Acute pyelonephritis occurs in 1–2 per cent of all pregnancies. The usual symptoms of discomfort on voiding with urgency and increased frequency of micturition are common in pregnancy even in the absence of UTI. Diagnosis is confirmed by the finding of pus cells with culture of a significant bacterial pathogen.

If *Proteus* or *Pseudomonas* species are isolated, a structural abnormality of the renal tract or a calculus is likely. Ultrasound scanning of the kidneys will identify upper tract lesions that might need immediate treatment.

Physiological dilatation of the urinary tract of pregnancy may be mistaken for obstruction. Cortical scarring may require micturating cysto-urethrography to identify vesico-ureteric reflux.

Differential diagnosis of acute pyelonephritis

Other urinary tract pathology, other causes of pyrexia; respiratory tract infection, viraemia or toxoplasmosis; other causes of acute abdominal pain such as acute appendicitis, biliary colic, gastro-enteritis, uterine fibroid degeneration, rectus abdomenis haematoma or abruptio placenta.

Treatment

Antibiotic sensitivity should be identified within 48 hours and an appropriate antibiotic commenced. For Gram-negative infection, use an **aminoglycoside** because they are effective against nearly all of the Gram-negative urinary bacteria. **Netilmicin** (4–6 mg/kg/day in divided doses eight hourly) is preferred to gentamicin because it is far less toxic to the eighth nerve and is not nephrotoxic. Do not use in the presence of renal impairment (creatinine >100 micromol/L) without adjusting the dose. Measure peak netilmicin levels $1\frac{1}{2}$ hours after the dose and trough levels immediately before the next dose is given.

Treatment should be continued for at least 2 weeks.

Follow up with a urine culture one week after finishing the antibiotic course and two weekly to monthly throughout the pregnancy.

Recurrent infection commonly occurs in up to 30 per cent of women. Fifteen per cent continue to have positive urinary cultures. These require long-term low dose antibiotics, either a cephalosporin, ampicillin or trimethoprim and folic acid as a single evening dose.

Further investigation

This should be considered post partum for any woman who develops acute pyelonephritis (particularly if it is recurrent). Carry out a renal ultrasound scan 6 weeks post partum. If a significant abnormality is found arrange an intravenous urogram for not earlier than four months post partum and refer to a nephrologist.

CHRONIC RENAL DISEASE

The significance of haematuria

Macroscopic or microscopic haematuria in the presence of casts and significant proteinuria suggests glomerulonephritis. Glomerular lesions (e.g. thin membrane disease) are the commonest cause of microscopic and macroscopic haematuria in this age group.

- Culture the urine for bacteria, tuberculosis and cytology.
- Refer to a nephrologist.
- The diagnosis may be confirmed by a renal biopsy, but in the absence of proteinuria, with morphologically abnormal red blood cells, 90 per cent will have a thin membrane disease and 10 per cent minor glomerular abnormalities.
- Renal ultrasound identifies structural abnormalities such as calculi or renal cysts.
- Neoplastic causes should also be excluded.

Prognosis of chronic renal disease (see Table 4.6.2)

Mild renal deficiency – plasma creatinine <125 micromol/L (1.4 mg/dL)

Usually the outcome of the pregnancy is successful and the disease course is not usually affected in the absence of severe hypertension and proteinuria (>1 g/day).

Table 4.6.2 The outcome of pregnancy according to severity of renal disease: per cent complications.

Prospects for the pregnancy	Disease severity		
	Mild	Moderate	Severe
Pregnancy complication (per cent)	??	41	84
Successive obstetric outcome (per cent)	95	90	47
Long term sequelae (per cent) (End stage renal failure)	<5	25	100

Moderate renal deficiency – plasma creatinine 125–250 micromol/L

This may progress into serious renal deterioration, with uncontrolled hypertension, increasing proteinuria resulting in a variable obstetric outcome. Post-partum a decline in renal function may be exacerbated.

Severe renal deficiency (end stage renal disease) – plasma creatinine greater than 250 micromol/L (2.8 mg/dL)

Most women will have amenorrhoea and/or are anovulatory. The aim should be to preserve what little renal function remains and/or to achieve renal rehabilitation with dialysis and transplant. Pregnancy may then be reconsidered.

In severe renal disease (i.e. creatinine >250 micromol/L) pregnancy is not realistic. End stage renal failure managed with dialysis and transplantation while the woman is pregnant may be possible (see Table 4.6.2).

Investigations

Chronic renal disease may present as urinary tract infections, proteinuria with or without haematuria and casts, or nephrotic syndrome.

- Measure renal function – urinary protein loss and creatinine clearance.
- Exclude lupus nephritis (investigations: anti-nuclear antibodies, complement levels and anti-DNA antibodies).
- Measure renal size by ultrasound.

ANTENATAL CARE OF PATIENTS WITH RENAL DISEASE

- Visits at least every two weeks until 32/40, then weekly.
- A 24 hour creatinine clearance and protein excretion should be done fortnightly if there is increased excretion on dipstick testing.
- Blood pressure monitoring may include domiciliary monitoring and ambulatory monitoring to obtain a profile.
- Uric acid and platelets should be measured at each visit from 26 weeks' gestation as an indicator of superimposed pre-eclampsia.

Fetal assessment: size, development, well-being

The aim is to maintain blood pressure at not greater than **150/90 mm Hg** because of the risk of renal damage with increases in intraglomerular pressure. The appropriate level of blood pressure needs to be determined by the woman's age, previous non-pregnancy blood pressure and previous blood pressure in pregnancy. Achieving a 'normal' blood pressure (e.g. <140/90 mm Hg) may reduce renal perfusion and cause renal function to deteriorate. The same may occur with utero placental blood flow. Consult with a nephrologist as necessary.

Treatment of hypertension with associated renal disease

Drug treatment in patients with hypertension and renal disease needs to be adjusted before conception. Angiotensin converting enzyme (ACE) inhibitors (e.g. captopril) are considered to be contraindicated, because of the risk of severe fetal abnormalities in the first trimester and because they cross the placenta and can cause severe acute renal failure in the premature infant.

The management of hypertension is discussed in Section 4.1.

Long-term effects of pregnancy on renal disease

Pregnancy does not appear to cause any deterioration or affect the rate of progression of renal disease beyond what might have been expected in the non-pregnant state, providing pre-pregnancy kidney dysfunction was minimal and hypertension is absent or controlled during pregnancy, without significant proteinuria.

Urolithiasis

This occurs rarely in pregnancy but must be considered in the presence of microscopic haematuria, recurrent urinary tract infection, sterile urine culture when pyelonephritis is suspected. Ultrasound of the renal tract should be carried out.

RENAL TRANSPLANTATION

Women of childbearing age with a functioning renal transplant are increasingly likely to become pregnant. Forty per cent may end in the first trimester in abortion. More than 90 per cent that go past the first trimester are successful.

Pre-pregnancy counselling with a renal transplant

For pregnancy to be considered optimistically the following conditions should be fulfilled:

- Good general health for 2 years following renal transplant.
- No proteinuria.
- Blood pressure well controlled on agents not contraindicated in pregnancy.
- No evidence of graft rejection. The level of renal function should be stable. The creatinine level should be <200 micromol/L for the previous 12 months.
- Drug therapy should be at maintenance levels, i.e. prednisolone <10 mg/day (usually 7.5 mg/day, cyclosporin A approximately 5 mg/kg/day, and azothiaprine 2 mg/kg/day or less. (There is no indication that this dosage causes an increase in developmental abnormalities.)
- Serious rejection occurs in about ten per cent of pregnant renal allograft recipients but is lower in those on cyclosporins. There is an increased incidence of pre-eclampsia with a renal graft.

POST-PARTUM ACUTE RENAL FAILURE

This condition should be *suspected* when the urine volume remains inadequate, following adequate fluid replacement.

There are three types of acute renal failure:
- pre-renal failure;
- acute tubular necrosis;
- acute cortical necrosis.

Acute renal failure occurs in pre-eclampsia, severe obstetric haemorrhage, and other causes of obstetric shock such as pulmonary embolism, amniotic fluid embolism, uterine inversion.

- The patient should be catheterised and an hourly urine volume measured. Fluid replacement should be appropriate.
- Following careful clinical assessment of intra-operative or post-partum blood loss and assuming the patient is euvolemic, give replacement at **1 mL/kg/hour** i.e. approximately **80 mL/hour**.
- Fluid replacement involves a clinical assessment of the patient for signs of overload or fluid depletion.

- If the patient is oliguric, a safe fluid challenge consists of 100 mL aliquots up to 5 times over two hours. It should only be repeated after careful assessment of the patient's overall fluid status (i.e. addition of input, losses and output over a time period). Once the patient is judged to be in ideal balance, then **oliguria is suggestive of acute renal failure if there is an output of <30 mL/hour (0.5 mL/kg/hour) which persists for eight hours**. Consultation with a nephrologist and transfer to a renal dialysis unit is then mandatory.
- The majority of patients who are oliguric will spontaneously resolve in 12 hours. Particularly post-operatively there is an antidiuretic hormone effect contributed to by syntocinon in labour.
- In assessing fluid overload, in pre-eclampsia, the O_2 saturation using a pulse oximeter is the best guide. A value of <95 per cent on air should be considered as indicative of early pulmonary oedema and require an immediate chest X-ray and may require invasive investigation such as a central venous pressure (CVP) line (see p. 271).

RENAL FAILURE AND SEPTIC SHOCK

- The commonest cause is septic abortion which can be spontaneous or induced.
- Septic abortion may be life-threatening particularly if due to clostridia or Gram-negative organisms. The syndrome is characterised by an abrupt rise in temperature (>40°C) together with myalgia, vomiting, bloody diarrhoea, jaundice, hypotension, oliguria and progression to shock.

Laboratory investigations

These reveal a severe anaemia, with markedly elevated bilirubin levels (due to haemolysis) evidence of DIC and a striking leucocytosis (>50 000 mm^3). Hypocalcaemia occurs.
- The oliguric phase in women with tubular necrosis due to septic abortion may be prolonged to three or more weeks and total anuria may occur in this period.

HAEMOLYTIC URAEMIC SYNDROME

This is an uncommon syndrome that presents with compromised renal function. It may be preceded by a prodromal illness manifested by diarrhoea and vomiting usually associated with a normal blood pressure and occurs either about two weeks prior to delivery or up to six weeks after delivery.

- Jaundice may be clinically evident.
- Biochemically, there is acute renal failure (markedly raised serum creatinine), deranged liver function tests and significant haemolysis.
- The outcome is fatal in approximately 60 per cent of cases.
- Two thirds of patients require dialysis in the acute stage and 15 per cent long term.
- The treatment is early delivery, with appropriate treatment of coagulation abnormalities and strict adherence to fluid replacement intravenously at 1 mL/kg/hour i.e. approximately 80 mL/hour.

4

4.7   Asthma in pregnancy

Asthma results from increased responsiveness of the bronchi causing widespread reversible narrowing of the airway. It is precipitated in susceptible individuals by exposure to allergens or other inhaled irritants. It may be acute or chronic (persistent). It complicates about one per cent of pregnancies.

SYMPTOMS

- Wheezing and/or persistent cough.
- Symptoms tend to be worse during the night and on first waking in the morning.
- Many pregnant women experience an increase in symptoms because they stop or reduce their medication due to mistaken fears about its safety during pregnancy.

COMPLICATIONS

- Recurrent maternal hypoxaemia can result in intrauterine growth retardation and even loss of the fetus.

- Severe attacks can lead to maternal death.

PRINCIPLES OF MANAGEMENT OF ASTHMA

- Pregnancy is an opportunity to review previously undiagnosed or inadequately managed asthma. **Do not stop or reduce asthma medication in pregnant patients**.
- All patients should have their own peak flow meter and keep regular records to give an objective measurement of the severity of their asthma.
- A clear written management plan of the action to be taken at varying levels of deterioration should reduce the morbidity from asthma.
- Smoking should be avoided.
- Medication aims to abolish symptoms and restore normal function of the airways.
- Medications commonly used in the management of asthma show no evidence of any teratogenic effect.
- There is less experience with the more recently introduced inhaled steroid budesonide and with the inhaled anticholinergic ipratropium, but they both appear safe.
- Oral steroids and oral beta-2 adrenoreceptor agonists may affect glucose metabolism. This is particularly important in those with impaired glucose tolerance.
- Neither oral nor inhaled beta-adrenoreceptor agonists delay the onset or slow the progress of labour and they should not be withheld.
- Ergometrine may cause bronchospasm and should be avoided after delivery.
- Breast feeding is safe with asthma medication.
- Avoid prostaglandins in women with a history of asthma because of the risk of severe bronchospasm.

TYPES OF MEDICATION FOR THE TREATMENT OF CHRONIC PERSISTENT ASTHMA

The following guidelines for therapy have been given in the guidelines for management of asthma in adults by the British Thoracic Society (British Thoracic Society, 1990a).

1 Bronchodilators

Inhaled beta-2 adrenoreceptor agonist (by inhalation) (such as salbu-tamol 100–200 micrograms or terbutaline 250–500 micrograms) should be used as required rather than regularly.

2 Inhaled anti-inflammatory agents

- Necessary for those who need to inhale a bronchodilator more than once daily, or who have night time symptoms.
- Prescribe them for use on a regular basis rather than as necessary. Alternatives are listed below.

3 Inhaled corticosteroids – beclomethasone dipropionate or budesonide 100–400 micrograms twice daily

Continue or increase medication for:

(i) persistent symptoms (especially nocturnal);

(ii) a continuing need for inhaled bronchodilators;

(iii) suboptimal peak flow (the woman's peak flow will usually be known).

Once symptoms and peak flow have improved, reduce the dose of inhaled steroid to the minimum that maintains control. If control with beta-2 agonist is not achieved, check compliance and method of administration. Maximum dose 2 mg.

Use a large volume spacer device to reduce oropharyngeal side effects and systemic absorption once the dose of inhaled steroids exceeds 800 micrograms daily, **or sodium cromoglycate 5–20 mg four times daily.**

Neodocromil sodium 4 mg four times daily.

4 Additional inhaled bronchodilators

Ipratropium bromide 80 micrograms four times daily.

Oral beta-2 agonists and methylxanthines should not be used as first line drugs. Main indication: night time symptoms, not controlled by high doses of anti-inflammatory drugs and standard doses of inhaled beta-2 agonists. A single, long acting night time dose of a slow release beta-2 agonist or methylxanthine may be used. Methylxanthines (e.g. aminophylline) have a narrow therapeutic/toxicity ratio. Levels need to be monitored.

5 High dose inhaled bronchodilators

Use only if the patient does not respond to standard doses. Beta-2 agonists and anticholinergics can be given from prediluted phials through a nebuliser:

- Salbutamol 2.5–5 mg
- Terbutaline $\leqslant 10$ mg
- Ipratropium 250–500 micrograms.

Oral steroids

A short course of oral steroids is indicated in the presence of:

- deteriorating peak respiratory flow;
- peak expiratory flow <60 per cent of patient's best result;
- sleep disturbance by asthma;
- morning symptoms persisting until mid-day.

Give prednisolone 30 mg daily, until two days after full recovery. (The dose of steroids does not need to be tapered if treatment has only been for one week.)

MANAGEMENT OF ACUTE SEVERE ASTHMA

A severe attack is defined by:

- high arterial carbon dioxide tension (P_{aCO_2}>6 kPa) in a breathless asthmatic patient;
- severe hypoxia: arterial oxygen tension (P_{aO_2}<8 kPa irrespective of treatment with oxygen);
- a low pH.

The following are potentially life threatening features which require expert medical assistance:

1 Clinical

- Increasing wheeze and breathlessness. Patient is unable to complete sentences in one breath or to get up from chair or bed.

- Respiratory rate $\geqslant 25$ breaths per minute, heart rate persistently greater than 110 beats per minute, peak expiratory flow <40 per cent of predicted normal, or of the best obtainable result if known (<200 L/minute if the best obtainable result is not known).

Imminently life threatening signs

- A silent chest on auscultation, cyanosis, bradycardia, exhaustion, confusion or unconsciousness.
- A rising P_{CO_2} despite medication

2 Investigations
Arterial blood gas measurements should be taken and repeated half an hour after treatment with bronchodilators, aminophylline and steroids. The woman's condition may become critical if the P_{CO_2} fails to come down with treatment.

Emergency treatment

1 Oxygen. Use the highest concentration available and set at a high flow rate.
2 High doses of inhaled beta-2 agonist, e.g. salbutamol 2.5–5 mg or terbutaline 5–10 mg and ipratropium bromide using a nebuliser. The two drugs may be combined and given in one nebuliser.
3 Give steroids, prednisolone 30 mg is effective given orally if the woman can swallow it or intravenous hydrocortisone 100 mg.

Ongoing treatment

Nursing staff must monitor the peak flow before and after medication is given. Medical staff must return to the woman and check the condition is improving. Repeat blood gases as necessary.
4 Intravenous bronchodilators, intravenous aminophylline 250 mg over 30 minutes or a beta-2 agonist salbutamol 200 micrograms or terbutaline 200 micrograms over 10 minutes.
5 Give a beta-2 agonist if the patient is already taking oral theophylline.
6 After the above give oral prednisolone 30 mg daily, or intravenous hydrocortisone 100 mg six hourly.
7 If the condition is improving give nebulised beta-2 agonist four hourly.
8 If not improved after 15–30 minutes repeat nebulisation and add ipratropium bromide 0.5 mg to the nebuliser solution.
9 If there still has not been improvement consider giving aminophylline or parenteral beta-2 agonist – aminophylline infusion 0.5–0.9 mg/kg/hour). If the woman is already on methylxanthines, check a level first to avoid toxicity.
▪ Alternatively give a salbutamol or terbutaline infusion (parenteral beta-2 agonist) 12.5 microgram/minute; range 3–20 microgram/minute.
▪ The rate of infusion should be adjusted according to the responses of the peak expiratory flow and heart rate.

Further investigations after treatment of the initial acute episode of asthma include a chest X-ray (to exclude a pneumothorax and to diagnose an exacerbating infection), plasma electrolytes, urea and full blood count.

Monitoring of treatment

- Measure peak expiratory flow every 15 minutes until the peak flow has almost reached normal for the woman. Measure and record the rate before and after the woman has taken nebulised or inhaled beta-2 agonist.
- Repeat blood gas analysis within two hours of starting treatment if either the initial P_{aO_2} was less than 8 kPa or the initial P_{aCO_2} was normal or raised or the patient's condition deteriorates.

Indications for artificial ventilation

Intermittent positive pressure ventilation is required if the P_{aO_2}<8 kPa and a P_{aCO_2}>6 kPa despite receiving 60 per cent oxygen, or if the woman is exhausted.

Subsequent management

Control of asthma is achieved when symptoms have cleared and lung function has stabilised or returned to normal or best level, identified by a peak expiratory flow of >75 per cent of the predicted level with less than a 25 per cent diurnal variation or deterioration, with no nocturnal symptoms.

- Commence inhaled steroids at least 48 hours before discharge. Discharge the woman taking one oral steroid (prednisolone 20 mg daily) for one week and inhaled bronchodilator (see above). Oral steroids can be stopped (or tailed off if the woman is on long term therapy and there is a risk of adrenosuppression) as long as the asthma is not worsening.
- Women may monitor their own treatment for asthma according to peak flow measurements as shown below.

Management of asthma according to peak flow

- **If peak flow greater than 70% of normal**

Continue maintenance treatment:

    (a) Bronchodilator twice daily or when needed.

    (b) Inhaled steroid twice daily.

- **If peak flow less than 70% of normal**

    (1) Double dose of inhaled steroid for number of days required to achieve previous baseline.

    (2) Continue on this increased dose for same number of days.

    (3) Return to previous dose of maintenance treatment.

- **If peak flow less than 50% of normal**

    (1) Start oral prednisolone 40 mg daily. Contact general practitioner.

    (2) Continue on this dose for the number of days required to achieve previous baseline.

    (3) Reduce to 20 mg daily for the same number of days.

    (4) Stop prednisolone.

- **If peak flow less than 30% of normal**

    (1) Contact general practitioner urgently or, if unavailable

    (2) Contact ambulance or, if unavailable

    (3) Go directly to hospital

(Peak flow self management plan from Fig. 1, Charlton *et al.* (1990).)

BIBLIOGRAPHY

British Thoracic Society, Research Unit of the Royal College of Physicians of London, King's Fund Centre, National Asthma Campaign. (1990a) Guidelines for management of asthma in adults: I – Chronic persistent asthma. *British Medical Journal*, **301**, 651–654.

British Thoracic Society, Research Unit of the Royal College of Physicians of London, King's Fund Centre, National Asthma Campaign. (1990b) Guidelines for management of asthma in adults: II – Acute severe asthma. *British Medical Journal*, **301**, 797–800.

Beasley, R., Cushley, M. & Holgate, S.T. (1989) A self-management plan in the treatment of adult asthma. *Thorax*, **44**, 200–204.

Charlton, I., Charlton, G., Broomfield, J. & Mullee, MA. (1990) Evaluation of peak flow and symptom only self management plans for control of asthma in general practice. *British Medical Journal*, **301**, 1355–1359.

4.8 Haemolytic disease of the newborn (HDN)

RHESUS DISEASE

The rhesus system has three alleles – C or c, D and E or e – which are inherited en bloc, e.g. CDE or cDe. D is the most potent of the Rh antigens and those possessing the D gene are termed rhesus-positive (DD homozygous, or D heterozygous).

A small number (perhaps 1 per cent) of pregnant Rh negative women develop immune anti-D in spite of anti-D prophylaxis. Clinically significant rhesus iso-immunisation is usually against the D antigen. It also occurs less often and usually less seriously against the c, and E and K antigens of the Kell blood group system.

Fifteen per cent of the population are Rh(D) negative and about 13 per cent of all partnerships (about 1 : 8) will be between a Rh positive man and a Rh negative woman. Forty per cent of men are heterozygous for D, so 67 per cent of children are Rh(D) positive.

In 10 per cent of pregnancies in which the mother is D negative the fetus will be D positive. After a mother has had one D negative fetus the chance of a second one being D negative is only 6:100.

The risk of sensitisation is less in women after a first trimester miscarriage. The risk of D immunisation following termination of the pregnancy in a D negative woman is four per cent.

Prophylaxis and treatment has meant that the incidence of neonatal deaths from HDN due to rhesus disease was 1/65 000 at the end of the 1980s compared to 1/2000 in the 1950s.

Spontaneous immunisation occurs in approximately 18/2000, i.e. approximately 1 per cent, usually detected by antibody screen in the last few weeks of pregnancy.

Pathophysiology of iso-immunisation

If Rh(D) fetal cells enter the circulation of a rhesus negative woman her immune system may become sensitised. The degree of sensitisation depends on the volume of the feto-maternal transfusion.

Subsequent challenge by Rh(D) erythrocytes (in the same or a later pregnancy) will result in a variable degree of IgG antibody formation.

IgG antibodies cross to the fetal circulation and cause fetal red blood cells to be destroyed by the reticuloendothelial system. This leads to haemolytic anaemia and, in severe cases, hydrops. Progressive fetal anaemia causes tissue hypoxia and extramedullary erythropiesis in the yolk sac, liver or medullary systems (depending on gestation). This can cause hepatomegaly, portal and umbilical venous obstruction, and hypertension. Impaired liver function results in decreased albumin production, ascites, generalised oedema and often pleural effusion (hydrops).

Management of the rhesus negative woman

All pregnant woman are grouped and tested for rhesus antibodies at booking. This is repeated in rhesus negative women at 26 and 32 weeks.

If the woman has Rh(D) antibodies, determine the Rh status of the father of the child. If he is Rh-negative, the fetus should be Rh-negative. If the father is Rh-positive, check his ABO group and Rh phenotype. Depending on his Rh phenotype, the likelihood of his Rh zygosity should be determined. If he is heterozygous, there is a 50 per cent chance that the fetus will be Rh-negative, halving the risk of Rh immunisation. If the father is ABO incompatible with his partner, there is about a 60 per cent chance that the baby will be ABO incompatible. If the fetus is ABO incompatible, the risk of Rh immunisation is reduced tenfold (16 per cent to <2 per cent).

Prophylaxis for rhesus disease

The incidence of rhesus sensitisation has declined due to effective prophylaxis using Rh(D) immunoglobulin (anti-D). **The standard UK dose of anti-D is 100 micrograms (500 IU) within 72 hours of the potentially sensitising event.**

American practice has been to use 300 microgram doses of anti-D.

(1) Antenatal prophylaxis

- Antepartum haemorrhage: give 50 micrograms (250 IU) as a standard dose or 100 micrograms (500 IU) or more if indicated by Kleihauer test.
- Give 100 micrograms (500 IU) to all Rh(D) negative mothers at 28 and 34 weeks, except those who already have antibodies.

(2) Postpartum prophylaxis

- **A Kleihauer test** identifies the volume of fetal cells in the maternal circulation and should be done for all women who are rhesus negative to check evidence of a greater than average maternal bleed, e.g. placental abruption, manual removal of the placenta or fulminating pre-eclampsia.

- After a normal delivery, 1/100 women have 3 mL or more of fetal red cells in their circulation; 1/300 have 10 mL or more; 1/1000 have a massive transplacental haemorrhage (25 mL of red cells).

- The dose of anti-D immunoglobulin is based on the ability of 100 micrograms (500 IU) to suppress immunisation by 4 mL of fetal cells.

- If the Kleihauer test showed a transplacental haemorrhage of more than 4 mL, additional anti-D should be given.

- Where a large dose of anti-D immunoglobulin is needed to combat massive feto-maternal transfusion, vials containing 2500 IU or 5000 IU should be used and the dose divided between two or more intramuscular sites. Doses of anti-D immunoglobulin should be limited to 10 IU intramuscularly per day. Further Kleihauer tests should be carried out every 48 hours to check the disappearance of fetal cells and to decide if further doses of anti-D immunoglobulin are required. Significant clearance may not be seen for 72 hours or more.

Anti-D immunoglobulin

Anti-D immunoglobulin is prepared from donor plasma mostly derived from deliberately immunised Rh-negative volunteers.

The intramuscular preparation of anti-D immunoglobulin used in the UK have shown no evidence of viral transmission in over 20 years of routine use.

Use of anti-D after miscarriage

Rh(D) negative women should be given anti-D immunoglobulin following abortion, 50 micrograms (250 IU) before 20 weeks and 100 micrograms (500 IU) after 20 weeks, depending on the result of the Kleihauer test. Give anti-D to all Rh(D) negative women with a threatened miscarriage after 12 weeks' gestation or an ectopic pregnancy.

Where bleeding continues intermittently the injection should be repeated at approximately six weekly intervals until delivery. During pregnancy some spontaneous transplacental haemorrhage occurs throughout, the but individual episodes rarely lead to an immune response. Recognised factors that may lead to a transplacental hae-morrhage causing allo-immunisation when 100 micrograms (500 IU) anti-D immunoglobulin should be administered are: chorion villus sampling, aminocentesis, external cephalic version, and ante-partum haemorrhage.

Failure rates of anti-D prophylaxis

Using 100–300 micrograms of anti-D immunoglobulin immediately after delivery, the number of D negative women who develop anti-D within the following six months is less than 5 per cent. This decreases to about 1.5 per cent after a second pregnancy.

Identifying the patient at risk of rhesus disease and assessing the severity of the maternal antibody level

Rhesus-negative mothers should have serum sampled for anti-D at the time of booking and again at 26 and 32 weeks to detect any antibodies induced by the index pregnancy.

A first sensitised pregnancy

In a first sensitised pregnancy, the risk of the fetus being affected is so low that they can be evaluated by monthly anti-D titres and serial ultrasound to identify any ascites. So long as the titre remains low, there is little risk of significant fetal anaemia and the pregnancy can usually be allowed to continue to term without other testing or intervention.

The severity of rhesus disease is not directly proportional to maternal serum anti-D levels.

Management of a subsequent pregnancy

If the maternal anti-D titre is 4 IU/mL, or greater, further assessment or referral is required. With maternal serum anti-D levels less than 4 IU/mL the fetus is likely to minimally affected with less than 5 per cent requiring neonatal exchange transfusion for hyperbilir-ubinaemia.

Levels between 4 and 8 IU/mL may lead to moderate disease and warrant further assessment and possibly delivery by 38 weeks.

Anti-D levels at or above 10 IU/mL need further investigation and delivery is likely to be necessary by 36 weeks. (Note: Levels can be high from a previous pregnancy and the index pregnancy may not be affected because the fetus is Rh-negative (identified from cordocentesis) as a result of the father being heterozygous).

Fewer than 20 per cent of rhesus patients have anti-D levels greater than 20 IU/mL. Levels at this range imply moderate to severe disease in the fetus.

Maternal serum antibody levels need to be measured fortnightly. The rate of rise of maternal antibody titres is important. Increases of 15 IU/mL or more suggest moderate or severe rhesus disease in the fetus.

Maternal anti-D titres do not accurately predict fetal status in a subsequent affected pregnancy. The rate of rise in anti-D titres may be much more helpful. The fetus tends to be more severely affected at the same or an earlier gestation. When previous fetuses have been moderately to severely affected cordocentesis in the current pregnancy can commence as early as 18–22 weeks' gestation.

Severity of iso-immunisation

The following indicate the severity of iso-immunisation in a previous pregnancy:
- The gestation at which fetal transfusion was necessary.
- The gestation at which delivery was necessary.
- The presence or absence of hydrops.
- the degree of neonatal jaundice, need for phototherapy, or exchange transfusion.
- The degree of anaemia: (haemoglobin level; (see Fig. 4.8.1 for haemoglobin levels and haematocrit for varying gestations). Severe anaemia is where there is a reduction in Hb of more than two standard deviations for gestational age at which the baby was delivered.
- Level of Rh antibodies in cord blood – the magnitude of antibody titre and the strength of reaction – whether 'Coombs' positive' or 'Coombs' negative'.

A direct Coombs' test is carried out on the baby's blood to test for antibodies to D on the fetal red blood cells. The baby's red blood cells are incubated with rabbit anti-human globulin. Haemagglutination takes place if Rh antibodies are present on the fetal red cells. An indirect Coombs' is used to identify maternal antibody against the rhesus red blood cell antigen (e.g. D), for which one is testing. Rhesus positive red cells are added to the maternal serum followed by rabbit anti-human globulin. If there is anti-D IgG in maternal serum it will be fixed to the Rh(D) positive cells which will be agglutinated by the second antibody.

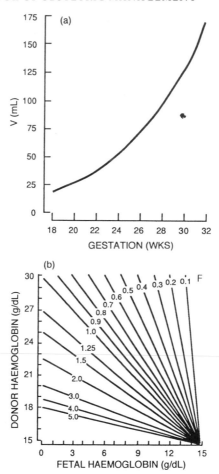

Fig. 4.8.1 A nomogram for intravascular transfusion. The value F is multiplied by the value V, e.g. for a fetus at 24 weeks the blood volume is 50 mL. If the pre-transfusion fetal haemoglobin is 5 g/dL, and the donor blood haemoglobin is 26 g/dL (value F = 0.9), then 45 mL donor blood will need to be transfused to achieve a post-transfusion fetal haemoglobin of 12.5 g/dL (normal mean for gestation). (Reproduced with permission from Nicolaides, K.H., Soothill, P.W., Clewell, W.H., Rodeck, C.H., Mibashan, R.S. & Campbell, S. (1988) Fetal haemoglobin measurement in the assessment of red cell isoimmunisation. *The Lancet*, **1**, 1074.)

Management principles of subsequent pregnancy

The presence of maternal Rh antibodies requires close surveillance in the next pregnancy. In general surveillance and possibly treatment is commenced **10 weeks** before the earliest gestation at which a previously affected baby required delivery (but not before 20 weeks). Every case needs to be individually assessed.

Management of rhesus disease in the fetus

The fetus is assessed initially by **ultrasound** to check for fetal hydrops: 'Doppler' studies may help to identify a hyperdynamic circulation associated with anaemia.

Amniocentesis Amniotic fluid bilirubin levels correlate with the severity of any haemolysis. Spectrophotometry to measure the optical density (OD) at 450 nanometres shows a peak directly proportional to the quantity of bilirubin. The amount of shift is called the delta (Δ) OD 450. The necessity for and an interval between amniocenteses are determined by the bilirubin levels.

Liley (1961) (Fig. 4.8.2) recommended management on the basis of the change in Δ OD 450 and neonatal outcome. He placed the Δ OD 450 in three zones:

- Zone I – fetus unaffected or with mild anaemia
- Zone II – moderately affected
- Zone III – severely affected.

    Management can be based on these zones as follows:

- Zone I: Await spontaneous delivery at term.
- Zone II: Repeat aminocentesis in 10–14 days: if still in Zone II induce labour at 37–38 weeks' gestation.

    If the Δ OD 450 is now in Zone III, deliver or perform a fetal blood sample and intrauterine transfusion, depending on the gestational age.

- Zone III: Repeat in 7-10 days. Consider a fetal blood sample. It is likely that transfusion will be required every two weeks until delivery.

    Note: False positives may occur in Zone III and false negatives in Zone II).

Cordocentesis

This provides a definitive diagnosis and a means of treatment. It is usually carried out

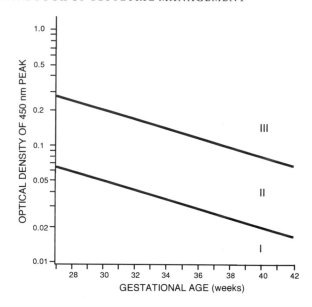

Fig. 4.8.2 The change in optical density at 450 nanometres: Zones I, II and III indicate treatment options. (Reproduced with permission from Liley, A.W. (1961) Liquor amnii analysis in the management of the pregnancy complicated by rhesus sensitization. *American Journal of Obstetrics & Gynecology*, **82**, 1362.

- 10 weeks before a previous fetal death, intrauterine transfusion or birth of a severely affected baby,
- if maternal antibody levels are >20 IU/mL.

It must only be carried out in specialist centres.

A 22 gauge spinal needle is used under direct ultrasound guidance. The fetal blood is collected into isotonic EDTA solution.

Fetal blood is identified by measuring red cell size in the Coulter counter and comparing the fetal mean corpuscular volume (118 to 135 femtolitres) with the maternal mean corpuscular volume (80–90 femtolitres).

The sample is tested for fetal blood group, direct Coombs' test, haemocrit and haemoglobin.

- Rh-negative fetuses require no further testing.
- Rh-positive fetuses with low haematocrits have treatment at the

same time as initial diagnosis: therefore fresh blood has to be organised and available for suspected cases.

Blood transfusion in the fetus

Donor blood should not be more than 72 hours old and ABO compatible, rhesus and Kell negative and screened for CMV, hepatitis and HIV. It is irradiated to kill leucocytes and packed to about 70 per cent of previous volume.

The quantity of blood to be transfused is calculated from an estimation of the feto-placental blood volume (Fig. 4.8.3), a pre-transfusion fetal haematocrit, and the haematocrit of transfused blood.

Transfusions need not be restricted to the second and early third trimesters of pregnancy, but once the fetus is 'viable' the risks of subsequent transfusion must be balanced against the chances of intact neonatal survival.

Complications of cordocentesis

The risk of loss in best centres is no higher than 1 per cent. Complications include haemorrhage from the umbilical vessels; tamponade

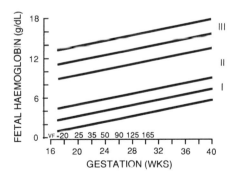

Fig. 4.8.3 Fetal haemoglobin concentration. Reference range with individual 95% confidence intervals of the normal haemoglobin for the gestation define Zone 1, and the individual 95% confidence intervals of the haemoglobin for gestation of the hydropic fetuses define Zone III. Zone II indicates moderate anaemia. (Reproduced with permission from Nicolaides, K.H., Soothill, P.W., Clewell, W.H., Rodeck, C.H., Mibashan, R.S. & Campbell, S. (1988) Fetal haemoglobin measurement in the assessment of red cell isoimmunisation. *The Lancet*, **1**, 1074.)

and thrombosis of the umbilical artery; infection, fetal bradycardia and stillbirth. Transplacental haemorrhage also occurs and may cause a considerable increase in the maternal antibody level.

Subsequent transfusions are determined by the need to prevent the haemoglobin dropping to cause hydrops in the fetus. This depends on:

- The fetal haematocrit achieved at the end of the previous transfusion.

- The rate of decrease in fetal haematocrit of approximately 1 per cent per day (0.3 g/day) (but can be greater in severe disease).

The rate of haemolysis depends on the activity of the disease. The interval between subsequent transfusions should successively increase because the fetal blood is being replaced by donor blood compatible with maternal blood. This means it is not prone to destruction by the antibodies. The aim is to maintain the fetal haematocrit and haemoglobin in the normal range of gestation (see Fig. 4.8.3).

Hydrops will not occur if the fetal haematocrit is greater than one third of the normal mean for gestation.

In general a repeat fetal transfusion is required every 2–3 weeks timed to the date of delivery and taking into account risks of the procedure and the overall fetal condition.

The significance of hyperbilirubinaemia at birth

Cord haemoglobin

Most babies with a cord haemoglobin concentration within the normal range do not require exchange transfusion.

Serum bilirubin level (see Fig. 4.8.4)

- Hyperbilirubinaemia is defined as a bilirubin level of 17 micromol/L or greater.

- Jaundice occurs when serum bilirubin levels exceed 85 micromol/L. Kernicterus is unlikely to develop with serum bilirubin concentrations below 342 micromol/L. This is the level for an exchange transfusion in a normal term baby.

- With haemolytic disease of the newborn management depends on whether the baby is term or preterm and on its overall clinical condition.

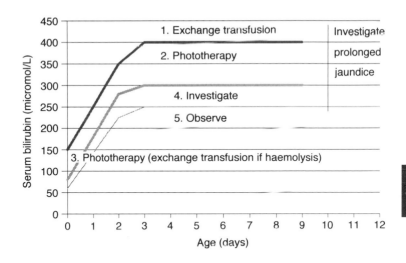

Fig. 4.8.4 Guidelines for the management of neonatal jaundice in term babies. (Courtesy Dr N. Marlow.)

Management

Measure Hb, haematocrit and bilirubin on cord blood taken at delivery. An exchange transfusion should be considered if:

- The cord haemoglobin is below 10 g/dL and/or the unconjugated bilirubin concentration is 80–100 micromol/dL. If immediate transfusion is not required and the baby is clinically jaundiced, start phototherapy. Repeat the serum bilirubin estimate on the baby every 4–6 hours.
- The rate of rise of the bilirubin is more than 20 micromol/L; this suggests extensive haemolysis, and an exchange transfusion is likely to be necessary within hours.

The baby who has had an intrauterine blood transfusion may have a cord bilirubin level higher than 100 micromol/dL suggesting the need for an exchange transfusion. However, since these babies have more donor and fewer sensitised fetal red blood cells, haemolysis will occur at a slower rate and exchange transfusion may not be necessary immediately.

HDN due to anti-Kell antibodies

HDN due to anti-Kell antibodies is uncommon but hydrops fetalis may develop quite rapidly in fetuses when anti-Kell antibodies are present. They can have a disproportionate effect on red cell precursors causing relatively more anaemia and less jaundice. There is a poor correlation between the severity of the disease and the antibody titre in the mother's serum. Low titres have been associated with hydrops.

ABO INCOMPATIBILITY

Anti-A and anti-B antibodies belong to a non-complement fixing subclass of IgG unable to mediate red cell destruction. Therefore high titres of anti-A or anti-B are not associated with severe cases of ABO haemolytic disease.

In 15 per cent of pregnancies the mother is blood group O and the baby is A or B, but this does not result in haemolytic disease *in utero*.

In HDN due to ABO incompatibility the haemoglobin concentration of cord blood may be below normal limits but is shortlived with an anaemia only lasting about two weeks. Rises in serum bilirubin can be controlled by phototherapy.

Management

Because ABO incompatibility seldom causes severe haemolytic disease, routine antenatal testing for anti-A and anti-B antibodies is not indicated. In women who have a history suggesting that a previous infant has been affected with ABO haemolytic disease, cord blood should be taken and tested after birth.

BIBLIOGRAPHY

Bowell, P.J., Wainscot, J.S., Peto, T.E.A. & Gunson, H.H. (1982) Maternal anti-D concentrations and outcome in rhesus haemolytic disease of the newborn. *British Medical Journal*, **285**, 327–329.

Caine, M.E. & Mueller-Heubach, E. (1986) Kell sensitization in pregnancy. *American Journal of Obstetrics & Gynecology*, **154**, 85–90.

Clarke, C.A. & Mollison P.L. (1989) Deaths from Rh haemolytic disease of the fetus and newborn, 1977–1987. *Journal of the Royal College of Physicians*, **23**, 181–184.

Hussey, R. & Clarke, C.A. (1991) Deaths from Rh haemolytic disease in England and Wales in 1988 and 1989. *British Medical Journal*, **303**, 445–446.

Liley, A.W. (1961) Liquor amnii analysis in management of pregnancy complicated by rhesus sensitization. *American Journal of Obstetrics & Gynecology*, **81**, 1359–1370.

Mayne, K.M., Bowell, P.J. & Pratt, G.A. (1990) The significance of anti-Kell sensitization in pregnancy. *Clinical & Laboratory Haematology*, **12**, 379–385.

Nicolaides, K.H., Rodeck, C.H., Millar, D.S. & Mibashan, R.S. (1985a) Fetal haematology in rhesus isoimmunization. *British Medical Journal*, **290**, 661–663.

Nicolaides, K.H., Warenski, J.C. & Rodeck, C.H. (1985b) The relationship of fetal plasma protein concentration in haemoglobin level to the development of hydrops in rhesus isoimmunization. *American Journal of Obstetrics & Gynecology*, **152**, 341–344.

Nicolaides, K.H., Rodeck, C.H., Mibashan, R.S. & Kemp, J.R. (1986) Have Liley charts outlived their usefulness? *American Journal of Obstetrics & Gynecology*, **155**, 90–94.

Nicolaides, K.H., Soothill, P.W., Clewell, W.H., Rodeck, C.H., Mibashan, R.S. & Campbell, S. (1988) Fetal haemoglobin measurement in the assessment of red cell immunisation. *The Lancet*, **i**, 1073–1075.

Osborn, L.M., Lenarsky, C., Oakes, R.C. & Reiff, M.I. (1984) Phototherapy in full-term infants with hemolytic disease secondary to ABO incompatibility. *Pediatrics*, **74**, 371–374.

Tovey, L.A.D. (1986) Haemolytic disease of the newborn – the changing scene. *British Journal of Obstetrics & Gynaecology*, **93**, 960–966.

4

4.9   Thromboembolism

INCIDENCE

Thromboembolism accounted for 33 deaths (16 per cent), 13 antepartum (over half before 20 weeks and most before 33 weeks gestation) and 11 post-partum (mostly after discharge from hospital) in the most recent triennial report on confidential enquiries into maternal death 1987–90 (Department of Health and Social Security, 1994).

Some women who died had unrecognised deep vein thrombosis or negative investigations; therefore the diagnosis was thought to have been excluded. Inadequate treatment of symptoms is an additional factor.

The incidence of deep vein thrombosis is almost 0.1 per cent during pregnancy and almost 2 per cent following caesarean section (i.e. 20 times greater).

The risk of fatal pulmonary embolus is at least ten times greater following caesarean section than vaginal delivery. A difficult instrumental delivery increases the risk.

REASONS FOR INCREASED RISK OF THROMBOSIS IN PREGNANCY

There is an increase in circulating coagulant factors in pregnancy. Factor VIII (the essential factor of the intrinsic system) and factor VII (the main component of the intrinsic system) are increased up to ten times. Fibrinogen (factor I) doubles from 2.4–4.0 g/L in the non-pregnant woman to 6.0 g/L in late pregnancy.

The naturally occurring anticoagulants antithrombin III, Protein C and its cofactor Protein S are increased in pregnancy. Physiological changes occur in pregnancy to alter the usual balance between the procoagulants and anticoagulants that achieve blood clotting. Antithrombin III is the essential heparin cofactor and exerts is main influence against factors Xa and thrombin. Protein C and Protein S balance activity in the procoagulant factors V and VIII. Occasionally, inherited deficiencies lead to a high risk of thromboembolism.

Fibrinolysis activity is reduced in pregnancy, due to placentally derived plasminogen activator.

DIAGNOSIS OF DEEP VEIN THROMBOSIS (DVT)

Clinical signs

The most consistent clinical sign of a deep vein thrombosis is an acutely tender swollen calf, but up to 50 per cent of women with this sign do not have a DVT. Therefore, if there is a serious suspicion of a deep vein thrombosis **anticoagulation with heparin** should be commenced and the diagnosis confirmed by investigations.

Pain in the leg, chest pain or dyspnoea in a pregnant or recently pregnant woman should be considered to be due to thrombosis or pulmonary embolism until proved otherwise.

In pregnancy thrombosis is much more common in the left femoral vein and tributaries than in the right.

Investigations

In diagnosing a DVT important features to establish are:
- its site and extent particularly the extension cephalad;
- whether it is free floating or not; and
- whether it is giving off emboli.

1 Contrast venography

Venography is the only diagnostic technique which looks at all levels of the vascular tree but it causes DVT in about 5 per cent of patients. The patient should be treated with intravenous heparin until the diagnosis is confirmed or refuted.

The fetus should be shielded from radiation.

2 Duplex ultrasonography

Non-invasive duplex sonography is being used increasingly to identify DVT, thus avoiding radiation exposure to the fetus. It produces a two dimensional image of the blood vessel and a wave form from the blood flowing through it (hence 'duplex' scanning).

It measures flow rates and hence detects clots. It is most useful for popliteal and femoral vessels. In pregnancy, imaging of the iliac vessels is more difficult. It is not useful for the lower calf.

Clinical signs of a pulmonary embolus

- **Major pulmonary embolus:** collapse, hypotension, central chest pain, breathlessness and cyanosis, shock, or cardiac arrest.
- **Minor pulmonary embolus:** pleuritic chest pain, breathlessness, haemoptysis, fever, confusion, or cardiac failure.

1 Examination

Auscultation – a third heart sign with a parasternal heave may be present. The jugular venous pressure (JVP) may be elevated which helps to distinguish the collapse from causes such as abruption, rupture of the uterus and amniotic fluid embolus.

2 Investigations

Blood gases

P_{aO_2}<70 mm Hg with a normal or reduced CO_2 suggests a pulmonary embolus.

Chest X-ray

This may show non-specific findings such as atelectasis or pleural effusion.

ECG

This may be normal or merely show changes of pregnancy (a deep S wave in lead I and Q wave and inverted R wave in lead III).

Perfusion scan

This will detect areas of decreased blood flow which may be suggestive of a pulmonary embolus. Radioactive technectium is injected intravenously. The distribution of radioactivity is visualised by a gamma camera. An abnormal result cannot confirm the diagnosis; however, a large perfusion defect is likely to be due to a pulmonary embolus if the chest X-ray is normal. The radiation dose to the fetus is minimal – approximately 59 mrem (approx 0.59 Sv) or one-tenth of the maximum gestational exposure recommended to radiation workers in the USA.

Ventilation scan

This is useful if both the perfusion scan and the chest X-ray are abnormal. Krypton is inhaled. A reduction in perfusion with maintenance of ventilation indicates a pulmonary embolus. If ventilation and perfusion are reduced, the condition is probably infective.

Management of massive pulmonary embolus

Notify the intensive care unit and obtain specialist help.

Treatment for cardiac arrest from pulmonary embolism

1 Prolonged external cardiac massage to break up clot and produce pulmonary blood flow.

2 Heparin Give 20 000 IU intravenously.

3 Hypotension Give noradrenaline infusion 2 mg in 500 mL of saline, titrated to a systolic blood pressure of at least 80 mm Hg.

4 Surgery (pulmonary embolectomy) may be needed in the acute phase:

- Indicated in the woman who does not die from massive PE, who remains shocked; systolic blood pressure <90 mm Hg; P_{aO_2} <60 mm Hg and urine output <20 mL/hour.

- Angiography (obtained only after the woman's condition is stable) confirms the diagnosis and localises the embolus.

- Thrombectomy in massive iliofemoral DVT may be considered, to reduce the incidence of post-phlebitic leg symptoms.

- The presence of recurrent pulmonary emboli following iliofemoral embolus is an indication for the percutaneous placement of an inferior cava umbrella by an expert.

5 Thrombolytic agents

- To be used only under the guidance of an expert.

- Give streptokinase as an infusion if a massive pulmonary embolus is confirmed on a pulmonary angiogram and the patient's condition is critical.

- Infuse directly into the pulmonary arterial tree, otherwise into a peripheral vein.

- Streptokinase is given as a loading dose of 600 000 IU and continued with 100 000 IU per hour or urokinase, or tissue plasminogen activator (TPA) which has the theoretical advantage of acting more rapidly and of not causing allergic reaction. Give 100 mg infused over two hours.

ANTICOAGULATION – TREATMENT OF VENOUS THROMBOEMBOLISM WITH HEPARIN

Heparin (molecular weight 10–30 kDa) is strongly polar and non-lipid soluble. It has a short circulating half-life (60 minutes) and does not cross the placenta.

Treat with 40 000 IU intravenously per day (see Table 4.9.1). Start treatment with an intravenous bolus of 5000 IU of heparin. The maintenance dose is by an intravenous infusion starting at 1400 IU per hour or two 12 hour boluses of 17 500 IU subcutaneously. (Maintenance regime 15–25 IU/kg/hour intravenously or 250 IU/kg 12 hourly subcutaneously.)

Table 4.9.1 Heparin infusion schedule. (Reproduced with permission from *Drug and Therapeutics Bulletin*, 28 September 1992, Consumers' Association, London; modified from Fennerty, A.G., Campbell, I.A. and Routledge, P.A. (1988) Anticoagulants in venous thromboembolism. *British Medical Journal*, **297**, 1285–1288.

(1) Loading dose   5000 IU i.v. over 5 minutes
(2) Initial infusion rate   25 000 IU heparin made up in saline in 50 mL gives a final concentration of 500 IU/mL to be started at 2.8 mL/hour (1400 IU/hour)

(3) Check APTT at 6 hours; adjust according to APTT ratio (APTT control) as follows:

APTT ratio	Infusion rate change
>7	Stop for 30 minutes to 1 hour and reduce by 500 IU/hour
5.1–7.0	Reduce by 500 IU/hour
4.1–5.0	Reduce by 300 IU/hour
3.1–4.0	Reduce by 100 IU/hour
2.6–3.0	Reduce by 50 IU/hour
1.5–2.5	No change
1.2–1.4	Increase by 200 IU/hour
<1.2	Increase by 400 IU/hour

(4) After each change wait 10 hours before the next APTT estimation unless the APTT ratio is >5.0, when estimates should be made more frequently, e.g. four-hourly.

Heparin acts instantaneously in contact with blood. It potentiates the effect of endogenous coagulation and antithrombin III (in particular the neutralisation of factor Xa and thrombin) and increases the permeability of the vascular endothelium and inhibits platelet function.

Pregnancy may reduce the sensitivity to heparin because of the changes in clotting factors. Therefore treatment needs careful monitoring.

Monitoring heparin anticoagulation

Monitoring is best done by the protamine sulphate neutralisation test (heparin assay). Aim to achieve 0.6–1.0 IU heparin per millilitre of blood.

The APTT may be used but is less sensitive. An APTT of 1.5 to 2.5 times the control is a necessary safe level of anticoagulation. With a previous history of thromboembolism, the APTT should be 3.5–4.0 times the control.

Heparin therapy

Give heparin for 3–7 days depending on the size of the clot and whether there is any evidence of a recurrence. Intravenous heparin is discontinued after seven days and subcutaneous heparin is given, 10 000 IU twice daily. Alternatively, a low molecular weight heparin (**40 mg/day** in pregnancy) may be used, e.g. enoxaparin, which has the advantage of being a once daily injection.

Give other parenteral medications intravenously, not intramuscularly, in patients on heparin to avoid bruising.

Subcutaneous heparin therapy is controlled by the heparin assay. Subcutaneous heparin therapy does not affect any of the conventional clotting tests. The heparin assay measures the anti-Xa activity of the heparin. The heparin level should be up to 0.4 IU/mL. If the heparin level is less than 0.4 IU/mL there is no risk from bleeding and subcutaneous heparin may be continued throughout labour. Because of concern about the possibility of epidural haematoma formation in women taking subcutaneous heparin, regional anaesthesia should not be used in patients on subcutaneous heparin within 24 hours of labour.

Heparin in small doses does not interfere with the activation of haemostatic mechanisms at the site of injury (e.g. episiotomy) nor does it interfere with platelet function.

After delivery the dose of subcutaneous heparin is reduced to 8000 IU twice daily, or once daily **enoxaparin 40 mg**. It should be continued for the first week of the puerperium. Patients may switch to oral warfarin on day 1 or continue subcutaneous heparin. If warfarin is used, stop heparin once the international normalised ratio (INR) is in the therapeutic range (see below).

Anticoagulate for a period of six weeks post-partum. Breastfeeding is safe in patients taking warfarin.

Complications of heparin therapy

Bone demineralisation can occur in patients taking only 20 000 IU heparin per day for three months.

Treatment of haemorrhage in an anticoagulated patient

Stopping heparin will usually suffice because of the short half life.

If bleeding is severe, give **protamine sulphate** 1 mg for every 100 IU heparin infused over the previous hour. Halve the dose if the heparin infusion has been stopped for one hour and reduce it to a quarter if the heparin has been stopped for two hours.

Do not give more than 50 mg of protamine sulphate in 10 minutes.

ORAL ANTICOAGULENT THERAPY – WARFARIN

Warfarin is best avoided antenatally because of the risks to the fetus. The only condition in which its antenatal use is justified is in the presence of prosthetic heart valves.

Effects of warfarin on the fetus

Warfarin crosses the placenta and effects on the fetus tend to be dose related. It can cause chondrodysplasia punctata (abnormal cartilage and bone formation), microcephaly and optic atrophy, retroplacental and intracerebral haemorrhage.

Mode of action

Warfarin competitively antagonises vitamin K, which is necessary for the production of the clotting factors II, VII, IX and X, and the inhibitors protein C and S, in the liver.

The plasma half-life of warfarin is 35 hours.

Managing warfarin therapy

Monitoring of warfarin dosage is via the international normalised ratio (INR). The treatment range is an **INR between 2 and 3**. It should be higher (3–4.5) in patients having systemic emboli from mechanical prosthetic heart valves or in patients with a current thromboembolic disease. There is a risk of bleeding if the INR is in excess of the treatment range.

Oral treatment with warfarin is started on the first day post-partum for venous thrombosis and on day 3–7 for massive ileofemoral thrombosis and pulmonary embolism.

Give the warfarin at the same time each day (17.00–19.00 hours). Measure the INR 16 hours later, i.e. 9.00–11.00 hours.

Commencement of warfarin therapy

To commence warfarin therapy (after initial heparin anticoagulation) see Table 4.9.2.

▪ Measure a baseline INR and titrate the dosage according to Table 4.9.2.

▪ A slightly lower dose initially may be required if the initial INR is greater than 1.4.

▪ Measure the INR daily. By day 3, half of the patients will be in the therapeutic INR range. The heparin can then be stopped. A steady anticoagulant state is usually achieved after about a week.

▪ Warfarin requirements are usually between 3 and 9 mg daily.

▪ Once the maintenance dose is stable in the therapeutic range the INR should be checked weekly.

▪ Continue warfarin for three months after the first venous thromboembolic episodes. It may be stopped immediately, without reduction in the dose.

4

Complications of warfarin therapy

▪ The major complication is haemorrhage.

▪ If the INR is above 4.5, stop warfarin for 2 days.

▪ For minor bleeding, give 1 mg of Vitamin K i.v.

▪ For life-threatening bleeding, give 5 mg of Vitamin K intravenously together with 1 litre of fresh frozen plasma.

PREVENTION OF THROMBOEMBOLISM IN PREGNANCY IN WOMEN WITH CARDIAC PROBLEMS

Warfarin should be stopped at 36 weeks' gestation, because of the risk of haemorrhage.

Should labour ensue or delivery be necessary, admit the mother to hospital. Give continuous intravenous heparin infusion to achieve a level of 0.4–0.6 IU/mL as measured by the heparin assay. The clotting system of the fetus will return to normal after the warfarin has been withheld for 7–9 days. Heparin therapy is reduced and when the heparin level is less than 0.2 IU/mL labour can be induced.

If the woman goes into labour while on warfarin, give fresh frozen plasma to correct her coagulopathy.

Table 4.9.2 Warfarin treatment – suggested warfarin schedule based on determination of the INR measured 16 hours after the dose of warfarin. (Reproduced with permission from *Drug and Therapeutics Bulletin*, 28 September 1992, Consumers' Association, London; modified from Fennerty, A.G., Campbell, I.A. and Routledge, P.A. (1988) Anticoagulants in venous thromboembolism. *British Medical Journal*, **297**, 1285–1288.

Day	INR 9.00–11.00 hours	Warfarin dose (mg) given at 17.00–19.00 hours
1st	<1.4	10
2nd	<1.8	10
	1.8	1
	>1.8	0.5
3rd	<2.0	10
	2.0–2.1	5
	2.2–2.3	4.5
	2.4–2.5	4
	2.6–2.7	3.5
	2.8–2.9	3
	3.0–3.1	2.5
	3.2–3.3	2
	3.4	1.5
	3.5	1
	3.6–4.0	0.5
	>4.0	0
		Predicted maintenance dose
4th	<1.4	>8
	1.4	8
	1.5	7.5
	1.6–1.7	7
	1.8	6.5
	1.9	6
	2.0–2.1	5.5
	2.2–2.3	5
	2.4–2.6	4.5
	2.7–3.0	4
	3.1–3.5	3.5
	3.6–4.0	3
	4.1–4.5	Miss out next day's dose then give 2 mg
	>4.5	Miss out 2 days' doses then give 1 mg

APTT should be within or below therapeutic range (1.5–2.5 times control). If APTT is above this range the heparin effect on INR should be neutralised by adding protamine (0.4 microgram/mL plasma) to the sample.

Prophylaxis to prevent either a first or recurrent thromboembolism

Prophylactic heparin may be given long term (the duration of the pregnancy) or short term (to cover the period of highest risk, i.e. delivery and the puerperium).

Before starting prophylactic heparin treatment the relative risks of a subsequent episode of thromboembolism and long-term heparin therapy (principally osteoporosis with heparin and fetal effects due to warfarin, if used) need to be considered.

Short term treatment is indicated if there has been a single episode of thromboembolism in or out of pregnancy, because of the relatively low risk of recurrences (12 per cent). It should be considered in the presence of gross obesity or after emergency caesarean section particularly for pre-eclampsia because of increased risk of thromboembolism. Other risk factors include maternal age over 35 years, parity >4, sickle cell trait, but prophylaxis is not routinely indicated in these women.

Women with SLE or antiphospholipid antibodies are also at increased risk.

Having a blood group O often gives some protection.

Short term heparin prophylaxis (in labour or before caesarean section)

Give 5000 IU 8 hourly subcutaneously. The half life of heparin injected subcutaneously is 18 hours in contrast to intravenously 1.5 hours. Plasma heparin levels of 0.02–0.2 IU/mL provide adequate prophylaxis against thromboembolism without the risk of bleeding.

Long term heparin therapy

- This is indicated for recurrent thromboembolism or in the presence of an inherited coagulopathy (see below).
- Give subcutaneous heparin as 10 000 IU b.d. for antenatal prophylaxis in high risk women. Reduce this to 7500 IU post-partum.
- Check heparin level the week before anticipated delivery if possible. If it is less than 0.2 IU with no prolongation of coagulation screening tests (APTT, prothombin time and thrombin time), epidural analgesia is not contraindicated.

• If there is a family history of thrombosis check for inherited coagulopathies by measuring Protein C, Protein S, and antithrombin III. If present treat as indicated below. If absent prophylaxis is not required.

INHERITED COAGULOPATHIES

Antithrombin III (ATIII)

The risk of recurrent thromboembolism is extremely high (approximately 80 per cent). The condition is autosomal dominant. Sites of thromboembolism include the deep leg veins, pulmonary circulation and mesenteric vein thrombosis or the arms.

• For episodes of thromboembolism use high dose intravenous heparin 20 000–45 000 IU/day to give a heparin level of 0.8–1.0 IU of heparin per millilitre of plasma and then change to subcutaneous heparin for the remainder of the pregnancy.

• Use heparin antenatally, prophylactically and a combination of ATIII concentrate or fresh frozen plasma and reduced heparin to cover labour, delivery and the immediate postpartum period.

• Infuse ATIII to maintain 80 per cent of normal levels. Start with 50–70 IU/kg of ATIII (1 IU = 1 mL normal plasma). The half-life is around 36 hours. Measure ATIII levels twice daily.

• Avoid venography in these patients because of the risk of thrombosis.

Proteins C and S

These are naturally occurring anticoagulants. Protein C selectively inhibits factors V and VIII. Protein S is a cofactor of C. Clinically significant deficiency occurs in up to 8 per cent of patients with recurrent thromboembolism.

OTHER ANTICOAGULANTS

Low molecular weight heparin (LMWH)

This is a new form of heparin and consequently there are few data as to its effectiveness in pregnancy. It is derived from standard heparin but has a longer half-life and greater bioavailability when injected subcutaneously. Its major advantage is that it can be given once daily and subcutaneous injection gives therapeutic levels within two hours with a peak of five hours. The dose is 40 mg in pregnancy.

Dextran

Dextran may be given as a prophylactic in labour, an induction or at caesarean section. As an alternative to heparin it has the advantage of not interfering with an epidural analgesia.

▪ Take blood for cross-match if required before giving the dextran because it causes rouleaux formation in red blood cells which makes cross-matching very difficult.

▪ Give a total of 750–1000 mL over 8–12 hours (initially slowly to reduce the risk of anaphylaxis).

▪ Prophylaxis can be continued as described earlier.

BIBLIOGRAPHY

Department of Health & Social Security. (1994) *Report on Confidential Enquiries into Maternal Deaths in England and Wales, 1987–1990.* Her Majesty's Stationery Office, London.

De Sweit, M. (1989) Thromboembolism, In: *Medical Disorders in Obstetric Practice*, 2nd edn., (Ed. by Michael de Sweit) pp 166–197. Blackwell Scientific, Oxford.

Drugs and Therapeutic Bulletin, Vol. 30, No. 28, 28 September 1992, Consumers' Association, London.

Fennerty, A., Dolben, J., Thomas, P., Backhouse, G., Nentley, D.P., Campbell, I.A. & Routledge, P.A. (1984) Flexible induction dose regimen for warfarin and prediction of maintenance dose. *British Medical Journal*, **288**, 1268–1270.

Fennerty, A.G., Thomas, P., Backhous, G., Bentley, P., Campbell, I.A. & Routledge, P.A. (1985) Audit of control of heparin treatment. *British Medical Journal*, **290**, 27–28.

Fennerty, A.G., Campbell, I.A. & Routledge, P.A. (1988) Anticoagulants in venous thromboembolism, *British Medical Journal*, **297**, 1285–1288.

Gallus, A., Jackaman, J., Tillett, J., Mills, W. & Wycherley, A. (1986) Safety and efficacy of warfarin started early after submissive venous thrombosis or pulmonary embolism. *The Lancet*, **ii**, 1293–1296.

Letsky, E. (1992) Thrombo-embolism. In: *High Risk Pregnancy*. (Ed. by A.A. Calder and W. Dunlop), pp 94–138. Butterworth Heinemann, Oxford.

Maternal and Neonatal Haemostasis Working Party of the Haemostasis and Thrombosis Task Force (1993) Guidelines on the prevention, investigation and management of thrombosis associated with pregnancy. *Journal of Clinical Pathology*, **46**, 489–496.

4.10   Thyroid disease in pregnancy

Hyperthyroidism occurs in about two per thousand pregnancies and hypothyroidism in nine per thousand.

HYPERTHYROIDISM

The commonest cause in this age group is Graves' disease diagnosed by an elevation in free and total T4 and a normal to elevated RT_3U and an elevated free thyroxine index.

- Treat either with propylthiouracil (PTU) or occasionally carbimazole. Both drugs cross the placenta and may suppress fetal thyroid function. Therefore, use the lowest possible dose. Commence PTU at 150 mg eight hourly. Doses up to 600 mg per day may be required. Alternatively, carbimazole 15 mg eight hourly.
- Test thyroid function every 6–8 weeks (a steady state needs to be achieved). The aim of therapy is to use the lowest does of PTU required to maintain the free thyroxine index or free T4 at the upper limit of normal. Usually, the dose can be reduced to about half the starting dose.
- If the woman has significant symptoms of thyrotoxicosis (tachycardia, tremulousness) treat with beta-blockers. Give propranolol 20–80 mg/day to keep the maternal heart rate slightly below 100 beats/minute.

HYPOTHYROIDISM

Most cases will be due to Hashimoto's thyroiditis.

- Monitor treatment for hypothyroidism by the thyroid stimulating hormone (TSH) level. It should be less than 6 mIU/L.
- Treat with 200–300 micrograms of thyroxine daily for three weeks. Adjust the dose until the TSH is around 1 mIU/L and the patient is asymptomatic. Usually the dose needs to be increased throughout pregnancy. Increase it by 50 microgram increments.
- Monitor the TSH every eight weeks. Women who are hypothyroid do not need to be seen in special clinics.
- Women with hypothyroidism may have a variety of thyroid block-

ing antibodies which pass across the placenta and can cause intrauterine and temporary neonatal hypothyroidism.

POST-PARTUM THYROIDITIS

Post-partum thyroid dysfunction (thyroiditis) occurs in 5–10 per cent of women. It is an immune disorder that may result in transient hyper- or hypothyroidism. Most women have anti-microsomal antibodies which may be screened for.

The clinical signs may not be typical of thyroid dysfunction and it may present as a postnatal depression. Thyroid function should therefore be tested in women who complain of symptoms suggestive of postnatal depression.

4

5 Obstetric Conditions

5

5.1   Labour

NORMAL LABOUR

This is characterised by:

- The spontaneous onset of contractions between 37 and 42 weeks' gestation.
- Normal maternal observations – pulse, blood pressure and temperature.
- A singleton fetus, cephalic presentation.
- Cervical effacement and dilatation (progress in labour) occurring at an average rate of at least 1 cm per hour.
- Descent of the presenting part through the birth canal.
- Clear liquor.
- Spontaneous vaginal delivery within one hour of adequate maternal pushing; less than one hour in the multiparous woman.
- Placental delivery within 30 minutes of delivery of the baby.
- Total blood loss of less than 500 mL.

The **onset of labour** is taken as that point at which uterine contractions become regular and cervical dilatation begins. It is difficult, however, to time the onset of labour accurately in practice.

The **first stage of labour** has a latent and an active phase (see Fig. 5.1.1). The latent phase starts from the onset of regular uterine contractions and ends when the cervix is 2–3 cm dilated and fully effaced. In the active phase the cervix dilates at up to 3 cm per hour in primigravidae and almost 6 cm per hour in multigravidae. The minimum acceptable rate is 1 cm per hour.

VAGINAL EXAMINATION IN LABOUR

This involves determination of the following features:

1 Cervical dilatation

The cervix starts off closed and uneffaced. In primigravid women the examiner cannot pass a finger through the cervical os, whereas in multiparous women it is just possible to do so ('multips os').

Cervical dilatation may be difficult to determine accurately. If the

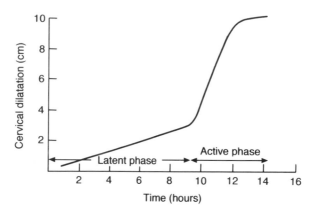

Fig. 5.1.1 Cervical dilatation time curve.

cervix is more than 5 cm dilated, this can be done by placing the index finger of the examining hand on the lateral vaginal wall and estimating (in centimetres) how much cervix remains. By multiplying this by two and subtracting from ten, the degree of cervical dilatation is obtained.

2 Effacement of the cervix

Effacement is the taking up of the cervix resulting in the loss of length. It usually starts at 2 cm in length and when there is no remaining cervical length, the cervix is said to be 'fully effaced'. The degree of effacement is expressed in terms of the percentage of the cervix affected, e.g. if the cervix was originally 2 cm long and it became 1 cm this is 50 per cent effaced.

3 Station

The station is the level of the presenting part in relation to the ischial spines.

The level of the ischial spines is designated 0. For each centimetre above or below the ischial spines the station is designated ± 1 to ± 4. For example at station –4, the presenting part may be only just felt. At station +2, the presenting part may be seen on parting the labia and at +4 it is probably just on the perineum.

A forceps or ventouse delivery should not be attempted unless the station of the head is at least station 0. The station of the **bony** part of the head must not be confused with caput. For most operative deliveries the head should be seen on parting the mother's labia – this is equivalent to station +2.

If the presenting part can neither be identified easily nor felt vaginally then a malpresentation should be suspected.

4 Position of the head

The position of the head is described using the position of the occiput in relation to the maternal pelvis.

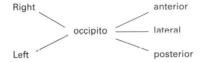

The occiput is that area from the posterior fontanelle to the foramen magnum. The posterior fontanelle can be differentiated from the anterior by the three sutures (fontal and two lambdoidal) emanating from the former and four (frontal, sagittal and two coronal) from the latter.

5 Degree of moulding

This is described as:
1+ The sutures are aligned
2+ The sutures are overlapping
3+ The sutures are not 'reducible' i.e. they cannot be moved in relation to each other with finger pressure on them.

This is most relevant in the second stage of labour and gives a clinical indicator of the 'tightness of the fit'.

6 Caput

This is the oedema of the subcutaneous tissue over the presenting part caused by pressure of the dilating cervix on it.

7 Amniotic fluid

Provided the membranes are ruptured the colour and consistency of the amniotic fluid should be observed at each vaginal examination. It is described as 'clear', 'blood stained' or 'meconium stained' (either thin or thick).

MANAGEMENT OF THE NORMAL PRIMIGRAVID WOMAN IN LABOUR

On admission to the delivery suite, the fetal heart should be assessed by a 30 minute cardiotocograph (CTG) recording, using an abdominal transducer. If it is normal, clinical intermittent monitoring with Pinards or ultrasound is satisfactory for labour (as long as it continues to be normal).

Establish whether or not the mother is in the 'active' phase of labour. In the active phase of labour the cervix is at least 3 cm dilated, effaced and two to three painful contractions occur every 10 minutes.

Management of the first stage of labour (see Fig. 5.1.2)

Women in early labour should be encouraged to mobilise and they may eat and drink.

Fluid balance

- Women in normal labour require approximately 200 mL of fluid per hour.
- If the woman is clinically dehydrated and labour is long up to 2000 mL Hartmann's solution and 1000 mL 5 per cent dextrose may be given over 24 hours. (Syntocinon can be used with either solution.)
- Fluid balance should be recorded on the partogram in all labours.
- Formal fluid balance sheets should be used in specific circumstances (e.g. major haemorrhage and pre-eclampsia).
- If significant ketonuria develops in labour treat with an i.v. infusion of normal saline (1 L) or Hartmann's solution (1 L) over 1 hour.

Further management of labour

- Once active labour has been identified, cervical dilatation should occur at a rate of at least 1 cm per hour.

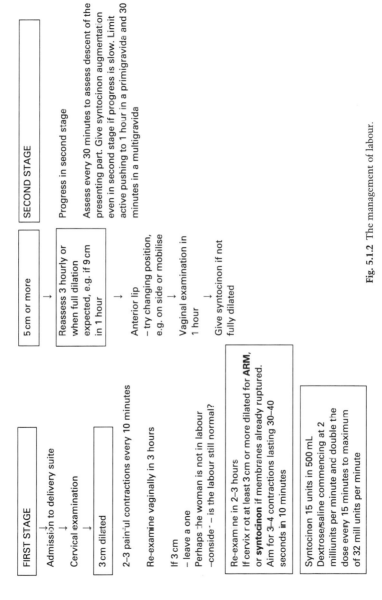

FIRST STAGE

Admission to delivery suite
↓
Cervical examination
↓
3 cm dilated

2–3 painful contractions every 10 minutes

Re-examine vaginally in 3 hours

If 3 cm
– leave a one
Perhaps the woman is not in labour
–consider – is the labour still normal?

Re-examine in 2–3 hours
If cervix r ot at least 3 cm or more dilated for **ARM**, or **syntocinon** if membranes already ruptured. Aim for 3–4 contractions lasting 30–40 seconds in 10 minutes

Syntocinon 15 units in 500 mL Dextrose/saline commencing at 2 milliunits per minute and double the dose every 15 minutes to maximum of 32 mill units per minute

5 cm or more
→
Reassess 3 hourly or when full dilation expected, e.g. if 9 cm in 1 hour
→
Anterior lip
– try changing position, e.g. on side or mobilise
→
Vaginal examination in 1 hour
→
Give syntocinon if not fully dilated

SECOND STAGE

Progress in second stage

Assess every 30 minutes to assess descent of the presenting part. Give syntocinon augmentation even in second stage if progress is slow. Limit active pushing to 1 hour in a primigravida and 30 minutes in a multigravida

Fig. 5.1.2 The management of labour.

5

- Vaginal examination to assess progress should be done every three hours but more regularly if clinically indicated (hourly or two hourly) and before the insertion of an epidural for analgesia, unless delivery is imminent.

Failure to progress in the first stage of labour

This may be due to either 'primary dysfunctional labour' or 'secondary arrest'.

- **Primary dysfunctional labour** is defined as cervical dilatation of less than 1 cm per hour in the active phase of labour (see Figs. 5.1.3 and 5.1.4).

- **Secondary arrest** is complete cessation of cervical dilatation over a period of three or more hours after a previously normal active stage (see Fig. 5.1.5).

The main cause of poor progress in the first stage of labour, particularly in the primigravid woman, is **occipito-posterior position** in which a larger diameter of the fetal head presents and a greater degree of rotation has to occur if the optimum position (occipito-anterior) for delivery is to be achieved.

Occipito-posterior position may be difficult to diagnose because caput and moulding often obscure the fetal sutures.

Use of oxytocin infusion

This can be used to augment or induce (see page 256) labour. Augmentation with oxytocin may be used:

- to encourage rotation and flexion of the fetal head from the occipito-posterior to enable either spontaneous or safe assisted vaginal delivery;
- to correct secondary arrest **as long as cephalo-pelvic disproportion has been excluded**;
- to achieve safe vaginal delivery in the second stage of labour (particularly if an epidural block has been used for analgesia).

In the primigravid woman it can result in fewer operative deliveries for failure to progress.

Augmentation should always be carried out with care and, in the following situations, only after consultation with an experienced obstetrician.

- A multiparous woman with secondary arrest at 5–6 cm of cervical dilatation.

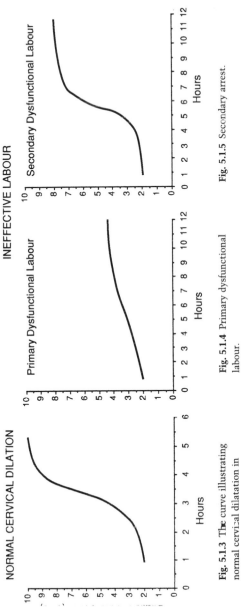

Fig. 5.1.3 The curve illustrating normal cervical dilatation in labour.

Fig. 5.1.4 Primary dysfunctional labour.

Fig. 5.1.5 Secondary arrest.

NORMAL CERVICAL DILATION

INEFFECTIVE LABOUR

Primary Dysfunctional Labour

Secondary Dysfunctional Labour

5

- A breech presentation.
- Previous caesarean section or history of myomectomy.

The multigravid woman is at risk of uterine rupture with injudicious use of oxytocin particularly if a malpresentation has not been identified.

Oxytocin infusion regimen

- Use an infusion pump with a paediatric giving set and 15 units syntocinon in 500 mL 5 per cent dextrose saline (see Table 5.1.1). This gives 60 drops or 30 milliunits per mL.
- The drop rates are increased at 15 minute intervals until contractions are considered adequate.
- If the contractions are not adequate at 64 drops per minute (32 milliunits per minute), an experienced obstetrician should be consulted.
- Once effective uterine contractions are established the syntocinon infusion should be reduced to the lowest dose that gives regular effective contractions to avoid too frequent and hypertonic uterine contractions.

Table 5.1.1 A regimen for the administration of oxytocin: 15 units of syntocinon in 500 mL.

Paediatric drops/minute 15 unit syntocinon/500 mL	Milliunits/minute
4	2
8	4
16	8
32	16
48	24
64	32

Management of the second stage of labour

The second stage is defined as the time from full dilatation until delivery.

Full dilatation of the cervix is suspected when there is anal dilatation and the vertex is visible. Confirm full dilatation with a vaginal examination. In uncomplicated labour the timing of the decision to encourage maternal effort is usually when the presenting part is 'on view' or there is obvious descent of the presenting part with an uncontrollable urge to push.

The second stage consists of a propulsive and expulsive phase. Epidural analgesia often lengthens the time it takes from full dilatation until the expulsive phase begins. Traditionally, the length of the second stage has been limited to one hour for the primigravid woman and half an hour in the multigravid woman. However, with epidural analgesia, it is safe to await descent of the presenting part **if there is no evidence of fetal compromise** until the mother has an urge to push and the fetal presenting part is visible.

Epidural analgesia complicates the management of the second stage because it obtunds the reflex to push. Pushing should be commenced when the presenting part is visible. If there is no descent one hour after active pushing is commenced a syntocinon infusion should be considered (see above).

Most women will become tired after one hour of active pushing and will need an operative delivery.

Poor progress in the second stage is defined as either

- poor descent of the presenting part, **or**
- a second stage with maternal pushing longer than one hour in a primigravid woman and half an hour in a multigravid woman.

> Intrapartum care is fraught with the problem of the rising caesarean section rate which in North America has increased from approximately 5 per cent in the late 1960s to over 20 per cent today (see Fig. 5.1.6). This is primarily due to a diagnosis of failure to progress in labour. Despite the increased incidence of caesarean section there is no associated improvement in perinatal outcome.
>
> Appropriately managed labour should give a normal vaginal delivery rate of over 80 per cent. The assisted delivery rate should be approximately 10 per cent. This leaves a caesarean section rate of about 10 per cent of which half will be elective and half during labour.

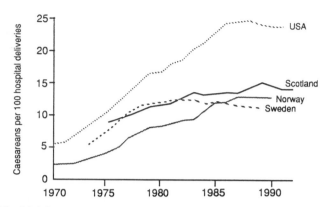

Fig. 5.1.6 Caesarean section rates for hospital births in selected countries. (Reproduced with permission from Macfarlane, A. & Chamberlain, G. (1993) What is happening to caesarean section rates? *The Lancet*, **342**, 1005–1006.)

ANALGESIA IN LABOUR

Entonox (50 per cent N_2O in O_2)

This should be used when necessary and may be continued through the first stage and into the second stage of labour if it is providing effective analgesia. Mothers should be instructed in the self administration of Entonox early in labour, so that they can use it when they need it.

It is given either via a mouthpiece or a mask with a good seal. Deep breaths are taken with the onset of contractions. The woman should stop breathing it when the peak of the contraction has passed. Nitrous oxide has a very rapid onset and offset.

Excess inhalation causes drowsiness. An inherent feature of delivery is that if this occurs, the mouthpiece falls away and N_2O levels drop.

Transcutaneous electrical nerve stimulation (TENS)

This instrument applies a low level electrical stimulus to the dermatome of spinal nerves supplying the lower abdomen, coming from the same spinal segment as those for uterine sensation, in an attempt to modify the transmission of painful stimuli along those same nerves.

Pethidine

Carry out a vaginal examination to determine cervical dilatation before pethidine is given, in case delivery is imminent. This avoids unnecessary sedation of the baby. Alternatively, cervical dilatation may not be occurring as rapidly as anticipated and an epidural block may be more appropriate, since in general only two doses of pethidine should be given in labour and its effects last only up to two hours.

The dose is 1–1.5 mg/kg.

The first dose of pethidine is normally not required until the mother has reached the active stage of labour (i.e. 3–4 cm dilated) but may be required, and should not be withheld, from those mothers who request it earlier.

A second dose may be required within the next three hours of active labour, the size and timing of such a dose being dependent upon the response to the first.

The baby may require naloxone (10 micrograms/kg) or initially half of an ampoule (40 micrograms in 2 mL) to reverse the respiratory depressant effects of pethidine if given late in labour.

Antiemetics

Antiemetics should only be given if vomiting becomes a problem. Extrapyramidal side effects (e.g. oculogyric crisis and opisthotonos) rarely occur even with small doses. They can be counteracted by promethazine ('Phenergan') 12.5 mg i.m. and 12.5 mg i.v. (titrated to response).

EPIDURAL ANAESTHESIA

The aim in the first stage of labour is to block the sensory nerve supply to the uterus (T_{10}–T_{12}). Later in the second stage of labour when perineal analgesia is required, S_2–S_4 need to be blocked.

Situations where an epidural block is useful/indicated for analgesia

- A mother likely to require an operative delivery
- The mother's request (with no contraindications)
- Maternal distress

- Difficult/prolonged labour (OP position, trial of labour)
- Hypertension
- Twins
- Operative deliveries
- Diabetics at risk of operative delivery. Fluctuations in the blood glucose may be due to circulating catecholamines that may be induced by pain. Appropriate control of pain by epidural analgesia may contribute to better diabetic control.

Contraindications include:

- Failure to obtain maternal consent
- Bleeding diathesis (including anticoagulant therapy). Check the coagulation status and review the need for an epidural.
- Local sepsis in the region of the block/septicaemia
- Shock and hypovolaemia
- Cardiac disease

Epidural anaesthesia may be used in patients with pre-existing neurological disease, provided they understand that coincidental relapses may occur, **unrelated** to the epidural.

A previous caesarean section is not necessarily a contraindication to epidural anaesthesia.

Drugs and dosages with regional analgesia

Bupivacaine ('Marcain')

- Slow in onset, long duration (1–2 hours).
- A variety of concentrations from 0.125 per cent to 0.5 per cent can be used for bolus injection. 0.75 per cent is contraindicated in pregnancy. The maximum dose is 2 mg/kg/4 hour period.

Note: Lower concentrations of bupivacaine (e.g. 0.0625 per cent) together with an opioid may be used for continuous infusions.

Lignocaine

- Rapid in onset, short duration ($\frac{3}{4}$ hours). Tachyphylaxis (increasing doses for same effect) occurs.
- Good for 'one off' procedures where speed is essential (e.g. forceps).
- Usually 1.5 per cent with or without adrenaline 1:200 000.
- Maximum dose 4 mg/kg (8 mg/kg with adrenaline).

See Table 5.1.2.

Table 5.1.2 Maximum doses of lignocaine (mL) for body weight.

Body weight	Strength of lignocaine (plain)	
(kg)	0.5%	1%
40	32	16
50	40	20
60	48	24
70	56	28

Insertion of an epidural block

A 14 or 16 G intravenous cannula must be in place and i.v. fluids must be running continuously to minimise the incidence of hypotension and/or reduced uterine blood flow, and be available should resuscitation be necessary. Up to 500 mL Hartmann's solution should be infused routinely increasing to up to 1.5 L if the block is being inserted before caesarean section.

The epidural space is, by definition, outside the dura. The epidural needle is inserted at the L_3–L_4 space and the ligamentum flavum is entered and slowly penetrated. Air or saline cannot be easily injected while the needle is within the ligamentum flavum, but as soon as it is penetrated resistance is overcome. The needle is now in the epidural space. Inadvertent puncture of the dura is usually recognised by backflow of cerebrospinal fluid (CSF) which can be identified by a positive glucose on a test stick (to differentiate it from the saline that was being injected). Occasionally a CSF leak may not be apparent, so a dural tap may be unrecognised until symptoms appear. For this reason a test dose of 3 mL of anaesthetic is given (see below).

The advantages of an epidural by infusion are

- Optimal analgesia with minimal motor block.
- Avoidance of 'top ups'.

An example of an infusion is 60 mL of 0.125% bupivacaine plus 3 mg of diamorphine run at 6–10 mL per hour.

'Top up' epidurals

As an alternative to continuous infusions, the appropriate dose of anaesthetic agent may be injected into the epidural space (L_3–L_4) via the indwelling catheter (see above). A 'top up' is given when the epidural has worn off in about $1-1\frac{1}{2}$ hours. The top up takes 10–15 minutes to work which can lead to undesirable swings in the level of analgesia.

There is a tendency to give more than is needed, producing an exaggerated cardiovascular response and a fall in blood pressure.

Top ups give greater motor block.

Peak blood levels of bupivacaine may affect the fetus causing CTG changes and autonomic block.

Method of inserting a 'top up' epidural for a woman in labour

For a 70 kg woman initially give a test dose of 3 mL of 0.5 per cent bupivacaine to establish that the catheter is indeed in the epidural and not the subarachnoid/intrathecal space. (3 mL of 0.5 per cent bupivacaine in the latter situation would result in a full block suitable for a caesarean section (T_4–T_6).)

The subsequent dose is given five to ten minutes later. The actual dose depends on the degree of analgesia needed but is usually about 8 mL of 0.25 per cent bupivacaine.

Management of women with an epidural block in situ

The management of an epidural anaesthetic is the responsibility of the anaesthetist who determines the frequency, volume and strength of 'top ups', or infusion strength and rate.

'Top ups' are normally given by an approved midwife.

To minimise hypotension and/or decreased uterine blood flow, due to pressure on the inferior vena cava and aorta, all women with an epidural block must at all times be nursed in the lateral, wedged supine, or proper sitting position (this is difficult to achieve and maintain). If the woman is in an inappropriate position, uterine blood flow may be diminished even if the blood pressure seems normal.

Check and record heart rate, respiratory rate, and height of block hourly during labour. The blood pressure is checked more frequently (see below).

Do this more frequently at the start of an infusion or after a 'top up'.

Bolus 'top ups'

'Top ups' are usually required every 1–2 hours in normal labour, but should be given when the sensation of contractions becomes painful.

After every top up the blood pressure is checked and recorded every five minutes for the first 15 minutes, and every 30 minutes thereafter.

The **level of block** should be checked and recorded hourly (see Table 5.1.3). This is done as follows:

▪ Drip ethyl chloride or ice onto the tip of the shoulder ($C_{5/6}$) to establish that it feels cold. Then start at the level of the thighs (levels L_3–L_4) and drip up until the mother recognises it as cold which is the upper limit of the block.

▪ Drip onto abdomen at the level to be tested, at least 6 cm from the midline bilaterally to establish that analgesia is independently present on both sides.

▪ The object is to achieve a patient who is comfortable (this does not imply devoid of all sensation), with a stable block (T_{10}).

Table 5.1.3 Identifying the level of the block and action to be taken should the block be less than ideal.

5

The dermatomes are

T_4 the nipple line	T_8 the umbilicus
T_7 the xiphoid process	T_{12} the groin

Check the level of the block hourly.
▪ If the block is at T_6 or above stop infusion and call anaesthetist immediately.
▪ If the block has gone up the body to T_6–T_8, decrease the infusion by 1 mL/hour.
▪ If the block is between T_8 and T_{10}, no action is required.
▪ If the block has not changed and the patient has no pain, no action is required.
▪ If the block has gone below T_{10} and the mother has pain, give smallest prescribed 'top up' and increase infusion by 1 mL/hour. Inform the anaesthetist if the 'top up' is unsuccessful after 20 minutes.

Check epidural prescription at 8 cm cervical dilatation and aim for lowest possible doses for further 'top ups' that will ensure the mother's comfort without producing a degree of motor block which reduces her ability to 'push' effectively. The use of lower concentrations of bupivacaine (e.g. 0.25 per cent or 0.375 per cent) should be considered just before the second stage.

The objective is to provide maximal analgesia and minimal interference with progress in the second stage.

The epidural block must not be allowed to 'wear off' so that the mother experiences uncontrollable pain in the second stage.

Loss of motor power with epidural analgesia can result in temporary leg weakness, so do not allow the mother to stand alone initially nor to be holding the baby when she first gets out of bed!

After delivery the epidural catheter is usually removed before the mother returns to the ward. In some cases (e.g. after lower segment caesarean section (LSCS)) the catheter can remain in situ for postoperative pain relief providing adequate nursing care is available.

Complications of epidural analgesia and their management

1 Hypotension
- Turn patient on to left side.
- Run in 500 mL Hartmann's solution (rapidly) i.v.
- Give O_2 (6 L/min) by face mask.
- Give colloid and ephedrine (multiples of 6 mg as necessary) i.v. if these measures are unsuccessful.

2 Dural puncture
Suspect if a mother complains of a severe incapacitating headache after delivery.

Management
- The epidural catheter is left in place and 50 mL of normal saline is administered through it over about 10 minutes and a further 1 L over the following 24 hours.
- In addition give up to 3 L of intravenous fluid per day and encourage oral intake.
- Prescribe regular analgesia (e.g. 10–15 mg of morphine 4 hourly i.m.) rather than intermittent, and give an anti-emetic e.g. prochlorperazine 12.5 mg i.m. six hourly. A stool softener (e.g. lactulose 5 mL daily) may be helpful because the headache can be made worse by straining at stool.
- There is no need for the woman to remain lying down but she may wish to if the headache is precipitated by assuming the upright posture.
- If there is no marked relief of headache within 48 hours an epidural blood patch can be offered in which up to 20 mL of autologous blood is injected into the epidural space. It should be carried out aseptically in theatre in the presence of two anaesthetists. Symptoms are usually relieved within 30 minutes and often in only five minutes.

3 Total spinal anaesthesia
Occurs when a large amount of local anaesthetic, intended for the

epidural space, is inadvertently injected into the subarachnoid space. It is rare, but potentially fatal and treatable (see Tables 5.1.4 and 5.1.5).

4 Haematoma or sepsis

These are rare complications, but if suspected the anaesthetic department must be notified immediately. They will, if necessary, arrange for an urgent neurosurgical opinion.

Table 5.1.4 Signs suggesting too high an epidural block – urgent anaesthetic action needed immediately.

Large fall in blood pressure
Pronounced maternal bradycardia (<50 beats/min)
Dyspnoea – difficulty, or abnormal awareness of breathing
Weakness in the arms
Sensory block (tested) found to be $>T_4$
Sudden onset of stuffy/runny nose (Horner's syndrome) is indicative of a high sympathetic block.

Table 5.1.5 First aid treatment in an emergency associated with regional anaesthesia.

A   Check airway
- Left lateral position
- Protect the airway
- Beware of gastric regurgitation

B   Check breathing

↓

If not breathing **start artificial respiration**.

C   Check circulation

↓

If no circulation **commence cardiopulmonary resuscitation**.

↓

If hypotensive place patient on side, head down
Increase rate of infusion of intravenous infusion
Give O_2 via a Hudson mask (6 L/min)
Give ephedrine (6–12 mg boluses) until blood pressure normal (Ephedrine comes as 30 mg diluted down to 5 or 10 mL so it is given in multiples of 3 or 6 mg.)

SPINAL ANAESTHESIA

This is a 'single shot' technique; thus if the block is ineffective other methods of anaesthesia will be required.

A free running i.v. drip via a 15 gauge or 14 gauge cannula must be inserted before the spinal block is established. Position the woman in the full lateral position (sometimes sitting). A lumbar puncture is performed at the L_3–L_4 interspace with a fine gauge non-cutting needle (e.g. 25 gauge Whitacre). The newer pencil point needles can markedly reduce the incidence and severity of post dural puncture headaches.

2.5 mL of 0.5 per cent 'heavy' bupivacaine (i.e. the solution contains glucose) are injected slowly (with or without 10 micrograms of fentanyl). The woman is immediately moved to a left lateral position with a 10–15° tilt and blood pressure is monitored. A block to T_5 is established within 5–10 minutes.

Occasionally a combined epidural/spinal technique may be used. This allows inadequate blocks to be topped up via the epidural catheter, and may be continued for post-operative analgesia.

Potential problems associated with spinal anaesthesia

Hypotension

This can be of rapid onset and profound. It is best prevented by use of the left wedged lateral or sitting position and by a fluid 'pre-load' of at least 1500 mL. It can also be treated using ephedrine 6 mg i.v. repeated as necessary or as an infusion (50–60 mg ephedrine in 500 mL Hartmann's solution after the pre-load has been given).

Total spinal anaesthesia

See above and Tables 5.1.4 and 5.1.5.

Headache

This is treated initially by copious oral fluids and simple analgesics. There is no need to confine all women who develop this complication to bed. If the headache does not improve epidural blood patch is the treatment of choice (see above).

Backache

There may be an increased incidence of backache in women who have had regional anaesthesia. It is minor and there is no long term sequelae.

Neurological deficit

Minor (usually short-lived) neurological sequelae such as VIth nerve palsy, temporary patches of numbness in the thigh, or even foot drop, may occur occasionally (see Table 5.1.6).

Table 5.1.6 Results from a postal questionnaire from 100 000 responses of complications of epidural analgesia in the United Kingdom. (Reproduced with permission from: Scott, B. & Hibbard, B.M. (1990) Serious non-fatal complications associated with extradural block in obstetric practice. *British Journal of Anaesthesia*, **64**, 537–541.)

Complications	No.	No. with permanent effects
Cardiac arrest	3	1 (brain damage)
Neuropathy involving the spinal cord	1	1 (paraplegia)
Neuropathy involving a single spinal nerve defect	38	1 (quadriceps weakness)
Extradural abscess	1	Improving
Extradural haematoma	1	Improving
Urinary problems	6	0
Severe backache	5	0
Memory loss	1	0
Dural tap with prolonged headache	16	0
Cranial nerve palsy	5	0
Subdural haemoatoma	1	0
Acute toxicity (convulsions)	20	0
High or total spinal anaesthesia	8	0
Anaphylaxis	1	0
Total	108	5

ANTACID THERAPY

It is used prophylactically to reduce the risk of aspiration of gastric contents due to slow gastric emptying in pregnancy and labour.

It may be used for elective procedures e.g. caesarean section (including those under epidural), tubal ligation and post-partum evacuation of the uterus. If the procedure is to be done in the morning give Ranitidine 150 mg orally the night before, plus Ranitidine 150 mg at 06.00 hours on the day of operation. If the procedure is to be done in the afternoon give Ranitidine 150 mg at 06.00 hours on the day of the procedure, plus Ranitidine 150 mg at 12.00 hours on the day of the procedure. Also give sodium citrate (0.3 M) 30 mL before giving the anaesthetic since its effects only last for approximately 20 minutes.

For emergency procedures (e.g. caesarean section, manual removal of placenta, trial of forceps and suture of cervical or third degree tear) give Ranitidine 50 mg intravenously slowly or i.m. and 30 mL of 0.3 M sodium citrate orally to neutralise existing gastric acid.

INSTRUMENTAL DELIVERY

Adequate analgesia must be achieved before application of forceps using one of the following:
- Local analgesia – involving pudendal and perineal blocks using up to 20 mL 1 per cent lignocaine hydrochloride (plain).
- An existing epidural block – ideally a 'top up' should be given before the forceps delivery.
- Spinal analgesia.
- General anaesthetic (see above).

Pre-requisites for an instrumental delivery

- A fully dilated cervix;
- no head palpable above the brim and no cephalopelvic disproportion;
- empty bladder and bowel;
- an active uterus.

Forceps delivery

The position of the fetal head should be clearly identified. Moulding may make this difficult. An occipito-posterior position is identified by the inverted Y shape described by the occipital bone on the parietal bones. The anterior fontanelle is identified by the overriding of the parietal bones on the frontal bones. It may be difficult to feel the division between the frontal bones with excessive moulding but it is possible to discriminate it by feeling with the right forefinger the fetal coronal suture and carefully moving 45° feeling for the frontal suture. It will then become apparent that there are four sutures which delineate the anterior fontanelle.

Before Keilland forceps are used, it is essential to identify abdominally which side the back of the baby is on. The forceps are applied with the 'knobs' facing towards the baby's occiput.

The posterior blade is applied first directly to the lateral aspect of the fetal head and the anterior blade is positioned either directly or by 'wandering'. The blades are locked. If the blades cannot be locked easily check the application of the forceps.

An abnormal position (e.g. occipito-transverse) is corrected by depressing the handles of the forcep blades and directing the fetal occiput to the anterior position in the direction of the side of the fetal back. The head is flexed at the same time. An excessive twisting force should not be necessary.

Delivery from the occipito-anterior position should be achieved within three pulls.

Ventouse delivery (vacuum extraction)

The same criteria should be met as for a forceps delivery except that delivery can be achieved without full cervical dilatation. It is preferable, but not critical, to identify the position of the fetal head.

It is associated with less maternal trauma.

A silastic cup is applied to the fetal occiput as posteriorly as possible to enable flexion of the fetal head. The pressure is pumped up to $0.2\,kg/cm^2$. The rim of the cup should be checked to make sure there is no other tissue inadvertently caught under the suction cup. The pressure is then increased to $0.8\,kg/cm^2$ and traction exerted with a uterine contraction.

Delivery should occur with three pulls.

BREECH DELIVERY

The appropriate clinical management of delivery with a breech presentation is suggested by the mother's past obstetric history, the size of the fetus (generally between 2000 g and 3500 g) and the attitude of the fetus (extended leg, flexed leg or footling breech). Ultrasound examination after 36 weeks is useful to confirm the attitude of the breech and give a fetal weight estimation.

The most important factor in determining whether or not a vaginal delivery is achieved is the efficiency of uterine activity producing cervical dilatation. There is little evidence that objective measurements of pelvic size correlates with the chance of vaginal delivery. If pelvimetry is required CT scanning may be preferable to X-ray because the radiation dose is less (see p. 252).

The breech in labour

Labour may fail to progress at any stage with a breech presentation and caesarean section needs to be considered in this situation.

In the second stage, especially if there is an epidural block present, the mother should be advised to push only when the presenting part is 'on view'. The length of active pushing should be confined to half an hour in the multigravid woman and one hour in the primigravid woman. A caesarean section may be required even at this stage.

The mechanism of delivery of the breech

An experienced obstetrician should supervise the breech labour and be present for the delivery.

Delivery should be achieved mainly by maternal effort with minimal assistance from the obstetrician. (Breech extraction is contra-indicated save occasionally for the delivery of a second twin or if the baby is *in extremis*.)

Ideally breech labour is best carried out without epidural block which can obtund the Fergusson reflex and cause failure to progress in the second stage.

Delivery of the breech precedes after the anus of the fetus is seen 'rising up' over the mother's perineum without retraction. This is the equivalent of crowning and an episiotomy may be required at this stage.

The accoucher delivers the legs (if flexed at the hip joints, extended at the knee joints) by inserting the thumb of the right hand into the baby's popliteal fossa, with the index finger on the anterior aspect of the thigh and the third finger on the anterior aspect of the lower leg. The leg is delivered by abducting the baby's hip joint and flexing the knee. The back is kept sacro-anterior and descent occurs until the scapulae are visible.

The baby's arms are delivered by the accoucher inserting a thumb into the baby's ante-cubital fossa, with index finger on the upper arm and third finger on the forearm. Delivery of the arms occurs by adduction at the shoulder and flexion at the elbow ('wiping the baby's hands across the face').

The Lovset manoeuvre is then carried out by holding the baby with the thumbs on the sacrum and index fingers on the anterior superior iliac spines. The baby is turned in an arc in a clockwise and then anticlockwise direction to enable descent of the shoulders. The nape of the neck usually becomes visible with the next contraction and delivery is achieved by either the Mauriceau–Smellie–Viet manoeuvre (where a finger is placed in the mouth and the head delivered by flexion) or by the application of Neville Barnes forceps for traction and flexion to achieve delivery.

Because the head does not have time to mould to the dimensions of the pelvis with a breech presentation, it is at increased risk of becoming stuck because the submentooccipital diameter of the head (dimension 13.5 cm) holds the baby's head up at the pelvic brim. This is a rare occurrence.

The main cause of a head being stuck is hyperextension. This is an obstetric emergency and skilled expertise is needed. The index finger of the left hand of the accoucheur is inserted into the baby's mouth and attempt made to flex the head by placing the right hand over the occipital region of the baby's head. The head is then flexed and turned obliquely to enter the pelvis at its widest diameter by downward pressure from the palm of the hand. If this is not successful symphysiotomy may be required (see below).

BROW PRESENTATION

The incidence is 1/1500 deliveries. In general delivery is by caesarean section. Occasionally a brow may extend to become a face and delivery spontaneously if it is mento-anterior.

If a conservative approach to labour is taken, then the mother should have a vaginal examination for degree of cervical dilatation every two hours to identify satisfactory progress. Syntocinon augmentation should not be used.

FACE PRESENTATION

Face presentation occurs in 1/500 deliveries. The diameters of the face are the normal hiparietal (9.5 cm) and submento-bregmatic which is the same as the occipito-frontal of a deflexed vertex.

A face presentation may deliver spontaneously as long as the chin is already anterior or is rotating forwards.

If the chin rotates posteriorly, then there is a large area of skull comprising the vertex and occiput which cannot follow the face out underneath the mother's symphysis pubis. Delivery is then required by caesarean section.

TRANSVERSE LIE

The incidence is 2 per cent early in the third trimester but only 0.3 per cent near term.

Placenta praevia, fibroids, ovarian cysts, fetal malformations, multiple pregnancy and abnormal uterus should be excluded.

Delivery is by caesarean section carried out by an experienced obstetrician who can best judge what approach to use. For example, a classical caesarean section is indicated for delivery of a transverse lie with ruptured membranes.

5

TWINS AND DELIVERY

The incidence of monozygotic twins is about 3.5 per 1000 births. Dizygotic twinning rates vary greatly according to age, parity, race and with assisted reproductive techniques. **Fetal risks include:**
- perinatal death (10 times the rate for singletons) of one or both twins
- pre-term delivery
- IUGR
- congenital malformation
- twin to twin transfusion syndrome
- hydramnios
- birth asphyxia
- need for operative delivery
- (rarely locked twins).

Induction of labour may be indicated for complications in a twin pregnancy. Induction at 38 weeks' gestation is not routinely indicated. During labour both twins should be monitored carefully. Intravenous access should be established and the mother's blood grouped and saved. Epidural analgesia provides excellent pain relief in labour and is of benefit in case there is difficulty in delivering the second twin.

The first twin should be delivered as for a singleton. After delivery of the first twin the lie of the second twin should if necessary be corrected to longitudinal by external cephalic version. Amniotomy is performed only when the presenting part of the second twin is clearly descending. Alternatively, if the lie is non-longitudinal, the foot of the second twin may be grasped and brought down to the introitus so that it is clearly identified ('internal podalic version'). It may then be delivered by gentle breech extraction. An infusion of syntocinon should be ready to administer in case uterine hypotonia occurs after delivery of the first twin.

Delivery of very premature twins by caesarean section may be very difficult since the lower segment may not be formed. A classical or lower vertical incision should be considered.

SHOULDER DYSTOCIA

This is most common with macrosomic babies who also have an increased risk of neonatal death, fractures of the clavicle and humerus, meconium aspiration and injuries to the brachial plexus and cervical cord injury.

Shoulder dystocia occurs in 9 per cent of babies >4000 g, 15 per cent >4500 g and 40 per cent above 5700 gm, compared to 1.5 per cent of all deliveries. However, 50 per cent of the cases of shoulder dystocia occur in babies who weigh less than 4000 g.

Shoulder dystocia may be heralded by the following:
- Slower progress in the second stage than expected.
- A second stage lasting longer than half an hour in a multiparous woman without an epidural with effective expulsive contractions.
- The head delivers, but there may be difficulty in suctioning out the mouth.
- If there is no further descent and/or delivery with the next contraction, then shoulder dystocia is diagnosed. **If this is the situation immediate assistance is required**.

1 Place the mother in lithotomy or the left lateral position and make a large episiotomy.

2 Exert suprapubic pressure and attempt to angle the baby's head downwards to deliver the anterior shoulder. (**Beware** as this can result in cervical cord injuries if extreme.) It may help to also apply pressure at the fundus of the uterus.

3 If the above does not release the anterior shoulder, attempt to rotate the body of the baby so that the posterior shoulder moves anteriorly.

4 If there is no rotation, deliver the posterior arm and deliver the trunk by flexion downwards.

5 If delivery does not occur within 10 minutes, seriously consider a symphysiotomy.

SYMPHYSIOTOMY

A symphysiotomy may be used in a desperate situation where the head of the breech fails to deliver or for shoulder dystocia and where, despite appropriate manipulations, there has been no progress in delivery for seven minutes or so.

A symphysiotomy is done by infiltrating the mons pubis with 1 per cent lignocaine. A catheter is inserted to displace the urethra from the midline. The superior and anterior fibres of the symphysis pubis are divided using a scalpel.

The mother's thighs are abducted slowly until approximately 2 cm separation of the symphysis occurs to enable descent of the fetal head into the pelvis. Delivery is expedited with forceps.

The suprapubic stab incision requires repair. The mother's legs are strapped together for 24 hours. Positioning on her side allows healing. Initially walking may require a frame but by 10 days post-partum walking should be unaided.

If the symphysis separates by more than 2 cm, nylon sutures are required inserted into the anterior periosteum on either side of the symphysis and tied across the front of the joint.

PELVIMETRY

The use of X-ray pelvimetry to measure the dimensions of the maternal pelvis has declined because of the possible risks of ionising radiation on the fetus. Conventional X-ray pelvimetry exposes the baby to 500–1100 mrad, compared to approximately 82 mrad for CT scanning. Normal pelvic measurements are shown in Table 5.1.7.

Table 5.1.7 'Adequacy' of pelvic dimensions.

Antero-posterior diameter of the inlet (cm)	>10
Transverse diameter of the inlet (cm)	>11.5
Transverse interspinous diameter of the mid-pelvis (cm)	>9.5
Antero-posterior dimension of the pelvic outlet (cm)	>11.5

The outcome of labour is determined more by efficient uterine activity than pelvic dimensions. Pelvimetry may be indicated with very short stature or by a congenital or traumatic pelvic deformity.

The lateral view pelvic inlet is measured from the anterior aspect of the sacral promontory to the posterior cephalic aspect of the symphysis pubis. The contour of the sacral body is assessed. The outlet is measured from the last fixed sacral segment to the posterior caudal aspect of the symphysis pubis. The antero-posterior view measures the maximum transverse diameter of the pelvic inlet. The interspinous distance is measured from the fovea capitalis of the femur taken on an axial view from a CT scan.

MANAGEMENT OF THE THIRD STAGE OF LABOUR

In most vaginal deliveries the third stage is managed actively to reduce the incidence of post-partum haemorrhage (approximately 5 per cent of all deliveries).

In the UK the commonest regimen involves the use of Syntometrine (5 units syntocinon with 0.5 mg ergometrine) 1 mL given i.m. with the birth of the anterior shoulder in a singleton pregnancy. However, syntocinon 5 units on its own may be as effective without producing the rise in blood pressure, nausea and vomiting associated with ergometrine. Syntometrine and ergometrine are relatively contraindicated in the presence of hypertension. In such cases syntocinon 5 units i.m. or i.v. may be given.

Once the baby is delivered and the cord clamped, the placenta can be delivered by controlled cord traction (CCT) when there are signs of separation and descent (uterine contraction, lengthening of cord, gush of blood). Occasionally at the mother's request and with the approval of the obstetrician the third stage may be managed passively/physiologically without oxytocics or CTT of the placenta.

At caesarean section defer giving any oxytocic agent (5 units syntocinon i.v.) until the cord has been clamped. With the delivery of a pre-term baby by caesarean section if at all possible neither the cord should be clamped nor an oxytocic given until the cord has stopped pulsating. This allows the placental and neonatal blood volume to equilibrate physiologically. Clamping the cord too early deprives the baby of vital blood volume. Giving an oxytocic before clamping risks overloading the baby's circulation.

5

EPISIOTOMY

Perineal repair

Polyglycolic acid is the preferred suture material. Use (for example) a 40 mm semicircular, multipurpose needle gauge 0 for the vagina and perineal body and a 30 mm semicircular multipurpose needle gauge 2/0 for closure of the perineal skin.

Alternatively, vicryl (polyglactin, braided, absorbable synthetic and undyed), e.g. on a 40 mm semicircular taper needle, may be used throughout the repair of the episiotomy.

- Commence the repair by carefully identifying the apex of the incision. Anchor the suture by inserting it and tying it 1 cm above the apex.
- Use a continuous suture to the vaginal wall. Tie this at the introitus just below the hymenal ring.
- The perineal body is repaired by deep interrupted sutures working from top to bottom and angling the sutures across at approximately 30°. Place the perineal suture as close to the skin edge as possible to give maximal closure of the wound.
- Close the skin layer subcutaneously, commencing at the apex (working bottom to top) and tying the suture to where the suture for the vaginal skin was tied just below the hymenal ring.

The maximum amounts of local anaesthetic that can be safely used for suturing are 4 mg/kg without adrenaline and 8 g/kg with adrenaline; e.g. for a 70 kg woman, using a 1 per cent solution of lignocaine, 4 mg/kg = 280 mg = 28 mL of a 1 per cent solution (see Table 5.1.2).

If an effective epidural is in place, use it ('topped up' if necessary) rather than local anaesthetic.

FETAL ASSESSMENT IN LABOUR

See Chapter 6 on cardiotocographs.

The indications for continuous electronic fetal heart rate monitoring are given in Table 5.1.8.

All other (normal/'low risk') pregnancies should have intermittent external CTG monitoring performed on admission to delivery suite for approximately 20 minutes; if it is normal thereafter usually every 2–3 hours. In between the fetal heart rate is monitored by regular

Table 5.1.8 Continuous fetal heart rate monitoring is suggested in the following women.

1 Those at risk of utero-placental vascular disease – including:
Maternal medical problems
Hypertension
Diabetes
Renal disease
Cyanotic heart disease
Haemoglobinopathy
Severe anaemia
Collagen disease
Hyperthyroidism

2 **Complications of pregnancy**
Vaginal bleeding in pregnancy
Prolonged pregnancy
Multiple pregnancy

3 **Those suspected of having a compromised fetus – including:**
Small for dates fetus
Poor fetal movements
Low score on biophysical profile (<6)

4 Fetal distress clinically
Meconium

5 **Complications of labour**
Prolonged labour (over 12 hours)
Pre-term labour (less than 37 weeks)
Epidural analgesia
Augmented and induced labour
Breech presentation
Prolonged rupture of membranes (over 12 hours)
Previous caesarean section
Intrauterine infection

auscultation. If it is normal and remains so for approximately 20 minutes thereafter, readings should be repeated every 2–3 hours.

FETAL BLOOD SAMPLING

Fetal scalp blood sampling is done in labour if it is necessary to assess the degree of fetal acidaemia (see Chapter 6). The fetus is at risk of asphyxial damage in the presence of significant metabolic acidaemia. This is difficult to identify by electronic fetal heart rate monitoring which is non-specific (i.e. there are many false positives).

The procedure for fetal scalp blood sampling is:

- Check that the analyser is ready to use.
- Set up all blood sampling equipment.
- Put the mother in the left lateral or wedge lithotomy position.
- Perform a vaginal examination; insert the amnioscope, visualise and clean the fetal scalp.
- Spray the scalp with ethyl chloride to create hyperaemia and smear silicone on that area.
- Make two controlled stabs and collect the blood into a pre-heparinised capillary tube.
- Ensure haemostasis before removing the amnioscope (pressure should be adequate).
- Measure pH and blood gases.

Difficulties in the interpretation of fetal scalp blood gas results occur because there is not a direct correlation between pH and base deficit and neonatal asphyxia or adverse outcome. Cord blood gas values at delivery provide a better correlation with asphyxia.

It is assumed that labour is an asphyxiating process and that an abnormal fetal blood scalp sample will only get worse in labour. This may not be the case where a healthy fetus is able to compensate and if the 'asphyxial episode' is short lived.

Traditionally, it has been suggested that a pH of less than 7.20 indicates the need for immediate delivery. However, the Dublin randomised controlled trial of electronic fetal heart rate monitoring versus auscultation (MacDonald et al., 1985) found fewer babies with a pH less than 7.1 in the electronic fetal heart rate monitored group, and of those fewer had neonatal seizures (1.4 versus 3.8 per 1000), although there were no differences in the longer term sequelae in either group. This suggests that, in the absence of other risk factors and given normal progress of labour, a pH of 7.20 does not necessarily indicate the need to deliver immediately but may be managed by close observation with further analyses (especially base deficit) up to half hourly.

Table 5.1.9 gives the blood gas criteria to allow labour to continue. Table 5.1.10 gives the mean blood gas values on cord blood at delivery.

INDUCTION OF LABOUR

Induction of labour may be achieved either with vaginal prostaglandins (PGs) (gel or pessaries) or artificial rupture of the mem-

Table 5.1.9 Fetal scalp blood gas values for labour to continue.

P_{O_2} (mm Hg)	>20
P_{CO_2} (mm Hg)	<50
Base deficit (mmol/L)	<9
pH	>7.16

Table 5.1.10 Normal values for cord blood gases at delivery.

	pH	P_{O_2}	P_{CO_2}	Base deficit
Mean arterial	7.26	221	253	4.5
Mean ± 1SD[a]	7.17	13	66	8.1
Mean venous	7.31	30	42	4
Mean ± 1SD[a]	7.25	22.5	51	6.7

[a] SD is standard deviation.

5

branes (ARM). It is indicated to avoid fetal or maternal compromise. The more 'favourable' the cervix is at induction the more likely is a vaginal delivery to be achieved. The 'favourability' of the cervix may be assessed by the modified Bishop score (see Table 5.1.11). A Bishop score of less than five is improved by administering PG gel or pessaries. For a primigravida 2 mg of PG gel or equivalent may be given into the posterior fornix and the cervix is assessed at 6 hours. If there is no change a further dose may be given to a total of 4 mg in 24 hours. If the Bishop score is > 5 the membranes may be ruptured to induce labour. Alternatively, if the score is < 6 a further dose of 1 mg PG gel may be given followed by ARM up to 6 hours later.

A multiparous woman with a Bishop score of <5 may have 1 mg of PG gel. If there is no cervical change and no contraction at 6 hours, the

Table 5.1.11 Bishop score – how it is derived.

Score	0	1	2
Position	Posterior	Mid	Anterior
Consistency	Firm	Intermediate	Soft
Length (cm)	3	1–2	<1
Dilatation (cm)	0	1–2	3
Station (cm)	−3	−2 to −1	0

dose may be repeated. The membranes are ruptured when the Bishop score is >6.

3 mg of prostaglandin E (PGE) pessaries are equivalent to 2 mg of PG gel.

Augmentation with syntocinon is required after ARM if contractions are not established within 2 hours for primigravid women and 3–4 hours for multigravid women.

PREMATURE RUPTURE OF THE MEMBRANES

Rupture of the membranes is premature when it occurs before the onset of uterine contractions. The management varies depending on whether the pregnancy is at term or pre-term.

Rupture of the membranes at term

Rupture of the membranes should be confirmed by observing liquor at the introitus or on vaginal examination using a sterile Cusco speculum and observing liquor coming through the cervix.

Providing there is no evidence of maternal or fetal infection or fetal compromise, allow 24 hours for the woman to go into labour before inducing labour. This approach results in fewer caesarean sections for failed induction.

If there are any signs of infection (e.g. offensive discharge, tense, tender uterus, decreased fetal movements, markedly decreased fetal heart rate, fetal heart rate variability or a fetal heart rate greater than 160 beats per minute) high vaginal swabs should be taken and labour induced or caesarean section considered for delivery.

There is no evidence to support the use of long term prophylactic antibiotics. They mask the early signs of intrauterine infection, prolonging fetal exposure. There are no benefits to the baby. Resistant strains may evolve.

If intrauterine infection is diagnosed give intravenous antibiotics (ampicillin or a cephalosporin and metranidazole) and deliver the baby.

At a gestation greater than 34 weeks, and certainly after 37 weeks, delivery may be expedited because the risk of sepsis outweighs the risks from fetal immaturity.

Premature rupture of the membranes before 34 weeks

With premature rupture of the membranes (uncomplicated) prior to 34 weeks' gestation it is appropriate to wait until spontaneous onset of labour to allow time for fetal maturation. The following observations and investigations are required:

- The administration of steroids to enhance fetal lung maturity is not necessarily contraindicated (see below).
- Twice weekly full blood count and mid-stream urine.
- Twice weekly liquor or low vaginal swab for Gram stain and culture. For accurate evidence of microorganisms in the liquor, an amniocentesis may be done.
- Four hourly maternal temperature and pulse.
- Daily cardiotocograph.

PRETERM DELIVERY

- Very low birth weight babies are defined as those weighing less than 1500 g.
- Extremely low birth weight babies are defined as those weighing less than 1000 g.
- Gestational age is the most important prognostic factor.
- Pre-term delivery occurs in 3–7 per cent of pregnancies.
- It may be due to:

Uncomplicated spontaneous preterm labour	28–40 per cent
Premature rupture of the membranes	20 per cent
Complicated or emergency delivery	25 per cent
Elective preterm delivery	16 per cent

Women in suspected preterm labour whose fetuses have absent breathing movements as observed on ultrasound scan usually progress to delivery within 48 hours. Those with fetal breathing tend not to go on to deliver.

Obstetric management of spontaneous uncomplicated preterm labour

- Diagnose labour by the change in the cervix in response to contractions, i.e. effacement or cervical dilatation.
- Accurately assess gestational age – compare date of last menstrual period and result of early ultrasound scan.

- Obtain an ultrasonically determined weight estimation (derived from the measurement of abdominal circumference).
- Exclude intrauterine infection. The following are associated with infection:

1 Maternal pyrexia, fetal tachycardia, decreased fetal movements and uterine tenderness.

2 On ultrasound the fetus may be observed in a deflexed attitude, in particular with a scaphoid spine rather than the normal flexed curvature of the spine.

- Consider Gram staining of amniotic fluid obtained by ultrasound guided amniocentesis.
- Take vaginal and rectal swabs for all women in pre-term labour to exclude infection with Group B streptococci, *Listeria monocytogenes* or *Haemophilus influenzae*.
- Decide on the mode of delivery.
- Give steroids for fetal pulmonary maturation.

Maternal steroid administration to enhance fetal lung maturity

Steroids are indicated between 24 and 32 weeks' gestation to reduce the incidence of respiratory distress syndrome and its sequelae (ultimately they reduce perinatal mortality by half). Steroids to use are:

- betamethasone 4 mg 12 hourly intramuscularly × 4 doses, **or**
- dexamethasone 12 mg intramuscularly × 2 doses 12 hours apart.

If uterine contractions are occurring and as long as there are no maternal contraindications to their use and no evidence of intrauterine infection, a beta-sympathomimetic agent (such as ritodrine) may be given with the aim of delaying labour until at least the steroids can begin to take effect (i.e. a minimum of 24 to 48 hours).

With the success rates of neonatal units **every woman considered for tocolysis must have intrauterine infection excluded as a likely cause of the preterm labour**, since unrecognised infection can have more devastating consequences on the mother and baby than respiratory distress syndrome.

Beta-sympathomimetic agents for tocolysis

Their use is contraindicated in the presence of:

- Cardiac disease
- Pre-eclampsia

- Intrauterine infection
- Intrauterine fetal death
- Ante-partum haemorrhage
- Placenta praevia.

The only true indication for tocolysis in pregnancy is to allow time for fetal pulmonary maturation to take place by suppressing preterm labour while steroids are given to facilitate fetal pulmonary maturation.

Regimen for the use of ritodrine hydrochloride

The use of beta-sympathomimetics has been associated with fatal maternal pulmonary oedema, so the mother's chest should be auscultated regularly to exclude pulmonary oedema and her fluid balance carefully monitored.

A controlled infusion device should be used for administering ritodrine. With a syringe pump the concentration of drug infused should be 3 mg/mL (150 mg ritodrine) solution in a total volume of 50 mL dextrose.

If a syringe pump is not available, the concentration should be 0.3 mg/mL (150 mg ritodrine in 500 mL of 5 per cent dextrose solution).

Saline dilutents should be reserved for women in whom dextrose solution is contraindicated such as those with diabetes mellitus.

BIBLIOGRAPHY

Bishop, E.H. (1964) Pelvic scoring for elective induction. *Obstetrics & Gynecology*, **24**, 266–268.

Cardozo, L. & Pearce, G.M. (1992) Oxytocin in active phase abnormalities of labour: a randomized study. *Obstetrics & Gynecology*, **75**, 152–157.

Crowley, P. (1989) Promoting pulmonary maturity. In: *Effective Care in Pregnancy and Childbirth* (Ed. by M. Inken, M.J.N.C. Kersey & Ian Chambers), pp 746–764. Oxford University Press, Oxford.

Friedman, E.A. (1954) The graphic analysis of labor. *American Journal of Obstetrics & Gynecology*, **68**, 1568–1575.

Gebbie, D. (1982) Symphysiotomy. *Clinics in Obstetrics & Gynaecology*, **9**, 663–683.

Liggins, G.C. & Howie, R.N. (1972) A controlled rial of antepartum glucocorticoid treatment for prevention of the respiratory distress syndrome in premature infants. *Pediatrics*, **50**, 515–525.

MacDonald, D., Grant, A., Sheridan-Pereira, M., Boylan, P. & Chalmers, I. (1985) The Dublin randomised trial of intrapartum fetal heart monitoring. *American Journal of Obstetrics & Gynecology*, **152**, 525–539.

McFarlane, A. & Chamberlain, G. (1993) What is happening to caesarean section rates? Editorial, *The Lancet*, **342**, 1005–1006.

O'Driscoll, K., Folly, M. & MacDonald, D. (1984) Active management of labor as an alternative to Caesarean section for dystocia. *Obstetrics & Gynecology*, **63**, 485–490.

O'Driscoll, K., Folly, M., MacDonald, D. & Stronge, J. (1988) Caesarean section and perinatal outcome: Response from the House of Horne. *American Journal of Obstetrics & Gynecology*, **158**, 449–452.

Philpott, R.H. & Castle, W.H.O. (1972) Cervicography in the management of labour on primigravidae: I. The alert-line for detecting abnormal labour. *Journal of Obstetrics & Gynaecology of the British Commonwealth*, **79**, 592–593.

Scott, D.B. & Hibbard, B.M. (1990) Serious non-fatal complications associated with extradural block in obstetric practice. *British Journal of Anaesthesia*, **64**, 537–541.

Spencer, J.A.D. (1988) Symphysiotomy for vaginal breech delivery: two case reports. *British Journal of Obstetrics and Gynaecology*, **94**, 716–718.

Turner, M.J., Webb, J.B. & Gordan, H. (1987) Active management of labour in primigravidae. *Journal of Obstetrics & Gynecology*, **7**, 79–83.

Thorpe-Beeston, G.J., Banfield, P.G. & Saunders, N.J. (1992) Outcome of breech delivery at term. *British Medical Journal*, **305**, 746–747.

5.2   Major obstetric haemorrhage

PRIMARY POST-PARTUM HAEMORRHAGE (PPH)

Primary PPH is blood loss of more than 500 mL within 24 hours of delivery. It occurs following 5 per cent of deliveries and major haemorrhage is still a major cause of maternal morbidity and mortality. Prophylaxis using oxytocics reduces the incidence of postpartum haemorrhage by one third.

Clinical estimations of blood loss tend to underestimate loss significantly (see below). Both continuous 'seepage' and the rate of loss may be underestimated. A **cupped double handful of blood clot** is very approximately equivalent to a loss of **500 mL**.

PRIMARY OBJECTIVES OF MANAGING OBSTETRIC HAEMORRHAGE

- Maintain normal intravascular blood volume.
- Control bleeding.
- Restore red cell mass once suitable compatibility tests have been done. See Tables 5.2.1 and 5.2.2.

MEDICAL CONTROL OF HAEMORRHAGE

1 Prophylaxis

Syntometrine (ergometrine maleate 500 micrograms and 5 units of oxytocin in 1 mL) combines the sustained oxytocic action of ergometrine with the more rapid action of oxytocin. **The routine dose is 1 mL intramuscularly**. It may be given intravenously under some circumstances (see below). It is used in the active management of the third stage of labour, usually given at delivery of the anterior shoulder in a normal singleton pregnancy.

2 Therapeutic measures to arrest further haemorrhage

Syntocinon

Syntocinon is a synthetic analogue of oxytocin, the posterior pituitary hormone. It is available as Oxytocin Injection BP containing 2 units in 2 mL, 5 units in 1 mL, 10 units in 1 mL or 50 units in 5 mL.

For post-partum haemorrhage due to uterine atony, **50 units in 500 mL** dextrose–saline may be infused intravenously over 3–4 hours. If more than 100 units over 24 hours is needed, because of the intrinsic antidiuretic effect, large volumes of dilute infusion fluid (e.g. 5 per cent dextrose) will cause water intoxication. Therefore if more than 100 units of oxytocin is required, delivery should be via high concentrations in a syringe pump.

Ergometrine 0.5–1 mg

Ergometrine alone is more likely to cause nausea, vomiting, headache or a rise in maternal arterial and ventral venous pressure. Avoid using in women with hypertension.

Syntocinon and ergometrine exert different cardiovascular effects. Syntocinon causes vasodilation, whereas ergometrine causes vasoconstriction. Therefore avoid ergometrine in hypertension or any

Table 5.2.1 Summary of management of obstetric haemorrhage. (Source with modifications courtesy of Dr T. Thomas.)

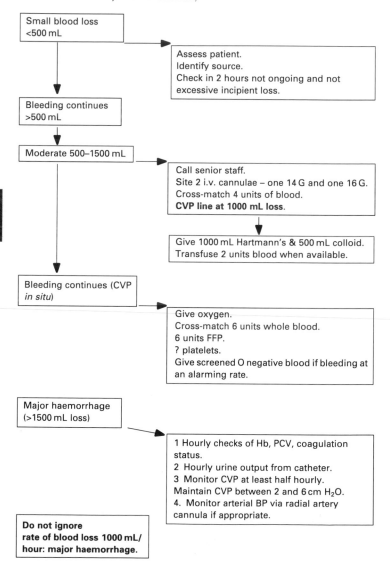

Small blood loss
<500 mL

Assess patient.
Identify source.
Check in 2 hours not ongoing and not excessive incipient loss.

Bleeding continues
>500 mL

Moderate 500–1500 mL

Call senior staff.
Site 2 i.v. cannulae – one 14 G and one 16 G.
Cross-match 4 units of blood.
CVP line at 1000 mL loss.

Give 1000 mL Hartmann's & 500 mL colloid.
Transfuse 2 units blood when available.

Bleeding continues (CVP *in situ*)

Give oxygen.
Cross-match 6 units whole blood.
6 units FFP.
? platelets.
Give screened O negative blood if bleeding at an alarming rate.

Major haemorrhage
(>1500 mL loss)

1 Hourly checks of Hb, PCV, coagulation status.
2 Hourly urine output from catheter.
3 Monitor CVP at least half hourly.
Maintain CVP between 2 and 6 cm H_2O.
4. Monitor arterial BP via radial artery cannula if appropriate.

**Do not ignore
rate of blood loss 1000 mL/
hour: major haemorrhage.**

Table 5.2.2 Persistent haemorrhage – medical treatment.

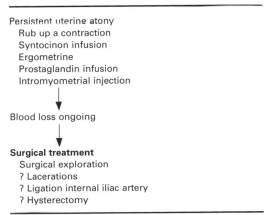

Persistent uterine atony
  Rub up a contraction
  Syntocinon infusion
  Ergometrine
  Prostaglandin infusion
  Intromyometrial injection

↓

Blood loss ongoing

↓

Surgical treatment
  Surgical exploration
  ? Lacerations
  ? Ligation internal iliac artery
  ? Hysterectomy

other condition to prevent increased systemic vascular resistance. Ergometrine is used in severe post-partum haemorrhage because it is long acting and because it does not have the vasodilatory effects of syntocinon.

Prostaglandin

A prostaglandin infusion in addition to a syntocinon infusion can be used when blood loss is in excess of 1500 mL and ongoing.

Give as an intravenous infusion of Prostaglandin E_2 5 mg in 500 mL of normal saline. Infuse at a rate of 10 micrograms/minute for 2 minutes and then 20 microgram/minute.

Carboprost (Hemabate™) 250 micrograms in 1 mL can also be used either by deep i.m. injection (using a tuberculin syringe) or preferably directly into the myometrium of an atonic uterus. Further doses of 250 micrograms can be given at intervals of approximately 1.5 hours but the total dose should not exceed 2 mg (8 doses).

Prostaglandin can cause severe pulmonary bronchoconstriction **and should be avoided in asthmatic women** or in those with cardiac disease.

CLINICAL ASSESSMENT OF BLOOD LOSS

The total blood volume of the average pregnant woman (weighing 75 kg) is 6 L. **Signs of significant blood loss are shown in Table 5.2.3.**

Table 5.2.3 The percentage blood loss and the clinical signs.

Blood loss		
Per cent	Volume (mL)	Clinical effects of blood loss
10	600	Pulse begins to rise.
15	900	Tachycardia and pallor due to vasoconstriction; cardiac output will have begun to fall but systolic BP is maintained by vasoconstriction e.g. tachycardia until 20% loss.
20	1200	Increase in pulse rate by more than 30 beats/minute compared with rate before haemorrhage; marked pallor; systemic blood pressure begins to fall.

Note: In pregnancy the above observations can be affected by aorto-caval compression, tachycardia as a result of pain in labour and the analgesia regimen which has been used.

- Do not ignore the rate of blood loss.
- Rise in pulse rate – a tachycardia or a rise of 20 per cent in pulse rate indicates major haemorrhage (1500 mL and over).
- Fall in blood pressure is a late sign.
- Skin pallor – occurs as a result of vasoconstriction (at about 15 per cent of blood volume loss) in order to maintain blood pressure.
- Decrease in urine output. Sometimes the significance of this is difficult to assess because some patients with major haemorrhage have other complicating factors of coagulopathies and pre-eclampsia.

MANAGEMENT OF MASSIVE HAEMORRHAGE

'Massive transfusion' is arbitrarily defined as that which requires replacement of the patient's total blood volume by stored homologous bank blood in less than 24 hours.

Volume replacement aims to maintain circulating blood volume, the oxygen carrying capacity of the blood, haemostasis, colloid osmotic pressure, and plasma biochemical balance.

Each centre should have written agreed protocols which are rigidly adhered to.

HOW TO REPLACE FLUIDS IN OBSTETRIC HAEMORRHAGE (see Table 5.2.4 for summary)

Types of synthetic replacement solutions

Crystalloids and colloids

These restore circulating blood volume. Crystalloids (e.g. Hartmann's solution) resemble extracellular fluid. The use of large volumes of crystalloids (particularly in pre-eclampsia) may contribute to the development of the adult respiratory distress syndrome. Infusion of albumin may be required if levels of albumin are low (<26 g/L).

Table 5.2.4 Suggested procedure for immediate resuscitation.

- Commence by **infusing crystalloid either Hartmann's solution or isotonic saline.** The circulation should show improvement after infusion of 1–2 L.
- Then **give 1 L of colloid (haemaccel or gelafusine) until blood arrives. Give 2 units of cross-matched blood.**
- After red cell replacement give colloid to replace removed albumin and fresh frozen plasma and platelets, depending on the extent of the blood loss.

Colloids

These are large molecules which increase the osmotic pressure. 25 per cent albumin draws fluid from the interstitial space into the circulation.

Albumin.   4.5 per cent human albumin solution (hAS) can rarely cause severe reactions. It is very expensive.

Other plasma substitutes.   These are cheaper than albumin but are more likely to produce severe reactions.

Dextran 70. Dextrans affect platelet function adversely and interfere with tests of blood grouping and cross matching. They therefore should not be used in obstetric haemorrhage because of the likelihood of coagulation deficit.

Modified gelatins, e.g. **Gelofusine** (a succinylated gelatin) and **haemaccel** (a urea-linked gelatin) have a half life in the circulation of 5–7 hours but a clinical effect of only 30 minutes to 2 hours. **Haemaccel** has a high calcium and potassium content. It does not interfere with cross matching of blood.

Heta starch (HESPAN) is a true plasma substitute that will increase osmotic pressure for several days but has a clinical effect of only 3 to 4 hours.

Blood transfusion

Blood transfusion is advised when 20 per cent or more blood volume has been lost (i.e. about 1200 mL calculated on 80 mL/kg) guided by haemoglobin measurements and circulatory variables.

If there is no time for full cross-match and there are no minor antibodies present, then grouped uncross-matched blood is preferable to (uncross-matched) O negative blood. **Only give uncross-matched O negative blood in an obstetric emergency if the woman's blood group is unknown, or type-specific blood is not available** because, since 85 per cent of women are Rh positive, there is a risk that transfusion with Rh(D) negative blood will cause the production of anti c antibodies. This could lead to haemolytic disease in a subsequent pregnancy, as well as causing cross-matching problems in any future blood transfusions.

Fresh whole blood has all the necessary coagulation factors required with massive haemorrhage. It cannot be used for transfusion because there is insufficient time for blood grouping tests and to exclude hepatitis surface antigen, HIV antibody, syphilis, and infections such as cytomegalovirus and Epstein–Barr virus. Fresh frozen plasma is probably the best plasma replacement therapy for obstetric haemorrhage because it has all coagulation factors – fibrinogen, factors V and VIII and the coagulation inhibitor antithrombin III.

Red blood cells are now packed in 100 mL of SAG-M (sodium chloride, adenine, glucose and mannitol), which contains no protein and no coagulation factors.

Give fresh frozen plasma after 4 units of such reconstituted red cells, and then 1 unit of plasma protein fraction (PPF) for every two further units of SAG-M blood used to maintain plasma osmotic pressure.

Cryoprecipitate is richer in fibrinogen than fresh frozen plasma, but it lacks antithrombin III (which is rapidly consumed in obstetric bleeding associated with DIC) and stored red blood cells provide all the necessary components and should be used.

Whole blood anticoagulated with citrate may contain complex calcium ions. Give 1 ampoule (10 mL of 10 per cent calcium gluconate) slowly over 10 minutes for every 6 units of blood infused. Alternatively, the serum calcium level should be checked and calcium given if it is low (corrected for reduced albumin levels).

Platelets

Give platelets after a blood transfusion of 8–10 units. The platelet count will drop to 50×10^9/L when one and a half to twice the blood volume has been replaced.

Each unit of platelets contains 0.55×10^9/L platelets and 50 mL plasma, and will raise the platelet count by 10×10^9/L.

The standard adult dose of six units of platelet concentrate should control the microvascular bleeding that results from low platelets, equivalent to 1 unit of platelet concentrate per 10 kg body weight.

Acute disseminated intravascular coagulation should be suspected when the thrombin time rises to more than double the control value. About 10 units of cryoprecipitate should then be given in addition to fresh frozen plasma to correct the deficiencies of fibrinogen and factor VIII.

Stored blood – disadvantages

Temperature – when rapid transfusion is necessary the blood should be warmed whenever possible by an in-line warmer.

Use blood that is less than 14 days old. Levels of 2,3-diphosphoglycerate (2,3-DPG) within the red blood cells fall with storage, shifting the oxygen–haemoglobin dissociation curve to the left. Thus haemoglobin in less efficient at releasing the oxygen for cellular consumption.

Platelets and neutrophils lose their function.

The labile clotting factors (V, VIII, IX and X) disappear.

The pH and calcium fall, the P_{CO_2} and potassium rise. ECG monitoring is mandatory. However, acidosis from a massive transfusion tends to be corrected because citrate in the stored blood produces an alkalosis.

THE RESUSCITATION TEAM

Teamwork is essential.

The overall policy should be directed by the senior staff in obstetrics and anaesthesia. All personnel must be fully informed about patients who require high dependency care from the outset. Duties may be divided as follows:

Resuscitation Manager	Duty anaesthetic registrar
Obstetric Manager	Duty obstetric registrar
Midwifery Manager	Midwife in charge of the case
Record Keeper	Obstetric senior house officer

Suggested roles for members of the resuscitation team

Resuscitation Manager

- Site peripheral i.v. cannulae and CVP line.
- Take 20 mL of venous blood and send to pathology laboratory for appropriate investigations (see Table 5.2.5). (Record Keeper to communicate with laboratory).
- Prescribe the manage i.v. fluid regimen.
- In conjunction with the Obstetric Manager order the appropriate quantities of blood products. Discuss haematological requirements of these patients with the haematology senior personnel.
- Dictate and sign an hourly resume in the notes.
- Ensure that the Record Keeper is fully informed as to all drugs and fluids prescribed, decisions made, laboratory contact (time) and requests.
- Prescribe H_2 antagonists (parenteral route) routinely for these patients (ranitidine 50 mg slowly i.v.).

Obstetric Manager

- Overall obstetric management (with the exception of resuscitation).
- Catheterise patient with indwelling catheter.

Table 5.2.5 Bloods to be taken with obstetric haemorrhage.

Investigation	Type of blood tube (in UK)
Cross-match	
Full blood count	EDTA (purple)
Platelet count	EDTA (purple)
APTT	Citrate (light blue)
Prothrombin time (extrinsic clotting time)	Citrate (light blue)
Activated partial thromboplastin time (intrinsic clotting time	Citrate (light blue)
Thrombin time (10–15 s)	Citrate (light blue)
Fibrinogen titre	Citrate (light blue)
Fibrin degradation products (FDPs) 2.0 mL	EDTA (purple)

- Pain relief in conjunction with Resuscitation Manager.
- Dictate and sign hourly resume notes if possible.
- Ensure that Record Keeper is fully informed.

Midwifery Manager

- General nursing care of mother.
- Give adequate explanations of events and procedures to patient and ensure relatives are informed.
- Measure blood loss, blood pressure, heart rate, CVP, temperature, urine output, urinalysis and dictate results to Record Keeper for recording on appropriate chart at 15 minute intervals (minimum) initially.
- Give i.v. fluids as prescribed.
- Physiotherapy – two hourly turning whenever possible.
- Record nursing procedures as required.

Record Keeper

- Responsible for recording and timing all events, results, telephone messages, particularly recording names against instructions.
- Ensure that a 'Special Observation Chart' is completed correctly.
- Remind the relevant clinician to write to dictate a summary following each visit and examination of the patient.
- Provide the communication link between members of the team, laboratory services and senior assistance.
- The Record Keeper should nominate a deputy if he/she has to leave the room.

INSERTION OF A CVP LINE

It is advisable to consider insertion of a CVP line when blood loss is over 1500 mL and ongoing (see Table 5.2.6).

Correct placement of the CVP line

The antecubital fossa should always be considered first. Check that the position of the tip of the catheter is correctly placed near the function of the superior vena cava and right atrium. Check the position by portable chest X-ray. If that is not possible, obtain a display of the pressure wave form on an oscilloscope. If the catheter is in the pulmonary artery, the CVP will be artificially raised.

Table 5.2.6 Subsequent monitoring and therapy after initial replacement.

Monitor the following:	Desired effect
CVP line	2–6 mm Hg
Venous access	Two 14 or 16 gauge cannulae
Catheterise	Urine output (0.5 mL/kg/hour)
	Restore systolic blood pressure to 80% of blood pressure before bleeding started.
Heart rate (ECG)	
Deliver oxygen at a concentration of 30%	Maintain the reading on the pulse oximeter at more than 96%. If the reading is abnormal do blood gases.

Measure the following: (initially every 15 minutes)
Haemoglobin
Haematocrit
Serum potassium
Clotting studies – platelets and fibrinogen level

Review the replacement fluids
Ratio of crystalloid to colloid 2:1
Clotting factors and platelets should be given on the advice of a haematologist
Ventilation is required if adequate pulmonary gas exchange cannot be maintained

Note: **Fresh frozen plasma** contains plasma, all coagulation factors but no platelets.
Cryoprecipitate contains fibrinogen, factor VIII, factor XIII, von Willebrand factor.

Using the external jugular vein has few complications but a lower success rate than the internal jugular vein.

Internal jugular or subclavian vein catheterisation should be performed only if other options have been rejected. This is because of the risk of puncture of the subclavian artery and pneumothorax, particularly when a coagulopathy or respiratory problems are present.

Reading the CVP

Ideally, the CVP should be measured by the same person on each occasion.

The zero of the water manometer should be on the same horizontal level as the right atrium, i.e. on the mid-axillary line in the supine position (with pelvic tilt). This position may be difficult to obtain in the labouring pregnant woman.

The normal value is 0–5 cm H_2O, and is reduced slightly by inferior vena cava compression from the gravid uterus.

Because of normal variation in the CVP, and the possibility of relatively large measurement errors, a useful test rather than treating absolute values, is to perform a fluid challenge: 200 mL 0.9 per cent saline or colloid solution is given as rapidly as possible and the CVP is monitored closely for the next 10–15 minutes. A normal response is for the CVP to rise by several centimetres of water and then return to baseline over 5–10 minutes. If the pressure stays above baseline, the circulation is overfilled. If the CVP hardly rises, then the circulation is underfilled and the challenge can be repeated.

Signs of adequate fluid replacement

- Hypotension and tachycardia are corrected.
- CVP returns to normal range or starting value. This will need to be checked repeatedly because, as compensatory vasoconstriction is reduced, the intravascular capacity will increase and CVP may fall again.
- Urine output should be 1–2 mL/kg/hour (70–100 mL/hour for the average woman).
- However, urine output may not accurately reflect intravascular volume replacement. The delay in onset of a physiological diuresis may be mediated through antidiuretic hormone operating post-surgically or post-partum.

SURGICAL CONTROL OF HAEMORRHAGE

General measures

Identify the site of bleeding from the genital tract. If the woman's general condition suggests a greater blood loss than is apparent inspect for concealed blood loss such as an intraperitoneal or a vulval haematoma.

Induce contractility of the uterus initially by 'rubbing up' a contraction and expelling any clot from the uterus. Maintain contractility with the use of oxytocics.

Consider manual internal or external aortic compression as a temporising measure for major haemorrhage.

Catheterise the patient and measure urine output hourly initially.

Beware of infusing too high a dose of oxytocin in a large volume of electrolyte free solution. Oxytocin has an antidiuretic effect and can cause water overload (headache, vomiting, drowsiness, blindness and convulsions), manifested by a low sodium (less than 125 mmol/L).

Exploration of the uterus

Make sure there are no retained products of conception due, for example, to delivery of an incomplete placenta or to a succenturiate lobe of the placenta.

Uterine scars, e.g. previous caesarean section or myomectomy. A previous caesarean section and anteriorly situated placenta identified in the lower segment in the current pregnancy puts the mother at a greater chance of having an abnormally adherent placenta ('placenta accreta') and of requiring a hysterectomy for the control of post-partum haemorrhage.

Techniques of exploration

Adequate analgesia/anaesthesia is vital.

Visualise the cervix using lateral wall vaginal retractors. Use sponge holding forceps to 'walk' around the circumference of the cervix inspecting carefully for bleeding.

Check the vaginal walls for spiral lacerations. Identify the apex of such lacerations and suture securely. Use 2/0 vicryl on a round bodied needle taking large bites of tissue, because it is likely to be very friable. Persistent vaginal bleeding puts the patient at risk of intractable bleeding and bleeding posteriorly to form a vulval haematoma, which can cause extensive concealed bleeding.

Explore the uterus digitally under anaesthesia and remove any retained products of conception.

Major surgical intervention

Ligation of the internal iliac (hypogastric) and/or hysterectomy should be considered in patients in whom haemorrhage is not controlled by conservative means. **These procedures should be performed neither too late nor too early.** They must only be carried out on the decision of and by an experienced obstetrician or surgeon.

Ligation of the internal iliac arteries

Both internal iliac arteries are ligated immediately below the bifur-cation of the common iliac artery **but only after positive identification**

and exclusion of the external iliac artery. The ureter and internal iliac vein can be identified readily. The internal iliac artery at this point is 1–3 cm in length and close to the pelvic brim.

The internal iliac artery is ligated immediately below the bifurcation of the common iliac artery.

No significant side effects have been reported after internal iliac artery ligation, except when the internal iliac artery has not been identified correctly and the external iliac artery has been ligated. Because of the wide collateral circulation of the pelvic tissue, necrosis or other damage from ischaemia does not occur.

Hysterectomy

Consider hysterectomy when bleeding is uncontrollable or after an 8–10 unit blood transfusion, before irreversible shock has set in. However, always try to repair uterine damage/rupture to preserve fertility.

This is necessary in less than 1 per cent of cases with a previous history of a caesarean section and in 2 per cent of those with a classical caesarean section due to scar rupture.

Predisposing factors to hysterectomy

Uterine atony due to multiple pregnancy, large baby, polyhydramnios or halothane anaesthesia; grand multiparity, antepartum haemorrhage (especially placental abruption); prolonged labour.

AMNIOTIC FLUID EMBOLISM

Incidence 1:8000 to 1:80 000. Mortality up to 90 per cent.

Clinical features

Respiratory distress, cyanosis, cardiovascular collapse, DIC or massive haemorrhage may be present. Sudden, extreme shock with cyanosis occurs due to shut down of the pulmonary circulation, possibly with secondary left ventricular dysfunction. This is followed by massive and intractable uterine bleeding and intravascular coagulation. Mortality occurs from respiratory and cardiac failure due to platelet fibrin thrombi formed which accumulate within the pulmonary blood vessels.

Management

- Circulatory support – may include inotropic agents/cardio-pulmonary resuscitation (CPR).
- Restore circulating blood volume – see p. 267.
- Insert a pulmonary artery flotation catheter as soon as possible because of possible left ventricular dysfunction.
- Maintain oxygenation – intermittent positive pressure ventilation (IPPV) may well be necessary.
- Correct coagulopathy on advice from a haematologist.
- Continue to monitor in an intensive therapy unit.

BIBLIOGRAPHY

Hewitt, P.E. & Machin, S.J. (1990) Massive blood transfusion. *British Medical Journal*, **300**, 107–109.

Prendiville, W.J., Elbourne, D.R. & Chalmers, I. (1988b) The effects of routine oxytocic administration in the management of the third stage of labour: an overview of the evidence from controlled trials. *British Journal of Obstetrics & Gynaecology*, **95**, 3–16.

Prendiville, W.J., Harding, J.E., Elbourne, D.R. & Stirrat, G.M. (1988a) The Bristol third stage trial: active versus physiological management of third stage of labour. *British Medical Journal*, **297**, 1295–1300.

Thomas, T.A. (1989) Resuscitation of the obstetric patient. In: *Cardiopulmonary Resuscitation* (Ed. by P.J.F. Baskett), pp. 275–294. Elsevier Science Publishers BV, Amsterdam.

6 Fetal Assessment

The purpose of fetal assessment is to try to determine the pattern of growth and the state of health of the fetus at the time of the examination. Tests allow inferences to be drawn about the presence or absence of **intrauterine growth retardation** and **fetal hypoxia**.

INTRAUTERINE GROWTH RETARDATION

Intrauterine growth retardation (IUGR) is the failure of the fetus to achieve its full growth potential. It is associated with increased perinatal morbidity and mortality (see Table 6.1). It is arbitrarily defined as being <10th centile of the birth weight for gestation (see Fig. 6.1 and Fig. 6.2). However, this definition will include infants who are normally grown but constitutionally small, and excludes larger infants who are truly growth retarded. The more rigorous definitions of less than the 5th or 3rd centiles include a greater number of babies at risk of complications (see below).

Table 6.1 Birth weight centiles and perinatal mortality rate per thousand.

Birth weight (centile)	Perinatal mortality/1000 total births
>10th	12
5–10th	22
<5th	190

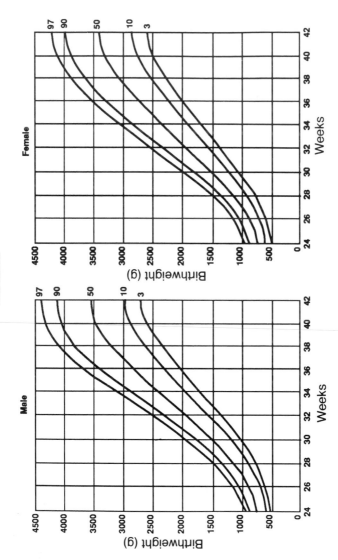

Fig. 6.1 Birthweight centiles by gestational age. (Reproduced with permission from Yudkin, P.L., Aboualfa, M., Eyre, J.A., Redman, C.W.G. & Wilkinson, A.R. (1987) New birthweight and head circumference centiles for gestational ages 24 to 42 weeks. *Early Human Development*, **15**, 49.)

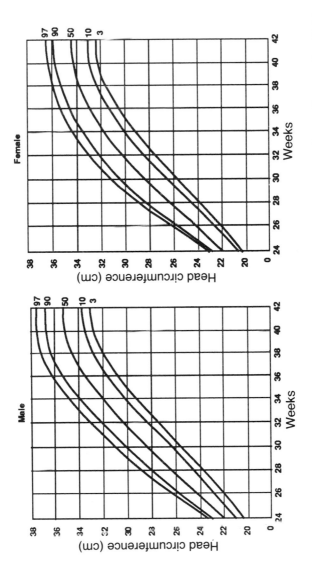

Fig. 6.2 Head circumference centiles at birth for individual gestations. (Reproduced with permission from Yudkin, P.L., Aboualfa, M., Eyre, J.A., Eedman, C.W.G. & Wilkinson, A.R. (1987) New birthweight and head circumference centiles for gestational ages 24 to 42 weeks. *Early Human Development*, **15**, 49.)

IUGR occurs as a result of impaired placental circulation causing fetal starvation. Head growth is relatively spared but depletion of the glycogen stores in the liver causes reduction in the expected abdominal circumference.

Antenatally, patterns of growth are determined by ultrasound scanning. Measuring the abdominal circumference at two week intervals identifies whether growth is appropriate (i.e. occurring along the centiles) for the individual baby (see abdominal circumference growth charts, Chapter 11).

After birth, the baby's **ponderal index**, a measure of soft tissue mass obtained by the formula (birth weight/length^3) × 100, is a better predictor of the complications of growth retardation than birth weight for gestation (see Table 6.2 and Fig. 6.3).

Table 6.2 Distribution of birth weight (g) for gestational age. 10th and 90th centiles = mean ± 1.28 standard deviation (SD); 50th centile is equivalent to the mean. (Reproduced with permission from Wilcox, M.A., Johnson, I.R., Maynard, P.V., Smith, S.J. & Chilvers, C.E.D. (1993) The individualised birthweight ratio: a more logical outcome measure of pregnancy than birthweight alone. *British Journal of Obstetrics & Gynaecology*, **100**, 344.)

Gestation (weeks)	Centile		
	10th	50th	90th
24	635	743	851
25	743	858	973
26	734	906	1078
27	843	1063	1283
28	833	1153	1473
29	960	1280	1600
30	1090	1507	1924
31	1308	1695	2082
32	1398	1906	2414
33	1745	2144	2543
34	1841	2324	2807
35	2023	2576	3129
36	2221	2774	3327
37	2418	2991	3564
38	2648	3197	3746
39	2828	3366	3904
40	2970	3522	4074
41	3090	3652	4214
42	3143	3750	4357

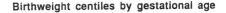

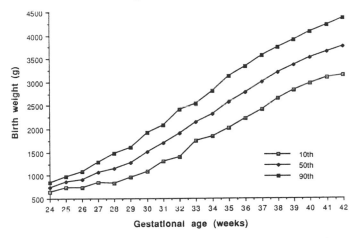

Fig. 6.3 Birthweight centiles by gestational age (corrected). (Reproduced with permission from Wilcox, M.A., Johnson, I.R., Maynard, P.V., Smith, S.J. & Chilvers, C.E.D. (1993) The individualised birthweight ratio: a more logical outcome measure of pregnancy than birthweight alone. *British Journal of Obstetrics & Gynaecology*, **100**, 344.)

6

Complications of growth retardation

1 Birth asphyxia (see below).

2 Hypoglycaemia: occurs in up to 30 per cent of growth retarded infants. It is due to reduced total glycogen stores. If not treated promptly it has a poor prognosis with serious neurological sequelae.

3 Meconium aspiration at birth occurs in up to 20 per cent.

4 Polycythaemia: occurs in up to 40 per cent of growth retarded infants. This may cause cerebral thrombosis and is associated with necrotising enterocolitis.

5 Hypothermia: a great deal of heat is lost through the skin because of reduced subcutaneous fat and an increased surface area:volume ratio.

6 Low birth weight infants remain at increased risk of death up to one year of age

FETAL HYPOXIA

In chronic hypoxia due to impaired placental function, the fetal circulation attempts to achieve perfusion of essential organs (e.g. brain, kidney, etc.) (see Table 6.3). Subcutaneous fat and tissue bulk are decreased producing the clinical picture of the scrawny growth retarded baby.

Table 6.3 Blood flow changes in organs associated with asphyxia.

Blood flow maintained in	Blood flow reduced in
Heart	Limbs
Brain	Gut
Placenta	Kidneys
Adrenal	Skin

Physical activity reduces, causing the changes in behaviour screened for by the biophysical profile (BPP); see below. Renal blood flow ultimately falls, causing a reduction in the production of amniotic fluid and, therefore, **oligohydramnios**.

As the fetus relies more and more on anaerobic metabolism, lactate is produced in increasing amounts and unbuffered HCO_3 diffuses out of the red blood cells, producing acidaemia. Cellular damage results if this is prolonged and severe. The following arterial cord blood gas levels are found in **severe acidaemia**:

pH<7.0

P_{O_2}<15 mm Hg

P_{CO_2}>75 mm Hg

The effects of acidaemia depend on its cause, duration and the ability of the fetus to compensate (this is poor in IUGR).

The well grown baby can withstand an acute hypoxia of short lived duration which will damage an already chronically stressed baby. For management of the fetus during labour see Chapter 5.

METHODS OF FETAL ASSESSMENT

Clinical assessment of pregnancy remains an important aspect of screening for fetal health and welfare.

The cardiotocograph (CTG)

The fetal heart rate and its components on the cardiotocograph have been used to try to identify the fetus at risk of asphyxia, both antenatally and intrapartum. A normal CTG identifies the fetus at low risk of asphyxia.

The components of the CTG are the baseline fetal heart rate (FHR) and its variability.

The baseline fetal heart rate (FHR)

The normal FHR lies between 120 and 160 beats/minute observed over a 5–10 minute period. **Bradycardia** is a FHR below 100 beats/minute. **Tachycardia** is a FHR over 160 beats/minute.

Variability

Short term variability is the changes that occur in the beat-to-beat interval. It cannot be defined adequately by the naked eye but can be usefully assessed by the computerised CTG. It is described in milliseconds, being the time interval from one heart beat to the next averaged over an epoch (3.75 ms). Short term variability is the difference in fetal heart rate from one epoch to the next averaged over one minute (16 in total). **Short term variability of 3 ms** or less indicates imminent fetal demise and appropriate action must be taken.

Long term variability is the oscillations of the FHR around its mean. Normal is 5–10 beats/minute for more than 40 minutes. If the baseline fetal heart rate fluctuates from 135 to 145 beats/minute with a baseline of 140 bpm, the long term variability is 10 bpm. When assessed by computerised CTG the lower limit of normal long term variability is about 30 ms. Readings of 20 ms or less are associated with a high incidence of chronic fetal hypoxemia.

FHR variability is influenced by fetal activity states and will be reduced when the fetus is asleep. Epidural analgesia is often associated with a rise in fetal heart rate and corresponding decrease in fetal heart rate variability.

Accelerations: A transient increase in the FHR of 15 beats/minute or more, lasting 15 s or over.

Decelerations: Transient episodes of slowing of the FHR below the baseline level of more than 15 beats/minute and lasting 10 s or more. They are further classified in relation to uterine contractions.

- **Early decelerations** are a drop in the baseline fetal heart rate where the nadir of the drop corresponds directly with the peak of the uterine contraction as observed on the tocograph recording.

- **Late declerations** occur when the nadir of the drop in the fetal heart rate occurs after the peak of the uterine contraction and fails to return to the baseline before the completion of the uterine contraction.

- **Variable decelerations** may be a more sinister feature.

CTG interpretation

Interpretation of the CTG to identify the compromised fetus is difficult for the following reasons.

- Both inter- and intra-observer error in interpretation are significant.

- It is difficult to interpret the significance of the magnitude and duration of FHR changes.

- Some combinations of components may be more important than others.

- Features of the CTG (decreased fetal heart rate variability) that characterise chronic hypoxaemia antenatally or identify the terminal fetus do not necessarily equate with acidaemia in labour.

- Although decreased FHR variability usually reflects central nervous system dysfunction secondary to asphyxia, it may be due to other factors such as intoxication, congenital malformations or other abnormalities.

- Certain features, particularly decelerations, can occur normally during the second stage of labour.

- Computerised analysis as an attempt at objective measurement of the components of the CTG has failed to correlate what are traditionally interpreted as abnormalities of the FHR on the CTG with acidaemia.

There are, however, certain patterns which are pathognomonic of severe fetal compromise. These are shown in Figs 6.4 to 6.8.

The predictive value of electronic fetal heart monitoring

The use of continuous CTG monitoring during labour at term in women at low risk of any adverse outcome does not result in any reduction in perinatal mortality or morbidity, save for a possible reduction in early neonatal seizures. However, longer term outcome is no better.

The biophysical profile (BPP)

This tries to determine fetal state by assessing a series of variable shown in Tables 6.4 and 6.5. A normal examination strongly suggests

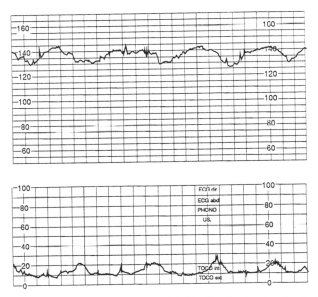

Fig. 6.4 CTG with no FHR variability and shallow late decelerations in relation to uterine contractions. A pre-terminal CTG resulting in a stillbirth. (Courtesy of Dr J. Westgate.)

that the fetus is well at that time and probably for up to 24 hours thereafter. However, the whole clinical picture must be taken into account, e.g. delivery may be indicated even in the presence of a normal score if the fetus is growth retarded, if the patient is beyond 42 weeks' gestation (i.e. post dates) or for maternal indications.

Even though assessment of amniotic fluid volume is subjective, significant oligohydramnios in the post dates' patient may be an indication for delivery even if all the other components of the biophysical score are normal.

Doppler ultrasound

When an ultrasound beam is directed at a moving structure the returning echo will have undergone a frequency shift – the Doppler effect. This can be used to calculate the velocity of flow of blood through blood vessels. **It does not measure flow directly.**

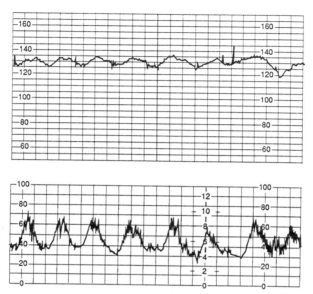

Fig. 6.5 CTG with the same pattern as above but very frequent uterine contractions due to placental abruption resulting in a stillbirth. (Courtesy of Dr J. Westgate.)

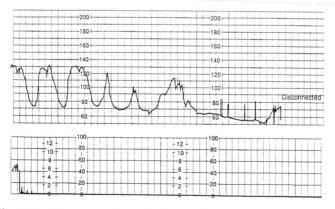

Fig. 6.6 Rapid increases in the length of time of the decelerations with decreasing baseline indicating imminent fetal death. (Courtesy of Dr K. Murphy.)

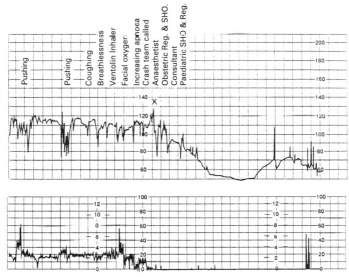

Fig. 6.7 A terminal fetal heart rate pattern. The mother collapsed and died at X (Courtesy of Dr E. Shellabear.)

6

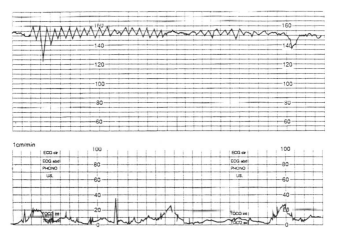

Fig. 6.8 A rarely seen sinusoidal CTG associated with fetal anaemia due to a large feto-maternal haemorrhage. The same pattern can occur in short bursts associated with thumb sucking.

Table 6.4 Biophysical profile scoring: technique and interpretation. (Source Manning *et al.* (1985).)

Biophysical variable	Normal (score = 2)	Abnormal (score = 0)
1 Fetal breathing movements	$\geqslant 1$ episode of $\geqslant 30$ s in 30 min	Absent or no episode of $\geqslant 30$ s in 30 min
2 Gross body movements	$\geqslant 3$ discrete body/limb movements in 30 min (episodes of active continuous movement considered as single movement)	$\geqslant 2$ episodes of body/limb movements in 30 min
3 Fetal tone	$\geqslant 1$ episode of active extension return to flexion of fetal limb(s) or trunk. Opening and closing of hand considered normal tone	Either slow extension with return to partial flexion or movement of limb in full extension or absent fetal movement
4 Reactive fetal heart rate	$\geqslant 2$ episodes of acceleration of $\geqslant 15$ beats/min and of $\geqslant 15$ s associated with fetal movement in 20 min	<2 episodes of acceleration of fetal heart rate or acceleration of <15 beats/min in 20 min
5 Qualitative amniotic fluid volume	$\geqslant 1$ pocket of fluid measuring $\geqslant 1$ cm in two perpendicular planes	Either no pockets or a pocket <1 cm in two perpendicular planes

The Doppler shifted signals from human vessels are converted to visual signals termed the flow velocity waveform (FVW). Doppler waveforms reflect cardiac contraction and peripheral resistance. The umbilical and utero-placental circulations have low peripheral resistance and therefore high frequency waveforms in diastole.

Findings can be expressed in several ways (where A is the systolic and B the diastolic measurement).

1 $\dfrac{A}{B}$ = A/B ratio

2 $\dfrac{A - B}{A}$ = Resistance index

3 $\dfrac{A - C}{\text{Mean}}$ = Pulsatility index

Table 6.5 Biophysical profile scoring: management protocol. (Source Manning *et al.* (1985).)

Score	Interpretation	Recommended management
10	Normal infant, low risk for chronic asphyxia	Repeat testing at weekly intervals. Repeat twice weekly in diabetic patients and patients $\geqslant$ 42 weeks.
8	Normal infant, low risk for chronic asphyxia	Repeat testing at weekly intervals. Repeat twice weekly in diabetic patients and patients $\geqslant$ 42 weeks. Indication for delivery = oligohydramnios.
6	Suspected chronic asphyxia	Repeat testing within 24 h. Indication for delivery = oligohydramnios or score $\geqslant$ 6.
4	Suspected chronic asphyxia	$\geqslant$ 36 weeks' score and favourable cervix – deliver. If <36 weeks see Fig. 6.5
0–2	Strong suspicion of chronic asphyxia	Extend testing time to 120 min. Indication for delivery = persistent score $\leqslant$ 4, regardless of gestational age.

All three indices decrease as gestation advances, as do the umbilical artery waveform indices due to a reduction in vascular resistance.

Waveforms obtained from compromised fetuses have low diastolic frequencies, reflecting an increase in vascular resistance (see Figs. 6.9 and 6.10). Loss of end diastolic frequency indicates that vascular resistance is so high that there is no forward flow through the umbilical artery to the placenta throughout the entire cardiac cycle. Further increase in placental resistance results in reversal of flow which is a poor prognostic factor. Abnormal flow velocity waveforms usually precede abnormalities in the CTG.

On present evidence delivery must be considered seriously where there is absent end diastolic flow, since this is associated with hypoxia and acidaemia in at least 50 per cent of cases. If the CTG becomes abnormal and end diastolic flow is absent there is a high risk of perinatal death.

Guidelines

The primary objective of antenatal fetal assessment is to discover the optimal time for delivery.

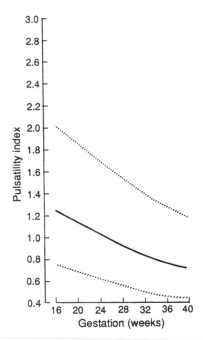

Fig. 6.9 Pulsatility index and 95 per cent confidence intervals for gestation. (Reproduced with permission from Pearce, J.M., Campbell, S., Cohen-Overbeek, T., Hackett, G., Hernandez, J. & Royston, J.P. (1988) Reference ranges and sources of variation for indices of pulsed Doppler flow velocity waveforms from the uteroplacental and fetal circulation. *British Journal of Obstetrics & Gynaecology*, **95**, 255.)

The results of fetal growth assessment (abdominal circumference), biophysical profile and umbilical artery Doppler recording may be combined in the context of the whole clinical situation, e.g. delivery is not indicated before 34 weeks' gestation on fetal grounds if the BPP is normal or if the sole adverse features are one reading suggesting a reduced abdominal circumference or one abnormal umbilical artery Doppler reading. However, beyond 34 weeks, delivery may be indicated in the presence of abnormal umbilical artery Doppler recording and reduced abdominal circumference **before** the BPP becomes abnormal.

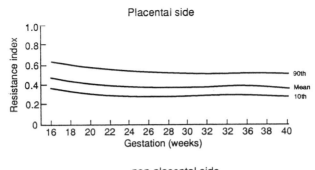

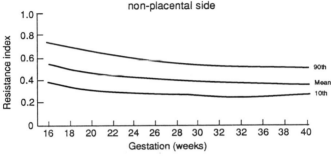

Fig. 6.10 Resistance index for gestational age and 95 per cent confidence intervals for gestation. (Reproduced with permission from Pearce, J.M., Campbell, S., Cohen-Overbeek, T., Hackett, G., Hernandez, J. & Royston, J.P. (1988) Reference ranges and sources of variation for indices of pulsed Doppler flow velocity waveforms from the uteroplacental and fetal circulation. *British Journal of Obstetrics & Gynaecology*, **95**, 254.)

Although normal antepartum fetal blood gas values have been established, (Fig. 6.11) they do not indicate when delivery is required.

INTRAPARTUM FETAL ASSESSMENT

1 Cardiotocography

See above.

2 Fetal ECG

This can be picked up using the same scalp clip as is used for CTG. It

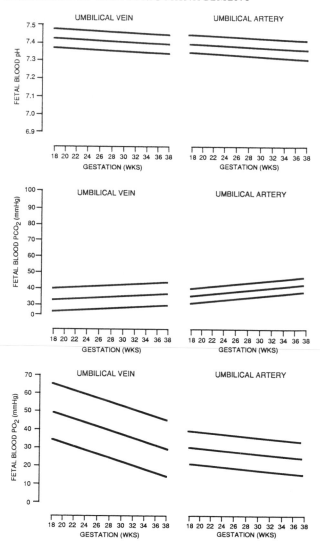

Fig. 6.11 Fetal blood pH, P_{CO_2} and P_{O_2} for gestational age. (Reproduced with permission from: Nicolaides, K.H., Economides, D.L. & Soothill, P.W. (1989) Blood gases pH and lactate in appropriate and small-for-gestational-age fetuses. *American Journal of Obstetrics & Gynecology*, **161**, 996–1001.)

depends on the analysis of the ST waveform. The following adverse features have been described:

- T/QRS ratio of greater than 0.25 or >0.5 over 15 minutes.
- a negative T wave.
- ST depression with T elevation.

These may help to discriminate better than CTG those fetuses requiring scalp sampling or delivery. The main benefit may be to reduce the operative delivery rate by giving reassurance in the presence of an abnormal CTG.

3 Fetal blood sampling

A fetal scalp pH of 7 or less is strongly associated with a poor outcome, particularly if the Apgar score (see below) is three or less at 5 minutes.

Although a pH of 7.2 has been used to indicate significant fetal acidaemia, it is within one standard deviation of the mean. A pH of 7.15 is, therefore, a clearer cut-off point suggesting the need to deliver.

However, since pH alone does not differentiate between metabolic or respiratory acidaemia, base deficit should also be measured. A base deficit of greater than 9 mmol/L is abnormal. The duration of the asphyxia and the ability of the baby to compensate are important determinants of outcome (e.g. IUGR is associated with poor outcome after asphyxia).

ASSESSMENT AT BIRTH

Apgar score – see Table 6.6.

The Apgar score was introduced in 1952 as an attempt at a systematic and objective assessment of the clinical condition of the newborn at birth (1 and 5 minutes and at 5 minute intervals thereafter if necessary) to direct attention to the need for resuscitation.

It is a global assessment of fetal state. Scores at 1 and 5 minutes do not correlate well with acidaemia or the incidence of cerebral palsy. However, if the Apgar score is still three or less at 20 minutes the incidence of cerebral palsy is almost 60 per cent among survivors.

Table 6.6 The components of the Apgar score applied to the newborn baby. (Reproduced with permission from Fleming, P.J., Speidel, B.D., Marlow, N. & Dunn, P.M. (Eds.) (1991) *A Neonatal Vade-Mecum*, 2nd edn., Edward Arnold, London.)

	Score		
Sign	0	1	2
Heart rate	Absent	<100 beats/min	>100 beats/min
Respiratory effort	Absent	Weak	Good, crying
Muscle tone	Flaccid	Some flexion of extremities	Well flexed
Relex irritability	No response	Grimace	Cough or sneeze
Colour	Blue	Blue peripheries	Pink

Cord venous blood gas analysis

This is another indication of fetal state at birth (see Table 6.7).

▪ The pH difference between the umbilical cord artery and vein should not be more than 0.02 pH unit.

▪ The larger the arterio-venous pH difference, the more acute the acidaemia, with mostly a respiratory component.

▪ The narrower the arterio-venous difference (usually associated with a higher base deficit), the more chronic the problem, indicating a metabolic acidaemia.

▪ The degree of acidaemia is a continuum. Very severe degrees of acidaemia are associated with a greater chance of complications (see Table 6.8).

Table 6.7 Mean cord arterial blood gases and range at delivery. (Courtesy of Professor Karl Rosen.)

	Mean	Range
pH	7.26	7.04–7.38
P_{CO_2} (mm Hg)	55	37–81
Base deficit (mmol/L)	2.3	(–2.8 to 9.4)

Table 6.8 Other complications (per cent) with degrees of acidaemia. (Adapted from Goldaber K.G. *et al.* (1991).)

	pH				
	<7.00	7.00–7.04	7.05–7.09	7.10–7.14	7.15–7.19
Admission to special care nursery	39.1	12.6	5.95	2.8	1.8
Intubation within first 48 h	13.8	6.3	1.7	0.6	0.6
Intraventricular haemorrhage	1.1	1.1	0	0.1	0
Apgar score ⩽3					
1 min	27.6	8.4	4.1	2.4	1.2
5 min	10.3	1.1	0.3	0	0.04

BIRTH ASPHYXIA

This is a non-specific descriptive term covering those babies born in a poor condition at birth. **It does not presuppose that it is caused by labour or delivery**.

'Birth asphyxia' is followed by neurological abnormalities of variable severity (see Table 6.9). A better term for this is **hypoxic ischaemic encephalopathy** (HIE) (see Table 6.10) which is described in three grades: mild, moderate and severe.

Mild (grade 1): increased reflexes with minor tone abnormalities, no seizures and recovery in less than 72 hours but mostly less than 48 hours.

Moderate (grade 2): semi-conscious, markedly irritable, areflexia, differential limb tone (upper less than lower), seizures.

Table 6.9 Clinical indicators of fetal asphyxia.

Abnormalities of fetal heart rate.
Low Apgar score (⩽3 at 5 minutes or at 5 minute intervals subsequently)
Delay in establishing respiration
Low fetal scalp or umbilical cord pH
Delayed onset of spontaneous breathing and/or need for resuscitation with positive pressure ventilation
Clinical signs of hypoxic ischaemic encephalopathy (HIE)
Multi-organ involvement

Table 6.10 Distinguishing features of the three clinical stages of postanoxic encephalopathy in the full-term newborn baby. (Source: Sarnat, H.B. & Sarnat, M.S. (1976), p. 700, Table 2.)

	Stage 1	Stage 2	Stage 3
Level of consciousness	Hyperalert	Lethargic or obtunded	Stuporous
Neuromuscular control			
Muscle tone	Normal	Mild hypotonia	Flaccid
Posture	Mild distal flexion	Strong distal flexion	Intermittent decerebration
Stretch reflexes	Overactive	Overactive	Decreased or absent
Segmental myoclonus	Present	Present	Absent
Complex reflexes			
Suck	Weak	Weak or absent	Absent
Moro	Strong; low threshold	Weak; incomplete high threshold	Absent
Oculovestibular	Normal	Overactive	Weak or absent
Tonic neck	Slight	Strong	Absent
Autonomic function	Generalised sympathetic	Generalised parasympathetic	Both systems depressed
Pupils	Mydriasis	Miosis unequal; poor light reflex	Variable; often
Heart rate	Tachycardia	Bradycardia	Variable
Bronchial and salivary secretions	Sparse	Profuse	Variable
Gastrointestinal motility	Normal or decreased	Increased; diarrhoea	Variable
Seizures	None	Common; focal or multifocal	Uncommon (excluding decerebration)
Electroencephalogram findings	Normal (awake)	Early: low voltage continuous delta and theta. Later: periodic pattern (awake) Seizures: focal 1 to $1\frac{1}{2}$ Hz spike-and-wave	Early: periodic pattern with isopotential phases. Later: totally isopotential
Duration	Less than 24 h	Two to 14 days	Hours to weeks

Severe (grade 3): coma, seizures, respiratory failure and profound hypotonia.

The severity of hypoxic ischaemic encephalopathy is a far more reliable predictor of adverse outcome than low Apgar score or acidaemia (cf. Tables 6.11 and 6.12).

Table 6.11 Longterm outcome (per cent) for each stage of hypoxic ischaemic encephalopathy (HIE).

	HIE		
Outcome	Mild (grade 1)	Moderate (grade 2)	Severe (grade 3)
Death/handicap	0	25	92

Table 6.12 A scoring system for postasphyxial morbidity. A score of six or more indicates severe morbidity while five or less moderate morbidity. (From Portman *et al.* (1990).)

	Score			
	0	1	2	3
5 min Apgar score	>6	5–6	3–4	0–2
Base deficit (mmol/L)	<10	10–14	15–19	$\geqslant 20$
Fetal monitoring	Normal	Variable decelerations	Severe or atypical variable or late decelerations	Prolonged bradycardia

Outcome after severe birth asphyxia

Most infants with very severe acidaemia at birth survive intact (see Table 6.13). Only very severe and prolonged asphyxia is associated with long-standing neurological deficits (see Table 6.12).

Predicting the severity of compromise after severe birth asphyxia is difficult because the duration of the insult and the intensity are not easily measured. The best predictor of longterm outcome is the clinical grade of HIE (see Table 6.11) but further clinical investigations should include: the electroencephalograph (EEG), ultrasound and CT scan, if available, and magnetic resonance imaging (MRI) of the baby's brain.

Table 6.13 Approximate frequency (per cent) of neonatal death, all seizures, and unexplained seizures according to pH cut off.

	pH				
	<7.00	7.00–7.04	7.05–7.09	7.10–7.14	7.15–7.19
Neonatal deaths	8	1.1	0	0.4	0.1
All seizures	12.6	4.2	0	0.3	0.2
Unexplained seizures	9.2	1.1	0	0.1	0.1
Neonatal death and seizures	2.3	0	0	0.05	

A good outcome is likely in infants in whom the clinical signs of mild encephalopathy disappear and the EEG reverts to normal within five days. The presence or absence of easily controlled seizures in the first two days does not seem to influence prognosis. The prognosis of neonates is good if they do not develop grade 3 HIE and if the total duration of grade 2 HIE is less than five days.

The number of deaths or neurological handicaps is low in babies with normal or mildly abnormal EEG. Outcome is poor in babies with severe EEG abnormalities.

ULTRASOUND

The incidence of handicap is directly related to the presence of intracerebral hypoechogenic areas of necrosis.

COMPUTERISED TOMOGRAPHY

If the CT scan is normal or only patchy hypodensities are present, the incidence of death or handicap is less than 20 per cent. Death or severe disabilities occur in up to 80 per cent of babies with marked hypodensities and haemorrhages on CT scan.

CEREBRAL PALSY

The incidence is about 2–4 cases per 1000 births. This has not decreased as obstetric standards have improved. There is a general assumption that this condition is 'caused' by intrapartum events. In fact less than 10 per cent of cases are associated with intrapartum events or birth asphyxia.

BIBLIOGRAPHY

Finer, N.N., Robertson, C.M., Peters, K.L. & Coward, J.H. (1983) Factors affecting outcome in hypoxic ischemic encephalopathy in term infants. *American Journal of Disease in Children*, **137**, 21–25.

Fleming, P.J., Speidel, B.D., Marlow, N. & Dunn, P.M. (Eds.) (1991) *A Neonatal Vade-Mecum*, 2nd edn., Edward Arnold, London.

Goldaber, K.G., Gilstrap, L.C., Leveno, K.J., Dax, J.S. & McIntire, D.D. (1991) Pathologic fetal acidemia. *Obstetrics & Gynecology*, **78**, 1103–1107.

Kramer, M., Olivier, M., McLean F., Willis, D. & Usher, R. (1990) Impact of intrauterine growth retardation and body proportionality on fetal and neonatal outcome. *Pedriatrics*, **86**, 707–713.

Low, J.A., Galbraith, R.S., Muir, D.W., Killen, H.L., Pater, E.A. & Karchmar, E.J. (1988) Motor and cognitive deficits after intrapartum asphyxia in the mature fetus. *American Journal of Obstetrics & Gynaecology*, **158**, 356–361.

Macdonald, H.M., Mulligan, J.C., Allen, A.C. & Taylor, P.M. (1980) Neonatal asphyxia: 1. Relationship of obstetric and neonatal complications to neonatal mortality in 38,405 consecutive deliveries. *Journal of Paediatrics*, **96**, 898–902.

MacDonald, D., Grant, A., Sheridan-Pereira, M., Boylan, P. & Chalmers, I. (1985) The Dublin randomised controlled trial of intrapartum fetal heart rate monitoring. *American Journal of Obstetrics and Gynecology*, **152**, 524–539.

Manning, F.A., Platt, L.D. & Cephos, L. (1980) Antepartum fetal evaluation: development of a fetal biophysical profile score. *American Journal of Obstetrics & Gynecology*, **136**, 787–795.

Manning, F.A., Morrison, I., Lange, I.R. & Harman, C.R. (1985) Fetal assessment based on fetal biophysical profile scoring: experience in 12,620 referred high-risk pregnancies 1. Perinatal mortality by frequency and etiology. *American Journal of Obstetrics & Gynecology*, **151**, 343–350.

Nelson, K. & Ellenberg, J. (1981) Apgar scores as predictors of chronic neurologic disability. *Pediatrics*, **68**, 36–44.

Nicolaides, K.H., Economides, D.L. & Soothill, P.W. (1989) Blood gases, pH and lactate in appropriate and small-for-gestational-age fetuses. *American Journal of Obstetrics and Gynecology*, **161**, 996–1101.

Portman, R.J., Carter, B.S., Gaylord, M.S., Murphy, M.G., Thieme, R.E. & Merenstein, G.B. (1990) Predicting neonatal morbidity after perinatal asphyxia: A scoring system. *American Journal of Obstetrics & Gynecology*, **162**, 174–182.

6

Pearce, J.M., Campbell, S., Cohen-Overbeck, T., Hackett, G., Hernandez, J. & Royston, J.P. (1988) Reference ranges and sources of variation for indices of pulsed Doppler flow velocity waveforms from the uteroplacental and fetal circulation. *British Journal of Obstetrics & Gynaecology*, **95**, 248–256.

Robertson, C. & Finer, N.N. (1985) Term infants with hypoxic-ischemic encephalopathy: outcome at 3.5 years. *Developmental Medicine and Child Neurology*, **21**, 473–484.

Robertson, C.M.T., Finer, N.N. & Grace, M.G.A. (1989) School performance of survivors of neonatal encephalopathy associated with birth asphyxia at term. *Journal of Paediatrics*, **114**, 753–760.

Sarnat, H.B. & Sarnat M.S. (1976) Neonatal encephalopathy following fetal distress. *Archives of Neurology*, **33**, 696–705.

Street, P., Dawes, G.S., Molden, M. & Redman, C.W.G. (1991) Short-term variation in abnormal antenatal fetal heart rate records. *American Journal of Obstetrics & Gynecology*, **165**, 515–523.

Sykes, G.S., Molloy, P.M., Johnson, P., Gu, W., Ashworth, F., Stirrat, G.M. & Turnbull, A.C. (1982) Do Apgar scores indicate asphyxia? *The Lancet*, **I**, 494–496.

Westgate, J., Harris, M., Curnow, J.S.H. & Greene, K.R. (1992) Randomised trial of cardiotocography alone or with ST waveform analysis for intraparum monitoring. *The Lancet*, **340**, 194–198.

Wilcox, M.A., Johnson, I.R., Maynard, P.V., Smith, S.J. & Chilvers, C.E.D. (1993) The individualised birthweight ratio: a more logical outcome measure of pregnancy than birthweight alone. *British Journal of Obstetrics & Gynaecology*, **100**, 342–347.

Yudkin, P.L., Aboualfa, M., Eyre, J.A., Redman, C.W.G. & Wilkinson, A.R. (1987) New birthweight and head circumference centiles for gestational ages 24 to 42 weeks. *Early Human Development*, **15**, 49.

6

7 The Neonate

7.1 Neonatal resuscitation

IDENTIFYING THE NEED FOR RESUSCITATION

Identification of which babies need resuscitation and which technique to use effectively is fundamental to successful resuscitation.

- Most babies do not require resuscitation.
- About 2 per cent of babies born after normal pregnancy and labour will require assistance at birth and one in five of these could not have been predicted.

- The identification of risk factors will predict most babies who need resuscitation.

Traditionally, paediatric staff attend deliveries on request on the basis of the obstetric risk factors, e.g.

- operative delivery;
- caesarean section;
- forceps or ventouse;
- the presence of meconium in the liquor;
- abnormalities of the fetal heart rate prior to delivery;
- abnormal presentation;
- obstructed labour;
- a technically difficult delivery;
- preterm delivery.

Each delivery unit should have

- All staff trained in basic resuscitation using bag and mask ventilation.
- Personnel trained in advanced resuscitation available in the hospital.
- Regular training sessions for all staff in immediate neonatal care and resuscitation.

Apgar scores should be recorded for each birth. The score indicates the need for resuscitation. The correlation of Apgar score with the degree of asphyxia is relatively poor, except for the extremes (see Chapter 6).

RESUSCITATION – ACTION AT BIRTH

The need for resuscitation is based on an assessment of breathing and heart rate.

At delivery a baby may manifest:

1 Normal breathing, colour (pink) and heart rate (>100 beats/minute)

2 Breathing irregular, cyanosed, but heart rate >100 beats/minute

3 Apnoea, not breathing or never breathed and heart rate may be over 100 beats/minute but rapidly drops to less than 100 beats/minute.

- **Dry the baby and put in a warm towel** – do not let the baby get cold, because cold stress compromises breathing.
- **Suction anterior nares and mouth** (maximum pressure 13.1 kPa (100 mm Hg), avoiding deep pharyngeal suction).
- **Assess clinical state at 1 minute.**

Airway – suction – and check patency.

Breathing

Regular breathing – Observe.

Irregular/absent – Call for assistance if advanced resuscitation is needed.

Bag and mask $\pm$ oral airway – Give 20 breaths; reassess after 20 breaths or half to one minute.

Heart rate falling –

Call for assistance.

Check ventilation.

Insert airway if necessary.

If advanced resuscitation insert an **endotracheal tube**.

Circulation

>100 beats/minute – Observe/stimulate.

60–100 beats/minute – Assess breathing.

<100 beats/minute – Commence **external cardiac compression** –

Rate: 100–120 compressions/minute; 3–5 compressions for every ventilation.

Position: One finger's breadth below the nipple line over the sternum. Encircling the chest may be more effective.

Drugs

Give if the baby's heart rate has failed to increase and the baby is still pale and blue despite ventilation and chest compressions.

- Adrenaline 10 microgram/kg intravenously (0.1 mL 1:10 000 solution. Repeat adrenaline 10 microgram/kg, then 100 microgram/kg may be given if there is no response.
- Insert intravenous catheter and give 10–20 mL of 4.5 per cent human albumin solution if two intravenous doses of adrenaline are ineffective with the presence of adequate ventilation.
- Do not use atropine.
- Give 1 mmol/kg of $NaHCO_3$ intravenously (use 4.2 per cent solution) if there is still no response; this may be of particular value if the baby is asystolic.
- **Opiate antagonist.** If the mother has received pethidine or other opiate within the previous 8 hours, give naloxone 10 microgram/kg. (One ampoule contains 40 micrograms in 2 mL.) Usually 1 mL is given initially, intramuscularly or intravenously. This will usually produce a response within two minutes. A repeat dose may be needed in 30–60 minutes.

7

Action if there is no response to resuscitation

- Check for technical fault, such as whether the oxygen is connected.
- Auscultate the baby's chest to check endotracheal tube position and patency.
- ? Effects of maternal opiate analgesia – give naloxone 10 microgram/kg.
- ? Anaemia – if there was fetal blood loss during delivery, give colloid e.g. 4.5 per cent albumin 20 mL/kg or blood group O negative blood.
- Consider pneumothorax (if present release the tension by inserting a 21 gauge butterfly needle through the second intercostal space, midclavicular line), place the end of the butterfly needle into saline and observe air bubbles if a pneumothorax is present).
- Check dextrostix and administer 0.5 g/kg glucose intravenously if the level is less than 1.8 mmol/L.
- Consider malformations, e.g. diaphragmatic hernia, congenital heart disease.

CONTROVERSIES IN RESUSCITATION

1 Bag and mask or endotracheal tube?

The endotracheal tube (ETT)

This is effective and efficient.

Use an ETT for babies of less than 30 weeks' gestation. The size is given as follows:

Baby's weight (g)	ETT size (mm)
<1000	2.5
1000–2000	3.0
2000–3000	3.0 or 3.5
>3000	3.5

Competent insertion requires skill and practice.

The bag and mask

The bag and mask are usually all that is required, especially in term babies.

- Their use should always precede use of an ETT.
- All staff should be proficient in their use.
- Use of an oral airway may be valuable.
- Use a bag and mask as initial resuscitation for all babies over 30 weeks' gestation.

- More than 80 per cent of babies will respond adequately to ventilation via a self-inflating bag and mask.
- Without a reservoir generally use a flow rate of 2 L/minute to give a F_{iO_2} of 40 per cent. Increase the flow to more than 5 L/minute if unsuccessful in establishing oxygenation (see Table 7.1.1).

Table 7.1.1 The percentage of oxygen given according to the flow rates.

Flow rate (L/minute)	Oxygen (per cent)
8	60–80
5	50–76
2	38–60

2 Use of 100 per cent oxygen

The potential advantages are that it is widely available, produces a rapid increase in P_{aO_2}, encourages ductal closure, relaxes the vascular pulmonary bed and increases energy supply to tissues.

The disadvantages are that it may cause an oxidative stress in the baby and a decrease in cerebral blood flow in preterm babies. It may also alter the N_2 reservoir in lungs, increasing the risk of atelectasis.

3 External cardiac compression

Cardiac compression is indicated if the baby is asystolic or if the heart rate is less than 60 beats/minute. It is conventionally given by two fingers placed on the sternum one finger's breadth below the nipple line, repeatedly depressing the sternum. A more effective technique may be to encircle the baby's thorax with both hands using the thumbs for cardiac compression over the same point as above.

The rate of cardiac compression should be 100–120 per minute in a ratio of 3–5 for every ventilation, i.e. 25–40 ventilations per minute.

Without cardiac compression the rate of ventilation is one per second or 60 per minute.

4 Drugs that may be given in neonatal resuscitation

Adrenaline

Asphyxiated babies already have very high catecholamine levels. Although there is little evidence that giving adrenaline (via an ETT) makes any difference it may be given. The conventional dose is 0.1 mL/kg of 1 in 10 000 solution intravenously or 0.2 mL via the ETT.

Plasma volume expanders

Use plasma protein fractions for the baby whose circulation has not responded to ventilation and adrenaline. Give 4.5 per cent human albumin solution.

Buffer – the use of bicarbonate at resuscitation

It may be of value when adrenaline has been given with no response. It is generally not used otherwise because of a negative inotropic action which may paradoxically increase intracellular acidosis.

Atropine

Counterproductive.

Calcium

Calcium gluconate is not now thought to be of value.

5 Management of meconium stained liquor

- Suction the baby's nares and mouth using deep suction via a mucus extractor when the baby's head has delivered.
- Direct visualisation of the airway and vocal cords on bed or resuscitaire using a laryngoscope enables suction of the posterior pharynx and larynx.
- If meconium is present in the posterior pharynx or larynx, intubate. Apply gentle suction to the endotracheal tube whilst removing the tube. If a plug of meconium is removed with this action, repeat the process.
- Do not use intermittent positive pressure ventilation in the presence of meconium until the airway is clear. Otherwise meconium may be forced into the baby's lungs with serious consequences.
- Do not intubate the crying baby. This only leads to mouth and tracheal trauma.

- Observe babies following aspiration of meconium from below the vocal cords for abnormal respiratory signs (tachypnoea, grunting, temperature instability, hypoglycaemia, cyanosis) for 4–6 hours. Later complications include infection and pneumothorax.

OUTCOME IN EXTREME CASES

As a general rule of thumb, the outcome for babies born with an Apgar score of zero known to have been alive shortly before birth who are not immature is that about 50 per cent survive intact. Of the remainder 50 per cent die and 50 per cent survive with significant disabilities.

Therefore, active attempts should be made at resuscitation if the circulation is established, followed by admission to the neonatal intensive care unit for further assessment and treatment. See Table 7.1.2 for when to stop resuscitation.

Table 7.1.2 When to stop resuscitation.

Major/lethal malformation (A senior member of the medical staff should be present to assess/confirm the severity of the malformation).
Gestation less than 25 weeks and not responding to resuscitation.

No heart beat by 10 minutes.
No respiration by 25 minutes.

7

The extremely preterm baby (less than 1000 g)

- The hospital policy should be laid down and made known.
- An experienced neonatal paediatrician should be present in the delivery room if at all possible.
- Resuscitation is probably not justified for babies of less than 25 weeks' gestation.
- If resuscitation is commenced it should initially be confined to assessment of response to endotracheal ventilation (see Fig. 7.1.1).
- Where support appears to be effective the baby should be admitted to the neonatal intensive care unit and reassessed.

VITAMIN K₁

Vitamin K_1 supplementation to the newborn is necessary because

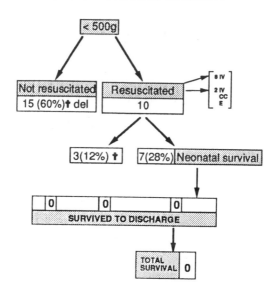

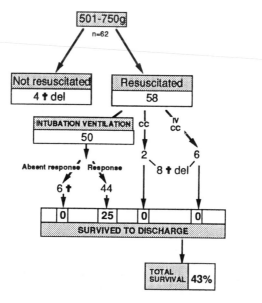

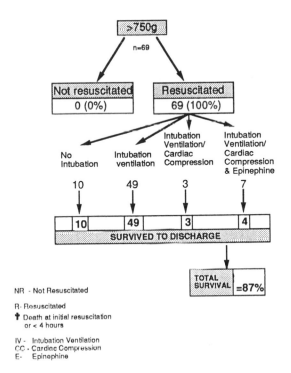

Fig. 7.1.1 Outcome for babies depending on gestational weight (less than 500 g, 500–750 g and 750–1000 g). (Source: Davies, D.J. (1993).)

stores of Vitamin K_1 essential for the activation of blood clotting factors II, VII, IX and X are small and rapidly depleted. The routine use of Vitamin K_1 1 mg i.m. or 2 mg orally (1 mg in 0.5 ml = 1 ampoule) prevents intracranial haemorrhage in about 40 term babies in the UK per year.

The risk of bleeding is 15–20 times higher in breastfed babies than in those fed with cows' milk formulae. Breastfed babies should therefore be given a further dose of 2 milligrams (2 ampoules) at 7–10 days and the same dose at the 6 week check.

A possible increase in childhood cancer associated with intramuscular injection of Vitamin K_1 has not been confirmed.

BIBLIOGRAPHY

Advanced Life Support Group (1993) *Advanced Paediatric Life Support. The Practical Approach.* British Medical Journal Publishing Group, London.

Davis, D.J. (1993) How aggressive should delivery room cardiopulmonary resuscitation be for extremely low birth weight neonates? *Pediatrics*, **92**, 447–449.

Fleming, P.J., Speidel, B.D., Marlow, N. & Dunn, P.M. (1991) *A Neonatal Vade-Mecum.* 2nd edn., Edward Arnold, London.

Marlow, N. (1992) Do we need an Apgar score? *Archives of Disease in Childhood*, **67**, 765–769.

Palme-Kilaner, C. (1992) Methods of resuscitation in low-Apgar-score newborn infants – a national survey. *Acta Paediatrica*, **81**, 739–744.

Peliowski, A. & Finer, N.N. (1992) Birth asphyxia in the term infant. In *Effective Care of the Newborn Infant* (Ed. by J.C. Sinclair & M.B. Bracken), Chapter 13, pp 250–279. Oxford University Press, Oxford.

7.2   Breast feeding

Breast milk should be every infant's right and society should allow mothers the opportunity to breast feed.

Advice on breast feeding should be given antenatally. Successful breast feeding relies on expectation of success, as the only method of feeding conferring unique benefits on the mother and baby. The best preparation for breast feeding is getting used to the idea. Antenatal education includes observation and discussion with a breast feeding mother, practical advice on optimal fixation and position, facts on the physiology of lactation, and awareness of the common problems encountered.

THE PRACTICE/MECHANISM OF BREAST FEEDING

1 Position of the baby (see Figs 7.2.1, 7.2.2)

Both head and shoulders should face the breast square on. The nose should be at the same level as the nipple. Avoid flexing the head onto the breast, i.e. keep the baby's head slightly extended and the spine straight. The baby's mouth appears asymmetrically placed on the nipple if the position is correct. More of the lower jaw and lip covers the lower areola than at the top.

2 Shaping the breast

Sustained hand/breast support may help to ensure effective milk delivery for many women.

Shape the breast in line with the baby's closed lips. The breast is supported underneath by the hand and fingers with the thumb on top.

3 Mouth – triggering the baby's rooting reflex

This is the key to positioning. Triggering the baby's rooting reflex will initiate a gaping, wide open mouth. Do not push the baby's chin down to get the mouth open.

Brush the baby's lips against the nipple to trigger the rooting reflex. This should result in the baby's mouth gaping wide open as much as a yawn. The baby plants the whole of the mouth onto the nipple, areola and breast. If the nipple is guided into the upper third of the baby's mouth, it will be correctly positioned.

Make sure the lower jaw is well away from the base of the nipple, i.e. it should be planted onto the areola.

The mother's breast is drawn into the baby's mouth so that it extends back to the soft palate when the baby is correctly attached to the breast. The nipple lies in a furrow formed by the baby's tongue and rhythmical action milks the breast, squeezing the milk into the mouth. Note that the lacteal sinuses (included in the areola) are drawn into the mouth along with the nipple.

There should be no friction of the baby's tongue on the nipple.

4 The mouthful of breast tissue

This means that the nipple plus the areola must be taken into the baby's mouth, which ensures that the breast is not traumatised and reduces the risk of sore nipples. This makes sure that the baby receives a balanced feed: (a) high volume, low fat foremilk; (b) low volume, high fat hindmilk.

The emptying of the breast is essential as hindmilk is important in ensuring slower gastric emptying. Therefore the baby will not need to be fed so frequently. It also maximises the intake of fat soluble vitamins and develops normal appetite control.

Do not use other oral objects, teats or dummies in the neonatal period. These may condition the baby to different oral actions that are inappropriate for breast feeding.

Figs 7.2.1–7.2.4 illustrate the baby before attachment (Fig. 7.2.1) with incorrect attachment (Fig. 7.2.2), and with improved attachment (Figs 7.2.3 and 7.2.4).

5 Initial feeding

In the first 30 hours after birth the breasts fill with colostrum, a high density low volume feed.

The nipple contains unmyelinated nerve endings (like the cornea) so it is extremely painful when traumatised by a baby that is suboptimally positioned. Stimulation of the nerve endings causes nipple erection and triggers the pituitary reflex mechanisms that release oxytocin and prolactin. Prolactin is involved with milk production and oxytocin the milk ejection reflex, contracting the myoepithelial cells forcing milk out into the ducts.

At 30–40 hours the amount of lactose produced increases (the most osmotically active component of milk).

6 Timing of feeds

Feed the baby on demand. This may be from $1\frac{1}{2}$ hours to 3 hour intervals.

The baby does not need any other foods until at least four months of age.

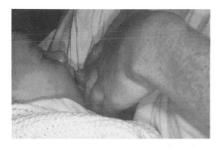

Fig. 7.2.1 The mother offering only the nipple. The baby has a small gape.

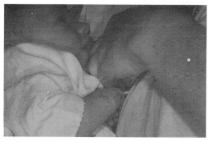

Fig. 7.2.2 The baby is just taking the nipple between the lips. The baby is not at the correct height for the breast.

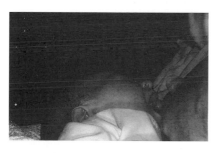

Fig. 7.2.3 Improved attachment with improved gape.

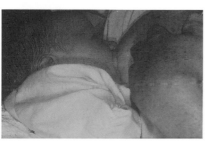

Fig. 7.2.4 Attachment with the lips well phlanged (curled) onto the breast.

7 Maintenance of milk production

This is effected by
- frequent afferent stimulation of the nipples by sucking;
- effective removal of freshly synthesized milk from the breast;
- the milk ejection reflex, mediated by oxytocin secretion.

Do not allow breasts to become over full during the first week. Gentle hand expression overcomes the outflow obstruction.

An adequate mouthful of breast tissue maximises the reflex milk release and extraction. Improving the mouthful may increase the let down release of milk due to an increase in oxytocin.

Failure to breast feed means that the breasts become engorged with milk stasis and involution of the mammary tissue. As long as there is frequent emptying of the breast, milk supply is adequate. This can be achieved by artificial means (hand or pump expulsion).

8 Breast feeding management

For the first few days feed 1–3 hourly. Later demand feeding will result in 5–7 feeds per day by one week. Feed the baby from the first breast until it comes off spontaneously. Then offer the second breast. If feeds are excessively long (greater than 40 minutes) or over frequent (less than one hourly) the baby's position may not be correct.

9 Electric pumps

These are efficient at establishing breast milk flow, though the suckling-induced surge of prolactin wanes with repeated use. It may be treated with dromperidone (10 mg t.d.s. orally) to offset any fall in milk supply associated with prolonged pump use, normally with the birth of a preterm infant.

10 Ways to encourage breast feeding

- Inform all pregnant women how and why to breast feed.
- Help mothers to initiate breast feeding soon after birth.
- Allow rooming-in 24 hours a day.
- Encourage breast feeding on demand.
- Give the infant no food or drink other than breast milk.
- Ensure continuity of breast feeding through support groups and health services.

Benefits of breast feeding

Immunoglobulins IgG, IgF, IgM are present in breast milk. There is also an adaptive anti-infective mechanism whereby enteromammary secretion may result in the secretion into milk of specific secretory IgA. It also stimulates the infant's immune system to mount its own response. Benefits include:

- **Decreased gastrointestinal symptoms**, decreased rate of **respiratory infection**, decreased urinary tract infection,
- **Increased IQ** (mean of 8.3 in preterm infants who received breast milk after controlling for other variables),
- **Infant colic**, improving positioning or removing the restrictions on feed duration may encourage the intake of more fat-laden hind milk that reduces the incidence of colic.
- **Reduced risk of sudden infant death syndrome.**
- **Reduced risk of autoimmune disease** particularly juvenile onset diabetes.
- Decrease in adult obesity.
- Decrease in eczema.
- Decrease in hypernatraemia and dehydration.
- Decrease in neonatal seizures.
- Decrease in dental caries.
- Psychological advantages for the baby.

Breast milk jaundice may develop after the first week of birth and persist for 6 to 8 weeks. Jaundice without any other explanation may raise the bilirubin level to 20 mg (to 340 micromol/L). A brief cessation of breast milk intake (for 24–48 hours) may be necessary to permit bilirubin levels to fall in prolonged cases. Express breast milk so that the mother is comfortable and discard.

Maternal advantages

The benefit for the mother is that breast feeding is a natural process that completes the natural hormonal cycle initiated at conception. It uses the reserves of the mother's body fat accumulated during gestation; it gives some lactational infertility, although due to the short half life of prolactin if the baby sleeps the whole night the mother is likely to ovulate. There is a reduced risk of maternal cancer (breast cancer and ovarian cancer) and a decreased risk of thromboembolism.

7

Physiology of lactation

Breast milk production is initiated by the removal of inhibition of the high circulating levels of prolactin by placental steroids (mainly oestrogens) following delivery of the placenta. Milk production occurs 2–5 days post-partum with an initial output of 200–900 mL/24 hours.

The infant's demand for breast milk regulates milk supply. Prolactin primes the system and determines the broad limits of milk supply in the first week post-partum, but then autocrine control may predominate.

Because the composition of breast milk varies it is important that the baby feeds by emptying one breast first before it is given the other as a result of an arbitrary time limit. This avoids giving the baby a high volume low fat diet since hindmilk is fat rich. A high volume low fat diet is associated with rapid gastric emptying and short gut transit time which may overwhelm the baby's lactase system with colonic bacterial overgrowth and symptoms of colic, flatus and loose stools. The fat rich hindmilk has a higher caloric quantity which is more satisfying for the baby.

Human milk is whey dominant, having a whey:casein ratio of 68:32. Cows' milk is casein dominated with a ratio of 23:77. Most formulae are now 'humanised' to achieve a ratio close to 60:40.

The newborn baby does not need any other food source apart from breast milk. The baby needs no other food for four months. The importance of breast milk is that it supplies the growing baby's entire needs, is immunologically competent against infection and diseases of infancy, biochemically triggers modulation of gut function, and supplies primed enzymes for digestion and utilisation of nutrients. It also enhances optimal oro-facial development and optimal ties of affection between mother and infant. Breast feeding is the safest form of feeding, particularly under unhygienic conditions.

Failure of lactation

Retained placental fragments may secrete sufficient oestrogen to continue inhibition of prolactin.

Problems of breast feeding

1 Breast milk insufficiency

Eighty five per cent of symptoms of insufficiency can be corrected by assessing and improving technique. A milk output of below 450 mL/

day at one month represents true insufficiency, for which supplementation will be necessary. Clinically this is detected by a 24 hour test weighing at home using electronic scales. Cumulated intake (post-feed weight – pre-feed weight for each feed in the 24 hour period) gives the output in millilitres (1 g = 1.03 mL).

2 *Impaired milk release*

Overcome by providing a relaxing familiar environment and reassuring skilled care.

3 *Incorrect positioning*

The baby is taking low fat foremilk resulting in volume or calorie depletion. It is only usually correctable at an early stage before the baby gets into the habit of poor feeding.

4 *Inappropriate pattern of breast usage*

Either exclusive single breast feeding or a rigid both breasts policy may result in inefficient feeding.

5 *Over efficient maternal physiology*

An over vigorous ejection reflex, particularly with incorrect positioning or inappropriate pattern of breast usage, may result in colic, overfeeding or symptoms of lactose malabsorption, i.e. flatus, wind, loose frothy acid stools, possibly because of rapid gastric emptying and spillage of lactose into the colon.

A temporary policy of only offering one breast at a feed, so long as optimal positioning can be assured, will best help to reduce supply to a manageable level.

MATERNAL COMPLICATIONS OF BREAST FEEDING

1 Engorgement

It is necessary to differentiate vascular engorgement from milk engorgement; the latter is usually caused by restricting the baby's access to the breast. If the baby is unable to remove the milk, then physical extraction is necessary, such as showers, manual expression, or the electric pump to draw off milk and reduce the areolar oedema.
■ Reduce prolonged engorgement of the breast by physical extraction if necessary.

- Wash the nipples with water only. Avoid soap or any other topical agents that may cause a skin reaction.
- Encourage the baby to take the nipple and areola tissue into the mouth.

2 Avoidance of sore or cracked nipples

- Identify the causative process which is most likely to be trauma due to the baby's sucking.
- Exclude an oral anomaly, e.g. tongue tie, by observing the length of the frenulum.
- If nipple soreness is due to an infective agent the commonest is *Candida*. The diagnosis is made empirically, being prolonged soreness after establishment of lactation.
- Treat *Candida* with **miconazole cream** – apply three time daily. Miconazole cream has the advantage of being both antifungal and antibacterial.
- Alternatively try putting breast milk on the lesion and leaving it to dry. Breast milk is the best agent to apply to the nipple because it has epidermal growth factors that have generalised effects of promoting skin repair.

3 Mastitis/blocked duct

This can be either infective or non-infective inflammation of the breast. The latter is caused by retrograde flow of milk under pressure from the lumen of the breast into the surrounding tissues with local and general immune responses.

It is difficult to discriminate between non-infective and infective inflammation of the breast. Both can have systemic symptoms of an infective illness. Open skin lesions are more likely to be infective.

If acute mastitis is infective or there is a breast abscess the infecting organism is probably *Staphylococcus*. Treat with flucoxacillin 250 mg three times daily, or erythromycin 500 mg q.d.s.

Advise the mother not to stop breast feeding from the infected breast as stopping will make the swelling worse and predispose to abscess formation, which will require surgical drainage.

ARTIFICIAL FEEDING

There are numerous products on the market with an overwhelming variety of constituents. It may be that the best product is that which approximates the make up of breast milk (see Table 7.2.2 below). The chief difference between breast milk and artificial feeds is the whey : casein ration (breast milk 68 : 32; artificial feeds approximate 60:40). This ratio affects the ability of the baby to digest proteins. Casein is the major nutritional protein and whey is a functional protein (e.g. its function is to prime the gut).

Each of the various brands are so similar that the only basis for preference should be cost. There is no evidence that less modified formulae with a higher casein content are more 'satisfying for the hungry and demanding infant'. Feed four hourly from birth and then feed on demand; recommended volumes are given in Table 7.2.1.

Table 7.2.1 Recommended volumes (mL) for artificial feeding.

Day 1	60–100
Day 2	90–120
Day 3	110–150
Day 4	130–180
Day 5	150–200
Day 6	150–200
Day 7	150–200
Day 8–13	150–200
Day 14–20	150–180
Day 21–27	150–180
>Day 28	150–160

BREAST MILK COMPOSITION (see Table 7.2.2)

Colostrum

Colostrum is secreted for the first 30–40 hours post-partum. Its average volume per feed is 30 ml. It is a high density, low volume feed which contains less lactose, fat and water soluble vitamins than mature milk but more protein, fat soluble vitamins (A, D, E, K) and more sodium and zinc. It is high in immunoglobulins.

Table 7.2.2 Composition of mature breast milk (units/L).

Energy	
MJ	2.93
kcal	700
Protein (g)	13
Casein:whey ratio	32:68
Carbohydrate (g)	70
Fat (g)	42
Na (mmol)[a]	6.5
K (mmol)[b]	15
Ca (mmol)[c]	8.7
P (mmol)[d]	4.8
Ca/P (mmol)	1.8
Fe (mg)[e]	0.8
Folate (micrograms)	52
Vitamins	
A (micrograms)	600
B_{12} (micrograms)	0.1
C (mg)	38
D (micrograms)	0.1
E (mg)	3.5
K (micrograms)	17

[a] Na is sodium.
[b] K is potassium.
[c] Ca is calcium.
[d] P is phosphorus.
[e] Fe is iron.

7

Protein

Human milk has the lowest protein concentration among mammals (1.15 g/100 mL).

Fat

There is 2.0 g/100 mL in colostrum compared with 4–4.5 g/100 mL 15 days post-partum. Variations occur with foremilk and hindmilk; the increased fat of hindmilk acts as a satiety regulator.

Lactose

Lactose is the major carbohydrate in breast milk. It facilitates calcium and iron absorption, and promotes intestinal colonisation with *Lac-*

tobacillus bifidus. Lactose intolerance can be avoided by letting the baby feed on the first breast until he/she comes off.

FOOD ADDITIVES

Vitamin K given at birth

If delivery was abnormal give 0.5 mg intramuscularly. For normal delivery give 1 mg orally with the first feed and a further 0.5 mg at one week.

Paediatric vitamin drops

The DHSS recommends all babies should receive 5 drops/day of children's vitamin drops from 6 months (see Table 7.2.3).

Table 7.2.3 Composition of paediatric vitamin drops.

	Vitamin A (micrograms (IU))	Vitamin C (mg)	Vitamin D (micrograms (IU))
Children's Vitamin Drops (5 drops)	214 (700)	21	7 (280)
Abidec[a] (Parke Davis) (0.6 mL)	1200 (400)	50	10 (400)
Adexolne Liquid (Glaxo) (0.2 mL)	210 (700)	21	7 (280)

[a] Also contains B vitamins.

7

Fluoride

Fluoride supplementation is recommended where the drinking water contains less than 0.33 ppm to reduce the incidence of dental caries. Give fluoride drops 0.25 mg daily, 2–5 drops. Reduced dosage may be given for water supplies containing 0.33–1 ppm fluoride. Information on the fluoride content of water in any area may be obtained from the local water authority.

NEWBORN ENERGY REQUIREMENTS

For normal growth 100–120 kcal/kg/day (420–504 kJ/kg/day) are required (see Table 7.2.4 for weight increase, Table 7.2.5 for age at teeth eruption, and Table 7.2.6 for basic nutrient requirements).

Table 7.2.4 Weight and weight gain of the baby.

Weight (kg)	
Average baby at birth	3.5
At 5 months	7
At 12 months	10.5
Weight gain (g/day)	
First four months of life	25
Fifth to eighth months	20
Ninth to twelfth months	12
Birthweight doubles at 5 months, trebles at 12 months.	

Table 7.2.5 Tooth eruption.

Teeth	Age (months)
Lower central incisors	6–10
Upper central incisors	8–11
Upper lateral incisors	10–13
Lower lateral incisors	10–14
First premolars	13–17
Canine	16–20
Second premolars	23–28

7

Table 7.2.6 Baby's basic nutrient requirements.

Fluid 150 (mL/kg body weight)	
Iron (mg)	
Full term infant	3–6
3 months of age	6–9
6 months	8–12
12 months	10–15
Calcium (mg/day)	600 (the amount in 300 mL milk)
Vitamins	
Vitamin C (mg)	15
Vitamin D (IU)	40
Protein (g/kg)	3
Energy (kcal/kg)	110
(kJ/kg)	462
Total feed (mL/kg)	150 reducing to 120

CESSATION OF LACTATION

This takes an average of 40 days. In abrupt weaning, it takes two days for immunoglobulin and lactoferrin levels to rise which leaves the breast vulnerable to infection. This is the reason for higher rates of abscess formation in women with mastitis who stop feeding from the affected breast.

THE CONTRACEPTIVE EFFECT OF BREAST FEEDING

Breast feeding gives good contraceptive effect, i.e. prevents ovulation as long as the baby is having at least five feeds per 24 hours with feeding throughout the night maintained. The total duration of suckling needs to be 65 minutes (>10 minutes per feed). The half life of prolactin is only 30 minutes. Therefore the mother is most at risk of losing the effect of prolactin levels on avoiding ovulation when the baby sleeps through the night. The failure rate for the contraceptive effect of breast feeding at six months with seven feeds a day is 2 per cent.

Oral contraceptives containing 2.5 mg or less of a 19-norprogestogen and 50 micrograms or less of ethinylestradiol or 100 micrograms of mestranol are safe and do not interfere with breast feeding.

7

RETURN OF MENSTRUATION

At the end of the third month post delivery, only 33 per cent of lactating women have a menstrual period, compared with 91 per cent of non-lactating women who have had at least one period.

By 9 months 65 per cent of women still lactating have had one period, and 30 per cent will become pregnant within one year (Table 7.2.7).

Table 7.2.7 The cumulative probability of pregnancy (per cent) at the end of six months in women exclusively breast feeding.

Amenorrheic	1.8
Return of menses	27.2
Partially breast feeding and return of menses	40.5

Of lactating women not using contraception, more than 50 per cent will become pregnant in the first nine months of lactation. A mother who breast feeds for 20 weeks will postpone menstruation for 12 weeks and ovulation for 18 weeks.

In the non-lactating woman, the earliest a period returns is 25 days post delivery. Ovulation occurs at 25–35 days with a 5 per cent chance of regaining fertility at six weeks post delivery.

BIBLIOGRAPHY

Consensus Statement (1988) Breast feeding as a family planning method. *The Lancet*, **2**, 1204–1205.

Dewey, K.G. & Lonnerdal, V. (1986) Infant self regulation of breast milk intake. *Acta Paediatrica Scandinavica*, **75**, 893–898.

Diaz, S., Perarta, O., Juez G., Salvatierra, A.M., Casado, M.E., Duran, E. & Croxatto, H.B. (1982) Fertility regulation in nursing women: I The probability of conception in full nursing women living in an urban setting. *Journal of the Biological Sciences*, **14**, 329–341.

Department of Health and Social Security (1980) *Present Day Practice in Infant Feeding*. Report on Health and Social Subjects. HMSO, London.

Gray, R.H., Campbell, O.M., Apello, R., Eslami, S.S., Zacur, H., Ramos, R.M., Gehret, J.C. & Labbok, M.H. (1990) Risk of ovulation during lactation. *The Lancet*, **335**, 25–29.

Howie, P.W., Forsyth, J.S., Ogston, S.A., Clark, A. & Florey, C. du V. (1990) Protective effect of breast feeding against infection. *British Medical Journal*, **300**, 11–16.

Lucas, A., Morley, R., Cole, T.G., Lister, G. & Leeson Payne, C. (1992) Breast milk and subsequent intelligence quotient in children born pre-term. *The Lancet*, **339**, 261–264.

Lucas, A., Brooke, O.G., Morley, R., Cole, T.J. & Bamford, M.F. (1990) Early diet of preterm infants and development of allergic or atopic disease: Randomised prospective study. *British Medical Journal*, **300**, 837–840.

Lucas, A. & Cole, T.J. (1990) Breast milk and neonatal necrotizing enterocolitis. *The Lancet*, **336**, 1519–1523.

Mitchell, E.A., Scragg, R., Stewart A.W., Becroft, D.M.O., Taylor, B.J., Ford, R.P.K., Hassall, I.B., Barry, D.M.J., Allen, E.M. & Roberts, A.P. (1991) Results from the first year of the New Zealand cot death study. *New Zealand Medical Journal*, **104**, 71–76.

Royal College of Midwives (1991) *Successful Breast Feeding*. 2nd edn. Churchill Livingstone, Edinburgh.

World Health Organisation (1989) Infant feeding: the physiological basis. *Bulletin of the World Health Organisation*, **67** (Suppl.), 19–40.

Woolridge, M.W. (1986) The 'anatomy' of infant sucking. *Midwifery*, **2**, 164–171.

Woolridge, M.W., & Baum, J.D. (1988) The regulation of human milk flow. In *Perinatal Nutrition*, (6th Bristol-Myers Nutrition Symposium) (Ed. by B.S. Lindblad), pp. 243–257. Academic Press, London.

Woolridge, M.W. & Fisher, C. (1988) Colic, 'overfeeding' and symptoms of lactose malabsorption: A possible artifact of feed management? *The Lancet*, **ii**, 382–384.

Woolridge, M.W., Ingram, J.C. & Baum, J.D. (1990) Do changes in pattern of breast usage alter the baby's nutrient intake? *The Lancet*, **336**, 395–397.

7

8 Drugs in Pregnancy and Lactation

PRINCIPLES OF PRESCRIBING DURING PREGNANCY AND LACTATION

The three major considerations in prescribing during pregnancy are changes in maternal physiology, transfer of drugs across the placenta and into breast milk, and possible adverse effects on the developing fetus.

Changes in maternal physiology

Total body water increases by as much as 8 litres in pregnancy which gives a substantially increased volume of distribution.

Serum proteins alter in concentration, in particular albumin which binds acidic drugs and decreases in concentration by up to 10 g/L. As a result, for example, levels of anticonvulsants should be monitored monthly and at one week and four weeks after delivery. The dose required usually increases as gestation progresses.

Liver metabolism increases in pregnancy. Therefore, drugs with a rate of elimination which depend on liver activity have a high rate of clearance in pregnancy.

Renal plasma flow has almost doubled by the last trimester of pregnancy. Drugs eliminated unchanged by the kidney are usually eliminated more rapidly. Ampicillin clearance doubles in pregnancy so the dose used in systemic infections should be doubled, but no change is necessary for urinary infections.

Transfer of drugs across the placenta and into breast milk

Lipid soluble, un-ionised, low molecular weight drugs cross the placenta easily and rapidly.

Most drugs cross the placenta and are excreted in breast milk at least to some extent. Dilution of the drug in the maternal circulation and the small volume of milk consumed by the baby usually means that the dose of drug the baby acquires is minimal (but see below).

Some drugs given close to delivery or during labour can affect the neonate.

Possible adverse effects on the developing fetus

The following milestones in **embryology** should, therefore, be noted:
- From conception until 17 days, implantation, blastocyst formation and gastrulation take place. Any insult during this time tends to result either in death and resorption or survival intact.
- Organogenesis takes place between 18 and 55 days after conception. The earlier in this period the insult occurs, the greater the likely effect.
- From 56 days onwards the effects of drugs, unless idiosyncratic, usually result in defects of growth and functional loss rather than gross structural abnormalities.

Fetal growth and development may be affected by drugs taken in the second and third trimester.

8

General principles

Taking note of these considerations the following general principles can be applied:
- **If possible avoid all drugs in the first trimester.** Although there is always a theoretical risk of malformations occurring at that time, proof is lacking for most and there is always a background risk for congenital malformations (3–5 per cent).
- **Drugs should only be used in pregnancy when the benefits to the mother are clear and are greater than the risk to the fetus.**
- **Only prescribe drugs in pregnancy which have established use in**

preference to newer drugs with less reliable data as to their use in pregnancy.

▪ Use the smallest effective dose taking into account the physiological changes of pregnancy that may affect drug absorption and dose, for the shortest therapeutic time.

The sections that follow provide only a general guide to prescribing in pregnancy. They are neither comprehensive nor definitive. It cannot be assumed that drugs not mentioned here are safe. For specific advice refer to the British National Formulary (or equivalent) or consult Regional Drug Centres. Potential drug interactions must also be considered.

DRUGS WITH KNOWN OR THEORETICAL RISK TO THE FETUS

Drug	Effect	Comment

Anti-infective agents

Drug	Effect	Comment
Tetracyclines	Tetracyclines cause discolouration of the deciduous teeth.	Use an alternative antibiotic in pregnancy.
Co-trimoxazole (trimethoprim & sulphamethoxazole)	Trimethoprim inhibits folic acid metabolism. Sulphonamides also interfere with folic acid synthesis. They compete with bilirubin for binding sites on albumin and therefore there is a **theoretical** risk of contributing to kernicterus.	No pregnancy-specific side effects have been noted. If it is necessary to use this combination at all, **avoid during the first trimester**. Main use in pregnancy will be for urinary infections where a single antibiotic is not felt to be sufficient and for toxoplasmosis.
Aminoglycosides (e.g. gentamicin tobramycin, netilimicin, amikacin, streptomycin, kanamycin)	All cross the placenta producing significant fetal levels. The main risk is of ototoxicity which may be increased 20 fold.	Use in severe infections in the mother if clinically indicated.
Metronidazole	Interferes with inosinic acid, an important nucleic acid precursor.	Although there have been no reported adverse effects it may be best to avoid in the first trimester.

Drug	Effect	Comment
Chloroquine	Causes fetal damage in high doses.	It can be used as an antimalarial in pregnancy but not for any other conditions.
Rifampicin	May increase the risk of bleeding in the neonate.	Isoniazid and ethambutol are drugs of choice for tuberculosis, but rifampicin can be used if a more potent drug is required. The neonate should be given Vitamin K.

Antihypertensives

ACE inhibitors	Cause congenital malformations in animal studies. May also adversely affect fetal and neonatal blood pressure control and renal function.	Contraindicated in women of reproductive age for the control of blood pressure.
Beta blocking drugs (e.g. atenolol, labetalol, oxprenolol)	Associated neonatal hypoglycaemia, and bradycardia. IUGR may be associated with use of atenolol.	Risks from severe maternal hypertension justifies anti-hypertensive therapy in pregnancy.
Ca channel blocking drugs (e.g. nifedipine)	Manufacturers do not recommend use in pregnancy because safety not fully established.	Nifedipine can be useful for control of severe hypertension. Main side effect is headache.
Methyldopa	Methyldopa may have unwanted side effects such as sedation, depression and postural hypotension that may require discontinuation of the drug.	Methyldopa is still the drug of first choice.

Anticoagulants

The indications for anticoagulation throughout pregnancy should be very clear. The risk of recurrence after one episode of pulmonary embolus or deep vein thrombosis is up to 12 per cent. Increasingly indications are only for recurrent thromboembolism and in those who have a hereditary predisposition to thromboembolism as indicated by activated Protein C resistance or deficiencies of Protein S, Protein C and anti-thrombin III.

Drug	Effect	Comment
Heparin	Heparin does not cross the placenta and it is not secreted in breast milk.	Bone demineralisation occurs in doses in excess of 10 000 units s.c. daily for greater than 3 months.
Warfarin	Warfarin crosses the placenta readily and may result in a syndrome characterised by nasal hypoplasia, chondroplasia punctata, stippled bone epiphyses, hydrocephalus, microcephaly, eye anomalies and postnatal developmental delay.	It is not excreted in significant quantities in breast milk.
Phenindione	Fetal and neonatal haemorrhage.	**Do not use in pregnancy**.

Anticonvulsants (for epilepsy)

	Anticonvulsants need to be continued throughout pregnancy because their benefits outweigh their risks	Monitor plasma concentrations frequently throughout pregnancy.
Hydantoins (e.g. phenytoin)	Associated with the 'fetal hydantoin syndrome' which includes craniofacial abnormalities such as cleft lip/palate, hypertelorism, broad nasal bridge, hypoplasia of the distal phalanges and nails, IUGR and mental deficiency. Minor cranio-facial abnormalities occur in approximately one third of babies born to mothers on phenytoin; 10 per cent have major congenital anomalites such as cardiac defects and cleft lip/palate.	
Carbamazepine	May be associated with neural tube defects (NTDs).	Women who become pregnant on carbamazepine or valproate should be counselled and offered ante-natal screening for NTD.

8

Drug	Effect	Comment
Valproic acid	It is also associated with an increased risk of NTDs.	It is unclear whether it is the epilepsy *per se*, the anticonvulsant medication or a combination of both or other factors that causes the embryopathy.

It may be that the embryopathy is due to effects on folate metabolism. Therefore, **offer folate supplements to all pregnant women on anticonvulsants**.

Corticosteroids

Prednisone, prednisolone	These should be used only when the benefit of the treatment outweighs the risk. High doses (>10 mg prednisone/day) may produce fetal and neonatal adrenal suppression.	Intravenous hydrocortisone cover may be necessary for the mother in labour.

Sex steroids

Oestrogens and progesterone	Maternal treatment with 19 norprogestogens, testosterone and diethylstilboestrol (DES) results in masculinisation of the female fetus. DES caused 'vaginal adenosis' and clear cell carcinoma of the vagina in daughters of mothers treated in early pregnancy.	**Avoid these drugs in pregnancy**.

Drugs acting on skin

Isotretinoin and tretinoin – derivatives of retinoic acid (Vitamin A)	The drug's half life is 96 hours. It is associated with such malformations as microcephaly, micrognathia, cleft palate, heart defects, eye and brain anomalies, hydrocephalus, and thymic agenesis.	In women who become pregnant while taking the drug (usually for the treatment of acne) up to 20 per cent will miscarry and in the remainder up to 20 per cent of the babies will have serious congenital malformations.

8

Drug	Effect	Comment
Isotretinoin and tretinoin *(Continued)*		Contraception should be used for one month before and one month after treatment. **Avoid even topical use during pregnancy**.
Etretinate and acitretin (also derivatives of Vitamin A)	Used for the treatment of psoriasis. The main association is with cranio-facial abnormalities.	They can persist in the circulation for a long time and **pregnancy should be avoided for at least 2 years after stopping treatment**.

Cytotoxic agents

Methotrexate	May be associated with short stature, cranio-synostosis, hydrocephalus, hyper-telorism, micrognathia and cleft palate.	Avoid conception for at least 6 months after stopping. Breast feeding is also best avoided.
Azathioprine	A derivative of 6-mercapto-purine. It is given in conjunction with corticosteroids for immunosuppression. When properly used, there is no good evidence of an increase in malformations.	The decision to continue in pregnancy depends on the condition being treated but, in general, it is best not initiated during pregnancy as a matter of principle.
Alkylating agents (e.g. busulfan: cyclophosphamide)	Used to treat some forms of leukaemia, they are associated with IUGR, cleft palate and eye defects.	Alkylating agents may be associated with up to a 15 per cent incidence of major congenital malformations.

Psycho-active drugs

Thalidomide	A hypnotic/sedative resulting in phocomelia if ingested between 27 and 42 days gestation.	**Must not be used** in the treatment of women of reproductive age.
Lithium	Used in the treatment of affective mental disorders. If used in early pregnancy there may be an increased risk of cardiovascular anomalies. May also cause neonatal goitre.	Therapeutic benefits must be carefully weighed.

8

COMMONLY PRESCRIBED DRUGS IN PREGNANCY

Drug	Effect	Comment
Anti-emetics	For nausea and vomiting. **Metoclopramide** lowers oesophageal sphincter pressure and accelerates gastric emptying.	**Meclozine** and **cyclizine** appear safe. Used in late pregnancy. There is no controlled data as to its use in early pregnancy.
Antacids	Non-absorbable antacids such as **aluminium hydroxide** or **magnesium trisilicate** may be used. Aluminium hydroxide used alone can cause constipation.	H2 receptor antagonists **cimetidine** and **ranitidine** are safe and effective for use before general anaesthesia (e.g. for caesarean section) to reduce harm from aspiration of gastric contents.
Antibiotics for asymptomatic bacteriuria	This occurs in up to 5 per cent of pregnancies and if it is not treated up to one third of women will develop pyelonephritis.	In general give **augmentin** unless sensitivities suggest otherwise. Women allergic to beta-lactams, can be given trimethoprim or nitrofurantoin.
Beta-agonist tocolytics	i.v. administration of **ritodrine**, **salbutamol** or **terbutaline** can cause pulmonary oedema. Risk factors include fluid overload, multiple pregnancy, pre-existing cardiac disease (may be covert) and maternal infection.	Use with care and only if absolutely necessary: administer via syringe pump using 5 per cent dextrose (not saline) as diluent.
NSAID	Regular use of powerful NSAIDs may result in closure of the fetal ductus arteriosus causing pulmonary hypertension. May also delay and prolong labour. When used for analgesia in women with severe pre-eclampsia they may cause renal failure and adult respiratory distress syndrome.	Use only if essential. **Do not use in presence of severe pre-eclampsia**.

8

Drug	Effect	Comment
Local anaesthetic agents	Large doses (e.g. for paracervical or epidural block) may cause neonatal respiratory depression, hypotonia, and bradycardia.	Neonatal methaemoglobinaemia may occur with **prilocaine** and **procaine**.
Thyroid replacement	Give **thyroxine** 100–200 microgram/day. The response is monitored by a fall in the TSH. Monitor thyroid function every 4–6 weeks in pregnancy as the dose may need to be increased.	Use the lowest possible dose to maintain euthyroidism in the mother. Measure serum free thyroxine and TSH monthly.
Anti-thyroid drugs	Either **propylthiouracil** (PTU) or **carbimazole** can be given. Both cross the placenta and, in high doses, may cause fetal goitre and hypothyroidism. PTU is preferred during breast-feeding (see below). Propanolol may be needed for the control of symptoms of thyrotoxicosis.	Fetal thyrotoxicosis may occur as the result of transplacental passage of thyroid stimulating antibodies even with control of maternal thyrotoxicosis.

DRUGS WHICH MAY CAUSE PROBLEMS DURING BREAST-FEEDING

As a matter of principle, the breast feeding mother should be prescribed only drugs which are essential.

Drugs given during lactation may cause toxicity to the baby if the drug enters the milk in pharmacologically significant quantities. Indeed, milk concentrations of some drugs exceed those of the maternal plasma so that therapeutic doses in the mother may cause toxicity in the baby (e.g. iodides).

Drugs in breast milk may cause hypersensitivity in the baby, even when the concentration is too low for a pharmacological effect.

Manufacturers often advise that a drug be not used in the breast feeding mother because there is insufficient evidence for safety.

The following list is not comprehensive and the absence of a drug from it cannot be taken to imply safety.

Acyclovir	Use with caution because a significant amount appears in milk.
ACE inhibitors	Manufacturers advise against use.
Amiodorone	Avoid if possible because of possible release of iodine (see below).
Amphetamines	Avoid; significant amount in milk.
Anticoagulants	**Warfarin** does not appear in milk in significant quantities and can be used. **Phenindione** should be avoided. **Heparin** does not appear in milk and can be used.
Aspirin	Avoid during breast feeding because of the risk of Reye's syndrome. Regular use of high doses theoretically can impair platelet function and produce hypoprothrombinaemia in the baby if neonatal Vitamin K stores are low.
Barbiturates	Avoid if possible because large doses may produce drowsiness.
Benzodiazepines	Avoid repeated doses.
Carbimazole	Neonatal hypothyroidism and goitre: if anti-thyroid drug needed propylthiouracil is preferred.
Chloramphenicol	Use another antibiotic: may cause bone marrow toxicity or the 'grey syndrome' in infants.
Oral contraceptives (or other oestrogens)	The combined oral contraceptive should be avoided for at least six weeks post partum for breast feeding to become established. Progestagen-only contraceptives do not affect lactation.
Cytotoxic drugs	Breast feeding is contraindicated
Ergotamine	Avoid.
Ethosuxaminde	Avoid; significant amount in milk.
Etretinate and isotretinoin	Avoid.
Fluconazole	Avoid.
Iodine based drugs	Either do not use or stop breast feeding: iodine is concentrated in milk and may cause hypothyroidism and goitre.
Lithium	Monitor infant carefully.
Mefloquine	Avoid: excreted in milk.
Methadone	Withdrawal symptoms in infant; breast feeding not necessarily contraindicated.

8

Metoclopramide	Avoid unless essential.
Metronidazole	Significant amount in milk: avoid single large doses.
Ofloxacin	Manufacturers advise against use.
Procainamide	Manufacturers advise against use.

BIBLIOGRAPHY

The British National Formulary, No. 29 (March 1995) pp 546–560, British Medical Association, London.

Rubin, P.C. (Ed.) (1987) *Prescribing in pregnancy*, British Medical Journal, London.

Briggs, G.G., Freeman, R.K. & Yaffe, S.J. (1990) *Drugs in Pregnancy and Lactation.* Williams and Wilkins, Baltimore, MD.

8

9 Contraception after Pregnancy and Post-partum Care

9

9.1 Contraception

EMERGENCY CONTRACEPTION

Hormonal

Between 2 and 4 per cent of women will become pregnant after a single act of unprotected intercourse. This risk can be reduced significantly by post-coital oestrogen/progestogen taken not later than 72 hours after intercourse.

The dose is **two tablets** 12 hours apart of 50 micrograms ethinyloestradiol + 250 micrograms of levonorgesterel (PC4 Schering) or Ovran (Wyeth). Ovran comes in packs of 21 tablets.

In the first half of the menstrual cycle this will inhibit or postpone ovulation. If taken in mid-cycle, treatment disrupts luteal function.

Side effects

Nausea (25–60 per cent) and vomiting (11–29 per cent); headaches, dizziness and breast tenderness. If the woman vomits within 3 hours of either dose she will need a further two tablets or possibly an IUCD fitted. To avoid a repeat visit, give **six** tablets at the initial visit. An antiemetic (e.g. metoclopramide) may be given.

Intrauterine device (IUD)

The estimated failure rate from an IUD inserted post-coitally is only 0.15 per cent. An IUD can be inserted up to 5 days after ovulation and is appropriate for women who present 3–5 days after unprotected sexual intercourse.

Follow-up advice

Emergency contraception may cause the next period not to be on time. The timing of the next ovulation is unpredictable. Therefore, make sure the woman has adequate contraceptive advice.

ORAL CONTRACEPTIVES

The 'mini' pill

This is a progestogen only containing pill (POP). It is suitable for use post-partum because the combined pill was thought to interfere with breast feeding and because of an increased risk of post-partum thrombosis with oestrogen.

Mini pills have a higher failure rate than combined preparations and must ideally be taken at the same time every day (e.g. 7 p.m.); maximum efficacy is three hours later. Commence one tablet daily.

A missed pill increases the risk of pregnancy and is defined as a pill taken over three hours after the usual time. In the event of a missed pill, continue with normal pill taking but use another method such as barrier methods for seven days.

Vomiting or diarrhoea may prevent absorption. Use additional precautions for seven days after recovery.

Breakthrough bleeding may occur with use of the mini pill at least initially.

Brand names of mini pills

Brand name	Active ingredient	Amount (micrograms)
Femulen	Ethynodiol diacetate	500
Micronor	Norethisterone	350
Microval	Levonorgestrel	30
Neogest	Norgestrel	75 (= Levonorgestrel 37.5 micrograms)
Norgeston	Levonorgestrel	30
Noriday	Norethisterone	350

The combined oral contraceptive (COC) pill

The combined oral contraceptive pill contains oestrogen (30–50 micrograms) and progestogen. It gives good cycle control and minimal side-effects. The two oestrogens used are ethinyloestradiol or mestranol. The progestogens are norethisterone, norethisterone acetate, ethynodiol diacetate, levonorgestrel, desogestrel or gestodene.

The benefits of the combined oral contraceptive pill are:

▪ High efficacy – the pregnancy rate if properly taken is 0.2 to 0.4 per 100 women years. In practice pills are often missed, leading to more failures.

▪ Suppression of menstrual disorders (menorrhagia and dysmenorrhoea), benign breast disease and functional ovarian cysts.

▪ Decreased risk of ovarian and endometrial cancer.

Among the minor side effects from the COC are nausea, headaches and breast tenderness. Migraine is a contraindication for use.

Biochemical changes include some degree of:

▪ Acceleration of the clotting of procoagulants in the extrinsic and intrinsic clotting systems, reduction of antithrombin III levels, increased fibrinogen levels, decreased fibrinolytic activity.

▪ Increase in fasting serum triglycerides and cholesterol. Some women have decreased glucose tolerance and a slight rise in systolic BP. Occasionally frank hypertension develops.

9

There is a slight dose related risk of venous thrombosis and embolism (particularly from pills containing desogestrel or gestodene), cerebro-vascular accident and acute myocardial infarction. These risks increase with age and are strongly associated with cigarette smoking.

There may be an increased risk of breast cancer, especially in women who have used the pill before the age of 25, and those who have used a high progestogen potency pill. After stopping the pill, fertility may be temporarily impaired for a month or so.

9.2   Medical termination of pregnancy

MIFEPRISTONE (RU 486)

Only use in compliance with the requirements of local abortion laws and in a licensed institution.

Mifepristone (RU 486) is used in combination with gemeprost to induce a medical abortion. Mifepristone in combination with a prostaglandin is an alternative to surgical termination of pregnancy of no more than nine weeks' gestation, and is effective in about 95 per cent of women. If used alone, it is effective in 60–85 per cent of women in inducing abortion.

Therapeutic use

- Do not use on a pregnancy after nine weeks' amenorrhoea (63 days).
- After careful counselling about the procedure, give the licensed dose of 600 mg of mifepristone (200 mg may be equally effective).
- Observe for two hours. Give advice on how to obtain emergency care when the woman returns home and ensure she has access to a companion.
- 36–48 hours later give a prostaglandin (e.g. gemeprost) pessary 1 mg vaginally. At this stage about 50 per cent of women will have already started to bleed, and 1–2 per cent will have already aborted, in which case the gemeprost is not given.

- 80 per cent will abort within four hours after the prostaglandin is given; 95 per cent within eight hours.
- The patient can be discharged once bleeding has subsided and the abortion is complete.
- Always follow up the patient within 8–12 days to verify that the abortion is complete.
- Advise use of appropriate contraception.
- Do not insert an IUCD until two weeks after complete abortion.

Contraindications

History of cardiovascular disease; renal or hepatic failure; asthma; smokers over 35 years of age, and in women with haemorrhagic disorders; long term corticosteroid users.

Clinical pharmacology

Pharmacokinetics

Mifepristone is well absorbed, peak plasma concentrations being reached within three hours after oral administration. It is metabolised in the liver and excreted in the bowel. Its half life is long (20–24 hours) because its clearance rate is slow.

Mechanism of action

Mifepristone is a 19-norsteroid like norethisterone. It acts by binding with high affinity to the progesterone receptor. Thus it inhibits the action of progesterone which is essential for establishing a normal pregnancy. By opposing the actions of progesterone, it increases the contractility of the myometrium and disrupts endometrial maturation. It also reduces the metabolism of prostaglandins, further stimulating uterine contraction.

Side effects

Among these are uterine haemorrhage and abdominal pain from uterine contractions. Abdominal pain usually responds to paracetamol but 30 per cent of women require opiate analgesia during the first few hours after the administration of the prostaglandin which may induce strong uterine contractions. Aspirin and non-steroid anti-inflammatory drugs inhibit the prostaglandin synthetase and could theoretically interfere with the efficacy of the mifepristone and prostaglandin. They should, therefore, be avoided until complete abortion has been confirmed 12 days after administration. Also avoid in women with asthma or other chronic obstructive airways disease, renal and hepatic failure.

Less than 1 per cent of women undergoing a medical abortion will require transfer or emergency evacuation of the uterus to control vaginal bleeding.

9.3   Second trimester loss, stillbirth and neonatal death

- If an intrauterine death is suspected it is best confirmed by real-time ultrasonic scan.
- If confirmed, discuss with the parents possible explanations, suggestions for labour, investigations and plans for future consultation.
- Parents need time to talk about the situation – give them the opportunity.
- Parents will probably like time to themselves.
- Mothers may feel guilty and that it is their fault.
- Only part of what is said is absorbed at any one time, and it will be necessary to repeat all key issues.

9

LABOUR AND DELIVERY

Choice of analgesia is important. Regional analgesia has many benefits, even if labour is short (i.e. only for an hour or so). It eliminates the memory of pain which may have its own psychological morbidity for the future and for future pregnancies. Opiate analgesia has sedative and disorientating effects, with specific hallucinatory effects in some women. Sedation of the mother may not be desirable. Consider giving an anxiolytic such as temazepam 20 mg.

The parents should be given the opportunity and encouraged to see and hold the baby.

The parents should be encouraged to name the baby and refer to the baby by his/her name.

A polaroid photograph of the baby should be taken. A copy should be available for the parents (they may not wish to have one initially and thus it should be kept in the notes in case they change their minds). A separate copy should be retained in the notes.

INVESTIGATIONS

1 Maternal blood

The following tests should be routine but consider others if suggested by the clinical circumstances, e.g. additional renal or bacterial serology; lupus inhibitor.

1 Full clotting screen and platelet count.
2 Kleihauer test to see if fetal haemorrhage has occurred.
3 'TORCH' screen.
4 Fructosamine and random blood sugar.
5 Thyroid function.
6 Repeat serological screen for syphilis.
7 Autoantibody screen.
8 If Rhesus negative repeat antibody screen.

2 Fetal

Post mortem examination

This examination is a vital part of the management. Sensitive counselling should be directed at obtaining parental consent to a full autopsy. If that cannot be achieved, much information can be gained by a more limited examination carried out by a perinatal pathologist. This can often be helpful if there are religious objections to autopsy. Fig. 9.1 shows a suggested pathology notification form.

Ward examination after second trimester loss or termination of pregnancy

This must be done in all cases even when a fetal anomaly is **not** suspected.

9

Baby

Name:

Registration no:

DOB:

Mother

Name:

Registration no:

DOB:

Previous pregnancy

	Date	Pregnancy	Labour	Birthweight	Sex	Outcome
1						
2						
3						
4						
5						

Present pregnancy

Date of LMP   Blood group   Rh
EDD
Amniocentesis   Yes/No (result   )
Ultrasound scan   Yes/No (result   )
Threatened abortion   Yes/No
APH   Yes/No
Hydramnios/Oligohydramnios   Yes/No
Hypertension   Yes/No
PET   Yes/No
Maternal pyrexia   Yes/No
IUGR   Yes/No

Labour

Spontaneous/Induced
Prostaglandins/Oxytocin
Indication   Liquor   ? Normal
First stage   hours
Second stage   min
Fetal distress   Yes/No
Time of delivery   Time of death
Date of delivery   Date of death
Presentation: Cephalic/Breech/Other
Delivery: Forceps/Caesarean/Other

Neonatal

Birth weight	g	Gestation	wks
Apgar score	at 1 min		at 5 min

Resuscitation: Nil

O$_2$

O$_2$ mask intubation

Neonatal problems	**Neonatal procedures**
1	
2	
3	
4	
5	

Suspected causes of death

1

2

3

4

5

Special points of interest to be looked for

Fig. 9.1 A suggested pathology notification form for fetal and perinatal deaths.

1 Record fetal and placental weights and fetal crown–rump and crown–heel length.
2 Carry out careful external examination:
- head – anencephaly, cleft lip or palate?
- thorax;
- abdomen – abdominal wall defect (exomphalos, gastroschisis?)'
- perineum – normal genitalia? anus?
- spine – neural tube defect?
- limbs – all present? abnormal length? extra digit on hands or feet?

9

Skin biopsy for cytogenetics

If this cannot be carried out routinely it **must** be performed if a cytogenetic anomaly is suspected.

If the fetus is macerated, the placenta can be biopsied (e.g. near the insertion of the cord) and sent for analysis.

A skin biopsy measuring 0.5–1 cm (together with some underlying muscle) is best taken aseptically from the upper fleshy part of the thigh. It should be placed in a sterile universal container with tissue culture medium or, if not available, sterile normal saline. **It must not be placed in formalin.** It should be despatched to the cytogenetics laboratory immediately with a fully completed request form. If necessary it may be refrigerated at 4°C overnight but **it must not be placed in a freezer.**

Cord or cardiac blood

This can be taken and sent for chromosomal examination, blood grouping, screening for infection (e.g. IgM, TORCH and VDRL).

CARE OF THE MOTHER BEFORE LEAVING HOSPITAL

1 Discuss further the possible causes, pending the results of investigations.

2 Explore emotional aspects and assist in the grieving process.

3 Offer any stillbirth literature to the parents.

4 Inform community midwives and general practitioners by phone of the outcome of the pregnancy and ensure that they receive written information.

5 Inform the antenatal clinic of the outcome.

6 It may be helpful to suppress lactation with bromocriptine (2.5 mg on day 1, followed by 2.5 mg twice daily for 14 days).

7 Discuss contraception.

8 Check for the need for anti-D gamma-globulin and rubella vaccination and give if appropriate.

9 Arrange referral to other specialists if appropriate (e.g. social worker, paediatrician, physician, geneticist).

10 Arrange an outpatient appointment for the lead obstetrician (usually the consultant) to see the couple in about six weeks to review the results of the investigation and discuss implications for the future.

Make sure the results of investigations are present in the case notes at this consultation.

9.4 Postnatal depression

Psychological complications of motherhood are frequent, diverse and often clinically unrecognised or poorly treated. Psychiatric conditions may arise from the complexity of the rapid biological, social and psychological transition that motherhood brings. There is a strong link with adverse social circumstances and pre-existing marital difficulties.

Post-partum psychological and psychiatric disturbance may have a far reaching effect on establishing breast feeding, attachment and bonding to the baby, relationship with the partner, other children and other family members.

Motherhood is an intrinsically stressful time because it often reveals a lot about a person psychologically, or about their background, particularly the relationship with the new mother's own mother. It challenges parenting skills and the relationship of responsibility and dependence.

Following delivery:

- 40–50 per cent of women may experience brief periods of 'the blues' lasting from a few hours to one week.
- 8–10 per cent may experience more substantial mood disturbances that persist for a week or more and which cause some impairment in functioning.
- In 3–7 per cent of women the depression may require treatment as an outpatient or in hospital.
- About 1 in 500 women may become psychotic after delivery and require intensive inpatient care in a mother and baby unit. It can pose severe problems for both mother and baby but treatment is usually effective.

There is a significant risk of recurrence of postnatal depression and psychosis in a future pregnancy.

9

AETIOLOGY OF POSTNATAL DEPRESSION AND PSYCHOSIS

- The role of hormones (e.g. oestrogen, progesterone, prolactin, androgens) and neurotransmitters (e.g. serotonin, catecholamines) in postnatal depression and psychosis is unclear, despite many claims for their significance.

IDENTIFYING FACTORS FOR POST-PARTUM DEPRESSION

- History taking is very important. Unless specific questions have been asked in relation to a psychiatric history, do not assume that there have been no episodes. There may be a history of post-partum depression in a previous pregnancy, or depression in the current pregnancy;
- a family history, particularly the mother or aunts.

Ask at the postnatal visit at six weeks whether the mother is enjoying the baby, by using an open ended question such as 'How are you feeling in yourself?' Depression is recognised by the fact that the woman feels miserable. She does not enjoy anything and has difficulty in coping, though this may not be obvious to observers and it is this group of women who are largely ignored. Those who are overtly emotionally labile get noticed and helped.

The standard classification for psychiatric disease comes from the DSM-III criteria for depression. In the year following birth of the baby it is difficult to use the criteria for weight gain and weight loss. Similarly, sleep is often disturbed because of the baby waking. Insomnia may be assessed by asking how easy it is to get back to sleep. Loss of libido is similarly difficult to assess because it is not uncommon, particularly with breast feeding.

Post-partum depression may be accompanied by a high level of anxiety, particularly in first time mothers.

Post-partum depression contrasts with 'maternity blues' which is emotional lability on the fourth or fifth day of post-partum experienced by most others. It lasts a matter of hours or days.

9

CRITERIA FOR A MAJOR DEPRESSIVE ILLNESS (DSM-III)

The following are features which typify a major depressive episode. They do not all have to be present, but many may have been present in the same two week period and show a change from the previous level of functioning; including one of the symptoms being depressed mood, or loss of interest or pleasure.

1 Depressed mood most of the day, either self reported or as observed by others.

2 Markedly diminished interest or pleasure in all, or almost all, activities most of the day, nearly every day as indicated by either a subjective account or observation by others of apathy most of the time.

3 Significant weight loss (when not dieting) or weight gain (e.g. 5 per cent in either direction) over one month, or decrease or increase in appetite nearly every day.

4 Insomnia or hypersomnia nearly every day.

5 Psychomotor agitation or retardation nearly every day which is observed by others and not subjective feelings of restlessness or being slowed down.

6 Fatigue and loss of energy nearly every day.

7 Feelings of worthlessness or excessive or inappropriate guilt (which may be delusional) nearly every day.

8 Diminished ability to think or concentrate, or indecisiveness, nearly every day (either by subjective account or as observed by others).

9 Recurrent thoughts of death (not just fear of dying), recurrent suicidal ideation without a specific plan, or a suicide attempt or a specific plan for committing suicide.

Other features

- It cannot be established that an organic factor initiated and maintained the disturbance.
- The disturbance is not a normal reaction to the death of a loved one.
- At no time during the disturbance have there been delusions or hallucinations for as long as two weeks in the absence of prominent mood symptoms (i.e. before the mood symptoms developed or after they have remitted).

■ Not superimposed on schizophrenia, schizophreniform disorder, delusional disorder, or psychotic disorder, non-specific in origin.

Depression may be mild, moderate or severe.

1 Mild

This is recognised as few or any symptoms in excess of those required to make the diagnosis. Symptoms result in only minor impairment in occupational functioning or in usual social activities, or relationships with others.

2 Moderate

Symptoms or functional impairment between 'mild' and 'severe'.

3 Severe, without psychotic features

Several symptoms in excess of those required to make the diagnosis, and symptoms markedly interfering with occupational functioning or with usual social activities or relationships with others.

4 With psychotic features

Delusions or hallucinations. Are they congruent with the mood?

Further enquiries

Once postpartum depression has been identified it is important to interview other significant family members – the partner and mother in particular.

A major degree of depression is identified by the fact that depressive reactions (e.g. in relation to stillbirth, congenital malformation or difficult delivery) shift to a pervasiveness of mood. There is a shift towards the vegetative features of depressive illness, with anergia (the inability to motivate oneself to do things), poor concentration and decision making and a general inability to enjoy life. The mood change is total: for instance the woman does not have the capacity to laugh at anything or to be motivated to any degree to show an interest in something.

■ Look at the social and physical circumstances.

■ Identify stress relieving factors, e.g. more help in the home.

■ Identify whether there are any thoughts of self-harm or harm to the baby. These may take the form of fantasies of getting out of the situation, e.g. not wanting to wake up. This is a dangerous situation for the mother and her baby. If such thoughts are present, they need 24 hour supervision on a one-to-one basis.

Puerperal psychosis

Psychosis that is due to the puerperium occurs within two weeks of delivery. It is a relatively severe disturbance of behaviour, mood, perception and thought. Puerperal psychosis has an incidence of one in five hundred women who are post-partum.

Symptoms may fluctuate. For instance it may be worse at night. Beware of night time manifestations of this condition that seem to resolve with appropriate behaviour in the morning. These women are at risk of being discharged from hospital without the follow up care necessary to their condition.

Psychosis has the potential to be very dangerous, because the mother may have delusions about herself or the baby; there may be bizarre behaviour that is dangerous to herself and the baby.

Other disorders of the mother–baby interaction

- Delayed attachment: It is not uncommon for mothers to experience some delay in affectionate feelings for their babies, or even hostility to the baby.
- Obsessional thoughts.
- Infanticide within 24 hours of the birth of the baby is almost always due to the baby being unwanted by mothers who did not seek an abortion or who made no preparations for the baby.
- Murder by the parent of the baby 24 hours or more after birth is usually associated with mental illness.

AETIOLOGICAL FACTORS IN POST-PARTUM DEPRESSION

9

Identifying risk factors is useful because the clinical occurrence of post-partum depression or psychosis may be prevented or reduced in severity by early and appropriate intervention.

Identifiable risk factors

- Any complicated pregnancy or delivery.

- Any problem with the baby.
- Bereavement during the pregnancy or just after the birth of the baby.
- A major stress in the mother's relationship with partner or family.
- A past history of poor parenting.
- The biggest risk factor is a past history of psychological or psychiatric illness or a family history to such.
- Depressive disorders are increasing world wide.
- There is an association between post-partum depression and premenstrual syndrome.

TREATMENT OF POST-PARTUM DEPRESSION

Women who meet the criteria for depression post-partum need specialised resources for support and adequate counselling.

Usually they need medication. A tricyclic antidepressant may be commenced at a dose of 50 mg per day titrated for the individual woman to a dose commensurate with an improvement in clinical symptoms. The tricyclic antidepressants are particularly useful because of their anxiolytic effect which is noted first, followed by an improvement in sleep. Mood improvement usually occurs two to three weeks later. Moclobemide, a monoamine oxidase inhibitor, is an alternative. It has fewer side effects. It is given in a dose of 300–600 mg. As yet there is little data on the suitability of the serotonin uptake inhibiting class of drugs in a breast feeding mother.

BIBLIOGRAPHY

Baird, D.T. (1992) Medical termination of pregnancy. *Review of Advances in Endocrinological Metabolism*, **4**, 83–94.

Consumer's Association (1993) Mifepristone/Gemeprost to abort early pregnancy. *Drug and Therapeutics Bulletin*, **31**, 5–6.

Kumar, R. & Brockington, I.F. (1988) *Motherhood and Mental Illness: Causes and Consequences*, Wright, London.

Norman, J.E., Thong, K.J. & Baird, G.T. (1991) Uterine contractility and induction of abortion in early pregnancy by misoprostol and mifepristone. *The Lancet*, **338**, 1233–1236.

Pike, M.C., Henderson, B.E., Krailo, M.D., Duke, A. & Roy, S. (1983) Breast cancer in young women and use of oral contraceptives: possible modifying accepted formulation of and age at use. *The Lancet*, **1**, 926–930.

Royal College of General Practitioners (1974) *Oral Contraceptives and Health*. Pitman, London.

9

UK Multicentre Trial (1990) The efficacy and tolerance of mifepristone and prostaglandin in first trimester termination of pregnancy. *British Journal of Obstetrics & Gynaecology*, **97**, 480–486.

10 Medico-legal Matters

The incidence of patients attempting to sue doctors, nurses and hospital authorities continues to rise exponentially. The reasons are complex. Among them are:

- Patients' expectations are greater than ever before but the money is limited.
- If things do not go as expected 'it must be someone's fault'.
- The new NHS climate of health care encourages patients to complain assuming that this can improve the service provided.
- Sometimes when things do go wrong they are handled badly by poor communication.
- The fear of litigation makes doctors and nurses defensive which increases the suspicion of patients.

Although medico-legal matters are now dealt with by NHS Trusts or Health Authorities, medical staff are advised to retain membership of a medical defence society.

PREVENTION OF MEDICO-LEGAL CASES

There are some things we must **always** do and some which should **never** be done.

Always

1 Maintain detailed, clear and legible records each time the patient is seen. Write down specific reasons for policies and decisions. **Poor note-keeping is the commonest cause of non-negligent cases being 'lost'.**

2 Make sure drug prescriptions are correctly recorded.

3 Make sure intravenous infusions (including blood) are properly recorded.

4 Recognise when you need to seek advice from senior colleagues and ask that they attend if you feel it necessary. Record this in the notes.

5 Write comprehensive, clear and accurate operation notes. Include a check for swabs and instruments.

6 Make sure that pre-operative consent is obtained well before surgery. In the case of sterilisation make sure that you explain (and record) that the operation, even when done properly, has a small risk of failure.

7 Record patient hypersensitivity to drugs.

8 Make particularly detailed records of any complications.

9 Record if patients refuse, or act against, your advice.

10 Tell the truth.

Never

1 Delete or revise a record in the case notes after the event. If a factual amendment is necessary write a full revised version giving the new time and date. Do not strike out the old record. If only a word needs to be changed annotate the change and initial it.

2 Remove any part of the medical records.

3 Criticise the work or conduct of a medical or nursing colleague in writing.

4 Write derogatory remarks about a patient in the notes.

5 Delegate a task to a junior unless satisfied that he/she is competent to do it and understands fully what is required.

WHAT TO DO IF A MEDICAL ACCIDENT OCCURS

1 Make sure that you and all involved write detailed notes of what happened and what has been said to the patient or the relatives.

2 Inform the consultant in charge (if he or she is not already involved) who should involve the clinical director.

3 Contact your medical defence society for advice.

If you have to appear in a civil or coroner's court as a witness make sure you have been given clear advice by your medical defence society.

10

11 Obstetric Data

11.1 Haematology

BLOOD TUBES AND THEIR USES

Table 11.1.1 shows blood tubes used according to United Kingdom universal colour coding. For reference the additives for each coloured blood tube are given. Table 11.1.2 shows which blood tube to use for what test.

Table 11.1 Universal colour coding of blood tubes used in the UK.

Blood tube	Colour coding
Serum separation tube	Yellow
Fluoride tube	Grey
Citrate tube	Light blue
Heparin tube	Green
EDTA (ethylenediaminetetra-acetic acid) tube	Purple
Plain tube (cross match)	Pink

Table 11.1.2 Whick UK colour coded blood tubes to use for what test.

Test	Bottle
Alphafetoprotein	Yellow
Australia antigen	Yellow
Grouping and cross match	Pink
B_{12}	Pink
Folate	Purple
Creatinine clearance	Yellow
Cytomegalovirus	Yellow
Chromosomes	Green
Clotting studies	Blue
Follicle stimulating hormone	Yellow
Fructosamine	Yellow
Glycosylated haemoglobin	Purple
Hb, full blood count	Purple
Kleihauer	Purplo
Luteinising hormone	Yellow
Liver function tests	Yellow
Prolactin	Yellow
Prothrombin	Blue
Plasma protein	Yellow
Rhesus	Pink
Rubella	Yellow
Serum progesterone	Yellow
Thyroid function	Yellow
Toxoplasmosis	Yellow
Urea and electrolytes	Yellow
Uric acid	Yellow
VDRL	Pink
Triglycerides	Yellow

HAEMATOLOGICAL AND BIOCHEMICAL INVESTIGATIONS

Table 11.1.3 shows ranges of values obtained for the pregnant woman at term.

11

Table 11.1.3 Ranges for haematological biochemical investigations in pregnancy; all values are given for term except where stated.

	Range
Haematology	
Haemoglobin (g/dL)	10.4–14.8
Haematocrit	0.31–0.44
Mean cell volume (femtolitres)	83–96
Mean cell haemoglobin (picograms)	27.0–32
Mean cell haemoglobin concentration (g/L)	32–36
Reticulocytes	0.02–0.12
Erythrocyte count ($\times 10^9$/L)	3.35–5.01
Red cell distribution width	0.126–0.158
Leukocyte count ($\times 10^9$/L)	4.0–15
Lymphocyte count (10^9/L)	1.0–4.0 (20–50%)
Monocyte count ($\times 10^9$/L)	0.02–0.08 (2–10%)
Eosinophils ($\times 10^9$/L)	0.04–0.4 (1–6%)
Basophils ($\times 10^9$/L)	0.01 (<1%)
Neutrophil count ($\times 10^9$/L)	4.8–13 (40–75%)
Platelets	
<36 weeks ($\times 10^9$/L)	140–370
>36 weeks ($\times 10^9$/L)	120–400
Mean platelet volume (femtolitres)	7.0–11.0 (mean = 9.0)
Coagulation tests	
Prothrombin time (s)	11.5–15
Activated partial thomboplastin time (s)	25–37
Fibrinogen (g/L)	1.5–4
Protein S (per cent)	60–140
Protein C (per cent)	70–150
Antithrombin III (per cent)	80–120
Heparin range	APTT should be 2.5–4.0 times control
Iron requirements and levels	
Iron	100 mg additional iron required in pregnancy
	2–3 mg/day in excess of normal requirements
Serum ferritin	>12 microgram/L indicates significant iron depletion in non-pregnant women
	Serum iron less than 10.7 nanomol/L implies iron depletion

Table 11.1.3 *Continued*

	Range
Serum ferritin *(continued)*	Hb <9.0 g/dL and Hct <0.29 indicate increased risk of fetal death, premature birth or low birth weight babies
Iron (micromol/L)	5–27
Iron binding capacity (micromol/L)	65–111
Transferrin saturation (micromol/L)	0.02–0.30
Ferritin (microgram/L)	15–300
Ions	
Sodium (mmol/L)	133–143
Potassium (mmol/L)	3.6–4.6
Chloride (mmol/L)	95–105
Bicarbonate (mmol/L)	18–26
Anion gap (mmol/L)[a]	6–14
Calcium (mmol/L)[b]	2.25–2.7
Magnesium (mmol/L)	0.65–1.0
Phosphate (mmol/L)	0.85–1.4
Nitrogenous compounds	
Urea (mmol/L)	1.5–5.2
Creatinine (mmol/L)	0.04–0.08
Uric acid (mmol/L)	
12 weeks	0.25
28 weeks	0.30
32 weeks	0.35
36 weeks	0.40
Term	0.45
Sugars	
Plasma glucose	10–15 per cent lower than serum
Post-prandial blood glucose (mmol/L)	7.2–7.8
Fasting blood glucose (mmol/L)	<5.8
Mean plasma glucose (mmol/L)	4.4–5.0
2 hours post-prandial 75 g load (mmol/L)	<6.1
Fasting (mmol/L)	<5.8
2 hour (mmol/L)	7.5
Fructosamine (micromol/L)	200–300
Glycosylated Hb (per cent)	5–8
Pigment	
Bilirubin (unconjugated) (micromol/L)	4–10

Table 11.1.3 *Continued*

	Range	
Enzymes		
Alanine aminotransferase (IU/L)	5–40	
Alkaline phosphatase (IU/L)	102–328	
Amylase (IU/L)	10–82	
Aspartate aminotransaminase (IU/L)	3–34	
Creatine kinase (IU/L)	0–227	
Gamma-glutamyl transferase (IU/L)	9–34	
Lactate dehydrogenase (IU/L)	342–686	
Total protein (g/L)	50–67	
Other proteins		
Albumin (g/L)	28–38	
Colloid osmotic pressure (cm H_2O)	19–31	
Alpha$_1$-antitrypsin (g/L)	1.1–2.1	
Ceruloplasmin (g/L)	0.2–0.6	
Complement C3 (g/L)	0.75–1.65	
Complement C4 (g/L)	0.25–0.65	
IgA (g/L)	0.8–2.8	
IgG (g/L)	5.4–16.1	
IgM (g/L)	0.5–2.0	
Metals		
Zinc (mmol/L)	6.0–10.8	
Copper (mmol/L)	25.6–44.5	
Selenium (mmol/L)	1.07–1.83	
Hormones		
Free T_3	3.3–8.2	
Total T_3 (nanomol/L)	1.3–3.3	
Free T_4 (picomol/L)	10–23	
Thyroid stimulating hormone (IU/L)	0.3–6.0	
Cortisol (nanomol/L) (09.00 hours)	150–700	
Aterial blood gases		
Normal		
P_{O_2} (mm Hg)	90–113	(10.6–13.3 kPa)
P_{CO_2} (mm Hg)	34–45	(4.6–6.0 kPa)
pH	7.37–7.42	
Standard bicarbonate (mmol/L)	22–28	
Oxygen saturation	0.95–1.0	

Table 11.1.3 *Continued*

	Range
Hypoxia (requiring transfer to intensive therapy unit (ITU) for intermittent positive pressure ventilation)	
P_{O_2} (mm Hg)	100 (13 kPa) (hourly downward trend – ITU)
P_{CO_2} (mm Hg)	34–40 (5.3 kPa)
pH	7.36–7.42 (normal – artificially higher in labour)

[a] (Sodium + Potassium) – (Chloride + Bicarbonate); it is high in acidaemic states.
[b] Corrected for albumin concentration of 42 g/L.

HAEMATOLOGY – VALUES IN PREGNANCY

Haemoglobin concentration

The lowest normal haemoglobin in a healthy woman living at sea level is 12.0 g/dL. Because of plasma volume expansion and red cell mass expansion the lowest haemoglobin in pregnancy should be 10.6 g/dL. The mean is usually between 11 and 12 g/dL. The lowest haemoglobin is at 34 weeks' gestation when the plasma volume expansion is maximal. After this there is a rise of 0.5 g/dL.

Haematocrit (packed cell volume) (PCV)

The haematocrit falls in parallel with the red cell count and the haemoglobin concentration due to haemodilution. The average non-pregnant figure is 0.40–0.42 and it falls to a minimum of 0.31–0.34.

The haematocrit of cord blood from a baby at term is 0.44–0.62.

Mean cell haemoglobin in concentration (MCHC)

This changes little in pregnancy.

Mean cell volume (MCV)

MCV declines in early pregnancy and increases in the latter half. There is a small physiological increase in red cell size (average 4 femtolitres), but the increase may be as high as 20 femtolitres.

11

White cell count

Total white cell count rises in pregnancy due to an increase in poly-morphonuclear leucocytes. The mean total white cell count is around 9×10^9/L.

Normal pregnant women may have up to 3 per cent myelocytes or metamyelocytes in their circulating blood. These decrease in the last month of pregnancy.

Increased blood volume

The total blood volume increases by up to 45 per cent maximum by the thirty-second week. The total plasma volume increase by 25–55 per cent, more than the 20–40 per cent increases in the red cell mass, resulting in the apparent anaemia of normal pregnancy with the haemoglobin concentration remaining above 10 g/dL.

Erythrocyte sedimentation rate (ESR)

This is up to 20 mm/h in normal pregnancy.

Red cell ageing

The normal red cell lifespan in humans is about 120 days.

Peripheral white blood cells

Range: 4×10^9/L to 10×10^9/L.

Platelets

The normal platelet count in pregnancy is between 120×10^9/L and 400×10^9/L.

A diagnosis of pre-eclampsia is suggested if the mean platelet volume exceeds 8.9 femtolitres (at least one standard deviation above the mean for normotensive women). Values below 8.0 femtolitres are consistent with essential hypertension or chronic hypertension. Increased platelet consumption leads to a greater proportion of young platelets in circulation which tend to be larger.

11

Iron metabolism

The total requirement for iron in pregnancy is 700–1400 mg. A normal mixed diet contains an average of 14 mg of iron per day. Only 1–2 mg (5–10%) is absorbed. Iron is absorbed either attached to haem in its inorganic iron or in its ferrous form. In most foods iron is in the ferric form and it is reduced to the ferrous form by substances such as Vitamin C and gastric secretions.

Pregnancy requires an additional 1000 mg or so of iron, i.e. about 4 mg/day in excess of normal daily requirements, which increases with increasing gestation. The daily intake needs to be increased by 15 mg because only a proportion is absorbed. The use of supplementation is to prevent depletion of iron stores.

The optimal maternal haemoglobin level is 11–12 g/dL and the haematocrit is 0.33–0.35. Women with a haemoglobin level <9.0 g/dL or >13.0 g/dL, or haematocrit <0.29 or >0.39 have an increased risk of pregnancy complication.

However, there is debate as to whether all pregnant women should have iron supplementation (iron prophylaxis) from 16 weeks' gestation or whether it should be confined to those in whom true iron deficiency anaemia has been diagnosed (microcytosis or hypochromia on blood film) (iron treatment). The 1972 WHO recommendations are 30–60 mg per day to those pregnant women with iron stores and 120–240 mg to those with none; 60–80 mg daily taken between meals is a compromise. Intramuscular injection of iron 1000 mg may be given in those who are non-compliant or unable to take oral iron.

Iron is important because iron deficiency is associated with a decrease in myoglobin responsible for oxygen transport. Iron deficiency results in alterations in dopaminergic and seratonergic neurotransmission.

Serum iron

The serum iron of non-pregnant women lies between 13 and 27 micromol/L (60–150 microgram/dL). It should be more than 12 micromol/L, but total iron concentration is less reliable than ferritin in assessing iron status.

The serum iron is higher in the early morning and lower in the afternoon due to fluctuating release of iron from reticuloendothelial cells. It is therefore recommended that all specimens be collected

11

between 09.00 hours and 10.00 hours. Erythropoiesis is decreased if the serum iron persists below 12.5 micromol/L.

The total serum iron-binding capacity is a measure of the serum concentration of **transferrin**, the specific iron-carrying protein. Transferrin is present in the serum at a concentration of 1.8–2.6 g/L and has a half-life of 8–11 days.

Ferritin is a stable compound not affected by recent ingestion of iron and the normal range in the plasma is 15–300 microgram/L. It reflects the iron stores accurately and quantitatively. A serum ferritin of less than 12 microgram/L in early pregnancy is an indication for daily iron supplement. Women with serum ferritin concentrations greater than 80 microgram/L are unlikely to require iron supplement. Ferritin levels fall from weeks 12 to 32 in pregnancy due to the expansion of the erythrocyte mass.

Total iron binding capacity (TIBC) in the non-pregnant state is 45–72 micromol/L (250–400 microgram/dL). The specific iron-binding protein transferrin is between 1.2 and 2.0 g/L (120–200 microgram/dL). At term the average serum iron concentration is reduced to about 35 per cent below the mean in non-pregnant women.

The total serum transferrin concentration rises from 1.2–2.0 g/L to 4.7 g/L by the second trimester. There is an increase in the TIBC to around 90 micromol/L. The raised TIBC returns to non-pregnant levels within three weeks of delivery. Serum iron of less than 12 micromol/L (70 microgram/dL) and a TIBC saturation of less than 15 per cent indicates deficiency of iron during pregnancy.

Measurements

Haemoglobin and mean cell volume should be measured at booking, 28 and 36 weeks' gestation. Should either be low, the serum ferritin should be measured if routine iron supplements are not being given and supplementation commenced if ferritin levels are low.

Plasma folate

Plasma folate falls in pregnancy. At term it is half the non-pregnant value. In the absence of any change, megaloblastic haemopoiesis should be suspected when there is not the expected response to adequate iron therapy.

A decline in serum folate levels from a mean of 6 microgram/L in the non-pregnant woman to 3.5 microgram/L at term is physiological.

The diagnosis of folate deficiency usually requires a bone-marrow aspirate.

The cause of megaloblastic anaemia in pregnancy is nearly always folate deficiency. Vitamin B_{12} is only very rarely the aetiological cause. The incidence is 0.2–5.5 per cent.

World Health Organisation recommendations for daily folate intake are as high as 800 micrograms in the antenatal period, 600 micrograms during lactation, and 400 micrograms in the non-pregnant state. The daily amount of folate given prophylactically in pregnancy varies from 30 micrograms to 500 micrograms. Supplements of 100 micrograms or more reduce the frequency of megaloblastic changes in the bone marrow. Daily supplementation needs to be of the order of 200–300 micrograms of pteroylglutamic acid. This should be given in combination with iron supplement.

Folate transfers single carbon units for the synthesis of nucleic acid. Cell division involves duplication of DNA chain. Folate is required for the synthesis of adenine, guanine and thymidine, three of the four bases constituting DNA. The increased requirement for folate in pregnancy arises from the accelerated cell division involved in pregnancy. Folate requirements are 100–500 micrograms daily, which approximates normal intake. A total folate intake of between 200 and 250 micrograms daily is required in uncomplicated pregnancy.

Folate status may be assessed by measuring serum and group cell folate. Supplementation for folate is 200–300 micrograms of pteroylglutamic acid daily.

It has recently been recommended that extra folate/folic acid is recommended for all women prior to conception and during the first twelve weeks of pregnancy. The recommendation is **0.4 mg (400 micrograms) folic acid when attempting to conceive until the twelfth week of pregnancy, to prevent a first occurrence of a neural tube defect.** To prevent a recurrence of a neural tube defect, folic acid supplementation: 5 mg (5000 micrograms) should be advised for all those women who wish to become pregnant or who are at risk of becoming pregnant. Supplementation should continue until the twelfth week of pregnancy.

Vitamin B_{12}

Muscle, red cell and serum Vitamin B_{12} concentrations fall during pregnancy. Non-pregnant serum levels of 205–1025 microgram/L fall to 20–510 microgram/L at term. The recommended daily intake is 3 micrograms per day during pregnancy.

Serum cobalamin (Vitamin B$_{12}$)

Daily requirement is 1–2 micrograms. Absorption requires binding to intrinsic factor, a glycoprotein present in gastric juice. The intrinsic-factor–cobalamin complex is taken up by the enterocytes in the ileum.

	Mean level of cobalamin (picogram/mL)
First trimester	320
Second trimester	250
Third trimester	190

There is active transfer of cobalamin to the fetus. The cord blood level is twice that of the mother. There are large cobalamin stores (3000 micrograms).

11.2   Fetal growth charts

NOTES FOR FIGURES AND TABLES

These notes give some background detail on the equations used to generate the data provided in Tables 11.2.1–11.2.6 and Figures 11.2.1–11.2.6. Each table contains both a lower and upper limit; these limits are also drawn on the figures. In each case the lower and upper limits represent approximate 5th and 95th percentiles. These are estimated by the actual estimate $\pm 2\sigma$ where σ is the standard error of the estimate. For further details readers should refer to the list of references.

Table and Figure 11.2.1

These data are based on the equation GA = [8.052 $\sqrt{\text{CRL}}$ + 23.73]/7 corrected by adding 1 mm and 3.7 per cent as suggested by Robinson and Fleming (1975), where GA (gestational age) is in weeks and CRL (crown–rump length) is in millimetres. The lower and upper limits are given by subtracting and adding 4.7 days to the estimated gestational age.

Table and Figure 11.2.2(a)

These data are based on the equation $BPD = -23.4 + 3.67GA - 0.000449GA^3$ where BPD (biparietal diameter) is in millimetres and GA is in weeks. The upper and lower limits were drawn by fitting a cubic function through the points $(BPD + 2\sigma)$ and $(BPD - 2\sigma)$ respectively where the 2σ is given in Table 1 of Hadlock *et al.* (1982a).

Table and Figure 11.2.2(b)

These data are based on the equation $GA = 6.8954 + 0.26345BPD + 0.000008771BPD^3$ where GA is in weeks and BPD is in millimetres. The lower and upper limits have been approximated by fitting smooth cubic functions through the error estimates given in Hadlock *et al.* (1982a).

Table and Figure 11.2.3

These data are based on the equation $HC = -103.4 + 14.8GA - 0.00226GA^3$, given in Hadlock *et al.* (1982b), where HC (head circumference) is in millimetres and GA in weeks. The standard error, σ, is estimated by a constant 9.7 millimetres.

Table and Figure 11.2.4

These data are based on the equation $AC = -69.3 + 10.985GA$, given in Deter *et al.* (1982), where AC (abdominal circumference) is in millimetres and GA is in weeks. The error term, 2σ, is estimated by $0.13 \times$ (predicted value of AC).

Table and Figure 11.2.5

These data are based on the equation
$$\log_e (BW) = -4.564 + 0.0282AC - 0.0000331AC^2 + \log_e(1000)$$
Where BW (birthweight) is in grams and AC is in millimetres. The lower and upper limits are drawn by fitting a smooth quadratic curve

11

(in the log scale) through the estimate $\pm\,2\sigma$ where the estimated values for σ are taken from Campbell and Wilkin (1975).

Table and Figure 11.2.6(a)

These data are based on the equation $FL = -38.929 + 4.2062GA - 0.034513GA^2$, given in Warda *et al.* (1985), where FL (femur length) is in millimetres and GA is in weeks. The error term 2σ is estimated by $0.14 \times$ (predicted value of FL).

Table and Figure 11.2.6(b)

These data are based on the equation $\log(GA) = 2.35301 + 0.023185 \times FL - 0.00007804FL^2$ where GA is in weeks and FL is in millimetres. The upper and lower limits are provided by using an estimate for 2σ of 0.103 in the log scale. Thus the upper limit is estimated by $e^{\log(GA) + 0.103}$ and the lower limit by $e^{\log(GA) - 0.103}$. Warda *et al.* (1985) refer to the exponentiation function as the antilog.

BIBLIOGRAPHY

Campbell, S. & Thoms, A. (1977) Ultrasound measurement of the fetal head to abdomen circumference ratio in the assessment of growth retardation. *British Journal of Obstetrics & Gynaecology*, **84**, 165–174.

Campbell, S. & Wilkin, D. (1975) Abdomen circumference in the estimation of fetal weight. *British Journal of Obstetrics & Gynaecology*, **82**, 689–697.

Deter, R.L., Harrist, R.B. Hadlock, F.P. & Carpenter, R.J. (1982) Fetal head and abdominal circumference: II. A critical re-evaluation of the relationship to menstrual age. *Journal of Clinical Ultrasound*, **10**, 365–372.

Hadlock, F.P., Deter, R.L. Harrist, R.B. & Park, K. (1982a) Fetal biparietal diameter: a critical re-evaluation of the relationship to menstrual age by means of real time ultrasound. *Journal of Ultrasound in Medicine*, **1**, 97–104.

Hadlock, F.P., Deter, R.L., Harrist, R.P. & Park, K. (1982b) Fetal head circumference: relation to menstrual age. *American Journal of Roentgenology*, **138**, 647–653.

Robinson, H.P. & Fleming, J.E.E. (1975) A critical evaluation of sonar crown–rump length measurements. *British Journal of Obstetrics & Gynaecology*, **82**, 702–710.

Warda, A.H., Deter, R.L. & Rossavik, I.K. (1985) Fetal femur length: a critical re-evaluation of the relationship to menstrual age. *Obstetrics & Gynaecology*, **66**, 69–75.

WHO (1972) Nutritional anaemias. *Technical Report Series No. 503*, World Health Organisation, Geneva.

Table 11.2.1 Gestational age for a given crown–rump length. (After Robinson and Fleming, 1975.)

Crown–rump length (mm)	Gestational age (weeks + days)	Lower limit (weeks + days)	Upper limit (weeks + days)
4	6 + 0	5 + 2	6 + 5
6	6 + 3	5 + 6	7 + 1
8	6 + 6	6 + 1	7 + 4
10	7 + 2	6 + 4	8 + 0
12	7 + 4	7 + 0	8 + 2
14	8 + 0	7 + 2	8 + 4
16	8 + 2	7 + 4	9 + 0
18	8 + 4	7 + 6	9 + 1
20	8 + 5	8 + 1	9 + 3
22	9 + 0	8 + 2	9 + 5
24	9 + 2	8 + 4	10 + 0
26	9 + 3	8 + 6	10 + 1
28	9 + 5	9 + 0	10 + 3
30	9 + 6	9 + 2	10 + 4
32	10 + 1	9 + 3	10 + 6
34	10 + 2	9 + 5	11 + 0
36	10 + 4	9 + 6	11 + 1
38	10 + 5	10 + 0	11 + 3
40	10 + 6	10 + 2	11 + 4
42	11 + 0	10 + 3	11 + 5
44	11 + 2	10 + 4	12 + 0
46	11 + 3	10 + 5	12 + 1
48	11 + 4	10 + 6	12 + 2
50	11 + 5	11 + 1	12 + 3
52	11 + 6	11 + 2	12 + 4
54	12 + 1	11 + 3	12 + 5
56	12 + 2	11 + 4	12 + 6
58	12 + 3	11 + 5	13 + 0
60	12 + 4	11 + 6	13 + 2
62	12 + 5	12 + 0	13 + 3
64	12 + 6	12 + 1	13 + 4
66	13 + 0	12 + 2	13 + 5
68	13 + 1	12 + 3	13 + 6
70	13 + 2	12 + 4	14 + 0
72	13 + 3	12 + 5	14 + 1
74	13 + 4	12 + 6	14 + 1
76	13 + 5	13 + 0	14 + 2
78	13 + 6	13 + 1	14 + 3
80	14 + 0	13 + 2	14 + 4

Fig. 11.2.1 Gestational age versus crown–rump length. (After Robinson & Fleming, 1975.)

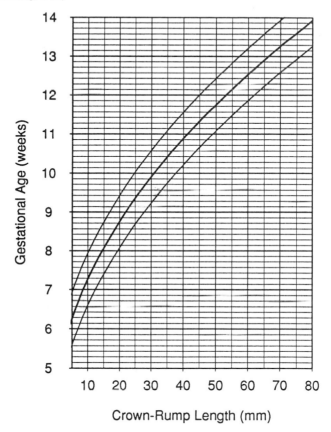

Table 11.2.2(a) Biparietal diameter for a given gestational age. (After Hadlock *et al.*, 1982a.)

Gestational age (weeks)	Biparietal diameter (mm)	Lower limit (mm)	Upper limit (mm)
10	13	11	15
11	16	14	19
12	20	17	22
13	23	22	25
14	27	24	30
15	30	27	33
16	33	31	36
17	37	33	40
18	40	37	43
19	43	38	48
20	46	42	51
21	50	45	54
22	53	48	57
23	56	50	61
24	58	54	63
25	61	58	65
26	64	59	69
27	67	63	71
28	70	66	73
29	72	69	75
30	75	70	80
31	77	73	81
32	79	74	85
33	82	77	86
34	84	81	87
35	86	82	90
36	88	84	91
37	90	85	94
38	91	86	97
39	93	84	102
40	95	89	101

Fig. 11.2.2(a) Biparietal diameter versus gestational age. (After Hadlock *et al.*, 1982a.)

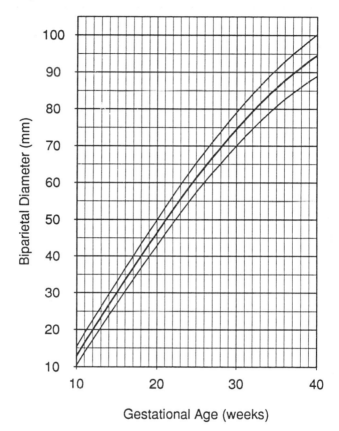

Gestational Age (weeks)

11

Table 11.2.2(b) Gestational age for a given biparietal diameter. (After Hadlock *et al.*, 1982a.)

Biparietal diameter (mm)	Gestational age (weeks + days)	Lower Limit (weeks + days)	Upper limit (weeks + days)
20	12 + 2	11 + 2	13 + 2
22	12 + 5	11 + 5	13 + 6
24	13 + 2	12 + 2	14 + 2
26	13 + 6	12 + 6	14 + 6
28	14 + 3	13 + 3	15 + 3
30	15 + 0	14 + 0	16 + 0
32	15 + 4	14 + 4	16 + 4
34	16 + 1	15 + 1	17 + 2
36	16 + 6	15 + 5	17 + 6
38	17 + 3	16 + 3	18 + 3
40	18 + 0	17 + 0	19 + 0
42	18 + 4	17 + 4	19 + 5
44	19 + 2	18 + 1	20 + 2
46	19 + 6	18 + 5	21 + 0
48	20 + 4	19 + 3	21 + 5
50	21 + 1	20 + 0	22 + 2
52	21 + 6	20 + 4	23 + 0
54	22 + 4	21 + 2	23 + 5
56	23 + 1	21 + 6	24 + 3
58	23 + 6	22 + 4	25 + 2
60	24 + 4	23 + 2	26 + 0
62	25 + 2	23 + 6	26 + 5
64	26 + 0	24 + 4	27 + 4
66	26 + 6	25 + 2	28 + 3
68	27 + 4	26 + 0	29 + 1
70	28 + 2	26 + 4	30 + 0
72	29 + 1	27 + 2	31 + 0
74	30 + 0	28 + 0	31 + 6
76	30 + 5	28 + 6	32 + 5
78	31 + 4	29 + 4	33 + 5
80	32 + 3	30 + 2	34 + 4
82	33 + 2	31 + 0	35 + 4
84	34 + 2	31 + 6	36 + 4
86	35 + 1	32 + 4	37 + 5
88	36 + 0	33 + 3	38 + 5
90	37 + 0	34 + 1	39 + 6
92	38 + 0	35 + 0	40 + 6
94	39 + 0	35 + 6	42 + 0
96	40 + 0	36 + 5	43 + 1
98	41 + 0	37 + 4	44 + 3
100	42 + 0	38 + 3	45 + 4

11

Fig. 11.2.2(b) Gestational age versus biparietal diameter. (After Hadlock *et al.*, 1982a.)

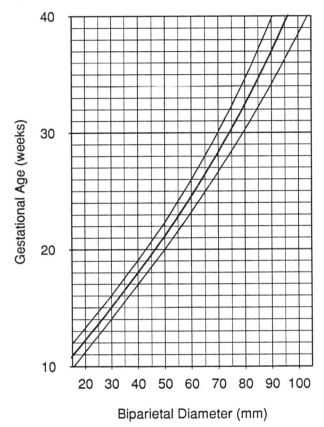

Table 11.2.3 Head circumference for a given gestational age. (After Hadlock *et al.*, 1982b.)

Gestational age (weeks)	Head circumference (mm)	Lower limit (mm)	Upper limit (mm)
10	42	23	62
11	56	37	76
12	70	51	90
13	84	65	103
14	98	78	117
15	111	92	130
16	124	105	143
17	137	118	156
18	149	130	169
19	162	143	182
20	174	155	194
21	186	167	206
22	198	179	217
23	209	190	229
24	221	201	240
25	231	212	251
26	242	222	261
27	252	232	271
28	261	242	281
29	271	251	290
30	280	260	299
31	288	269	307
32	296	277	315
33	304	284	323
34	311	292	330
35	318	298	337
36	324	305	343
37	330	310	349
38	335	316	354
39	340	320	359
40	344	325	363

11

Fig. 11.2.3 Head circumference versus gestational age. (After Hadlock *et al.*, 1982b.)

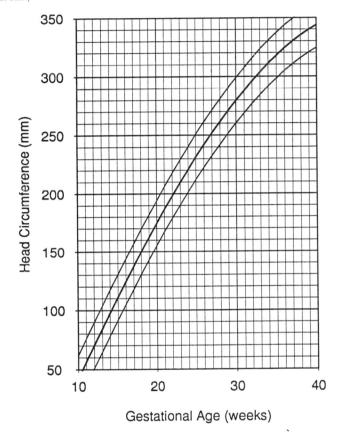

Table 11.2.4 Abdominal circumference for a given gestational age. (After Deter *et al.*, 1982.)

Gestational age (weeks)	Abdominal circumference (mm)	Lower limit (mm)	Upper limit (mm)
10	35	30	39
11	46	40	52
12	63	54	71
13	74	64	83
14	84	74	95
15	95	83	108
16	106	93	120
17	117	102	133
18	128	112	145
19	139	121	157
20	150	131	170
21	161	140	182
22	172	150	195
23	183	160	207
24	194	169	220
25	205	179	232
26	216	188	244
27	227	198	257
28	238	207	269
29	249	217	282
30	260	226	294
31	271	236	306
32	282	246	319
33	293	255	331
34	304	265	344
35	315	274	356
36	326	284	369
37	337	293	381
38	348	303	393
39	359	312	406
40	370	322	418

11

Fig. 11.2.4 Abdominal circumference versus gestational age. (After Deter *et al.*, 1982.)

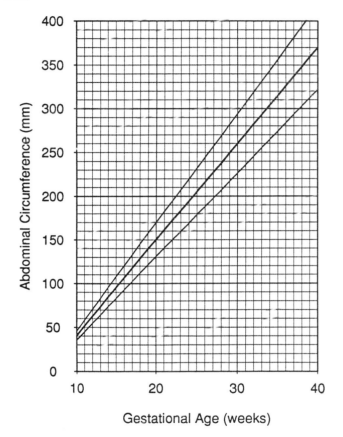

Abdominal Circumference (mm)

Gestational Age (weeks)

Table 11.2.5 Birthweight for a given abdominal circumference. (After Campbell and Wilkin, 1975.)

Abdominal circumference (mm)	Birth weight (g)	Lower limit (g)	Upper limit (g)
200	780	690	870
205	840	740	940
210	903	793	1013
215	969	844	1094
220	1039	899	1179
225	1111	961	1261
230	1187	1027	1347
235	1265	1090	1440
240	1346	1156	1536
245	1431	1231	1631
250	1518	1308	1728
255	1607	1387	1827
260	1700	1470	1930
265	1794	1554	2034
270	1891	1641	2141
275	1989	1724	2254
280	2090	1810	2370
285	2191	1901	2481
290	2294	1994	2594
295	2398	2068	2718
300	2502	2162	2842
305	2606	2251	2961
310	2710	2340	3080
315	2814	2429	3199
320	2917	2517	3317
325	3019	2609	3429
330	3119	2699	3539
335	3217	2787	3647
340	3312	2872	3762
345	3405	2950	3860
350	3495	3025	3965
355	3581	3101	4061
360	3663	3173	4153
365	3741	3241	4241
370	3814	3304	4324
375	3882	3362	4402
380	3945	3415	4475
385	4002	3462	4542
390	4053	3453	4603
395	4099	3539	4659
400	4137	3567	4707

11

Fig. 11.2.5 Birthweight versus abdominal circumference. (After Campbell & Wilkin, 1975.)

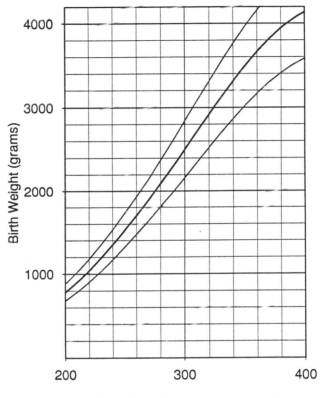

Abdominal Circumference (mm)

Table 11.2.6(a) Femur length for a given-gestational age. (After Warda *et al.*, 1985.)

Gestational age (weeks)	Femur length (mm)	Lower limit (mm)	Upper limit (mm)
13	10	9	11
14	13	11	15
15	16	14	19
16	20	17	22
17	23	19	26
18	26	22	29
19	29	25	33
20	31	27	36
21	34	29	39
22	37	32	42
23	40	34	45
24	42	36	48
25	45	38	51
26	47	41	54
27	49	43	56
28	52	45	59
29	54	46	62
30	56	48	64
31	58	50	66
32	60	52	69
33	62	54	71
34	64	55	73
35	66	57	75
36	68	58	77
37	69	60	79
38	71	61	81
39	73	62	83
40	74	64	84

Fig. 11.2.6(a) Femur length versus gestational age. (After Warda *et al.*, 1985.)

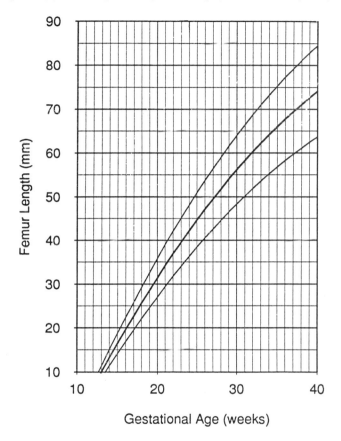

Gestational Age (weeks)

Table 11.2.6(b) Gestational age for a given femur length. (After Warda *et al.*, 1985.)

Femur length (mm)	Gestational age (weeks + days)	Lower limit (weeks + days)	Upper limit (weeks + days)
10	13 + 1	11 + 6	14 + 4
12	13 + 5	12 + 3	15 + 2
14	14 + 2	13 + 0	15 + 6
16	15 + 0	13 + 3	16 + 4
18	15 + 4	14 + 0	17 + 2
20	16 + 1	14 + 4	18 + 0
22	16 + 6	15 + 2	18 + 5
24	17 + 4	15 + 6	19 + 3
26	18 + 2	16 + 3	20 + 1
28	19 + 0	17 + 1	21 + 0
30	19 + 5	17 + 5	21 + 6
32	20 + 3	18 + 3	22 + 4
34	21 + 1	19 + 0	23 + 3
36	21 + 6	19 + 5	24 + 2
38	22 + 5	20 + 3	25 + 1
40	23 + 3	21 + 1	26 + 0
42	24 + 2	21 + 6	26 + 6
44	25 + 1	22 + 4	27 + 6
46	25 + 6	23 + 3	28 + 5
48	26 + 5	24 + 1	29 + 4
50	27 + 4	24 + 6	30 + 4
52	28 + 3	25 + 5	31 + 4
54	29 + 2	26 + 3	32 + 3
56	30 + 1	27 + 1	33 + 3
58	31 + 0	28 + 0	34 + 3
60	31 + 6	28 + 6	35 + 3
62	32 + 6	29 + 4	36 + 3
64	33 + 5	30 + 3	37 + 2
66	34 + 4	31 + 1	38 + 2
68	35 + 3	32 + 0	39 + 2
70	36 + 3	32 + 6	40 + 2
72	37 + 2	33 + 4	41 + 2
74	38 + 1	34 + 3	42 + 2
76	39 + 0	35 + 1	43 + 2
78	39 + 6	36 + 0	44 + 2
80	40 + 6	36 + 6	45 + 1
82	41 + 5	37 + 4	46 + 1
84	42 + 4	38 + 3	47 + 1
86	43 + 3	39 + 1	48 + 0
88	44 + 1	39 + 6	49 + 0
90	45 + 0	40 + 4	50 + 0

11

Fig. 11.2.6(b) Gestational age versus femur length. (After Warda *et al.*, 1985.)

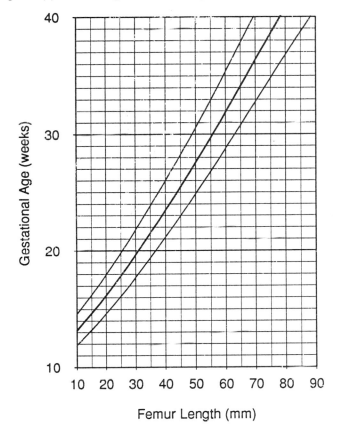

Index